Nursing Education: Foundations for Practice Excellence

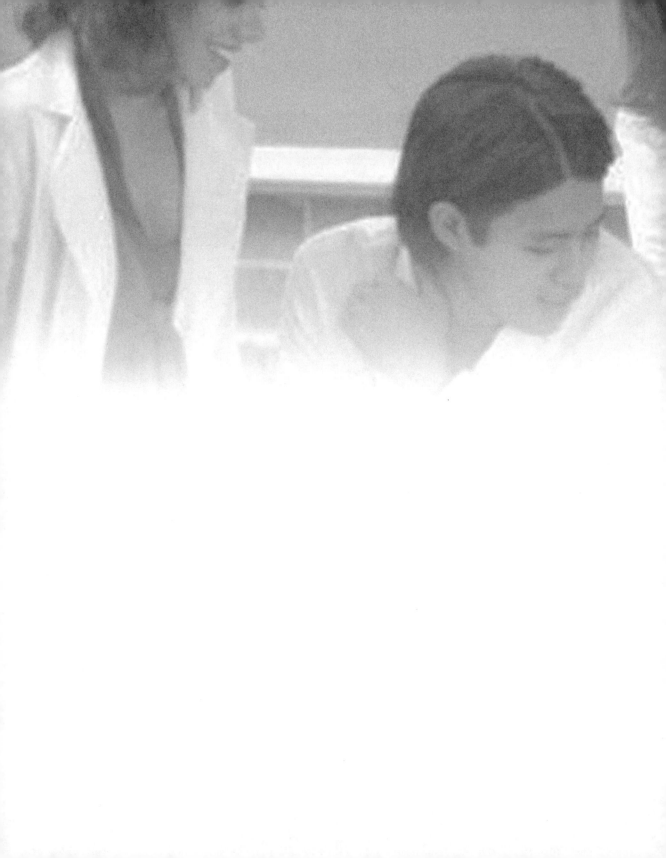

NURSING EDUCATION: FOUNDATIONS FOR PRACTICE EXCELLENCE

By
Barbara A. Moyer
and
Ruth A. Wittmann-Price

F. A. DAVIS COMPANY • Philadelphia

F. A. Davis Company
1915 Arch Street
Philadelphia, PA 19103
www.fadavis.com

Copyright © 2008 by F. A. Davis Company

Printed in the United States of America

Last digit indicates print number: 10 9 8 7 6 5 4 3 2 1

Acquisitions Editor: Joanne Patzek DaCunha, RN, MSN
Developmental Editor: Caryn Abramowitz
Project Editor: Kristin L. Kern
Art and Design Manager: Carolyn O'Brien

Library of Congress Cataloging-in-Publication Data

Nursing education : foundations for practice excellence / [edited] by Barbara A. Moyer and Ruth A. Whitman-
Price.
  p. ; cm.
  Includes bibliographical references.
  ISBN-13: 978-0-8036-1404-8
  ISBN-10: 0-8036-1404-7
1. Nursing—Study and teaching. I. Moyer, Barbara A. II. Whitman-Price, Ruth A.
  [DNLM: 1. Education, Nursing—methods. 2. Teaching—methods. WY 18 N97363 2007]
  RT71.N76 2007
  610.73071′1—dc22   2007012509

This book has exceeded our expectations, not only because of the wonderful work that the contributing authors have provided but also because they have embellished the text with the concept of caring for each educator to impart on every future nursing student. We are thankful for each contribution to this book and believe that the pieces, as well as the totality of it, will have a positive impact on nursing education and ultimately on thousands of patients who will benefit from the expertise provided within its pages.

Thank you.

In Memoriam

"Every action of our lives touches on some chord that will vibrate in eternity."
—Sean O'Casey

Dr. Susan Leddy's contributions to nursing research, knowledge, education, and practice will touch the lives of nurses for eternity.

PREFACE

This book was developed as our small way to help offset the increasing nursing shortage. Without nurse educators the well-documented shortage cannot be addressed appropriately. Nursing graduate programs, such as the one at DeSales University, have risen to the call and are doing a phenomenal job of educating nurses from all walks of practice to become educators. During the planning of the Graduate Nurse Educator track at DeSales, we recognized a need for a book about nursing education that would not only be philosophically sound but contain information on the current technological world we teach in, address the needs of the diverse learners that we teach, and have a vision for the future of nursing education. This unique book fills that need; it offers experience in nursing education to new educators as well as innovative strategies to experienced educators who are now faced with increased numbers of diverse students that must be prepared to function in a world of nursing that is technologically complicated yet calls for humanistic, culturally competent care.

This book is a patchwork of pieces carefully crafted to fit together from different nurse educators who are all artists in their field. They have produced a beautiful quilt that covers not only the foundations of nursing education but is filled with threads of wisdom about educational methodologies, technology, and strategies to help all nurse educators become innovative facilitators of the art and science of nursing. The contributing authors of this book are all educators who are passionate about education and have an acute awareness and understanding of the social and global implications of their work. They are in the forefront of nursing education and know the demands of being an educator today. They have used that experience to produce a blanket of knowledge that can be immediately and effectively implemented in the development of curriculum and strategies for today's classroom, in whatever forms that may be, physical or virtual.

The pieces of this book have been woven together to take the nurse educator on a journey. It begins by a thoughtful and reflective discussion of nursing education from a philosophical standpoint and then lays the groundwork for achieving excellence in the field of nursing education. The art and science of nursing education is addressed before the journey continues to a pivotal point where the discussion focuses on why a professional chooses the path of nursing education as a career. The road then becomes one of signature signposts that speak of curriculum development and the needs of the learner infused with practical management strategies. The landscape then quickly turns to the mountains of information about technology, learning labs, instructional methodologies, and evaluation strategies, as well as clinical education. All of the topics that are relevant to our positions as educators and are so often discussed at faculty meetings and conferences are included with thorough explanations, recent research findings, and practical "how tos". Next, the journey pauses at a reflective pool to develop the cognitive realizations about how a nurse makes the role transition from clinician to educator. The discussion focuses on the human resources and caring needed to ensure self-efficacy as an educator. Finally, the book ends with a vision, a journey into the future. What we know as nursing educators today cannot be taken for granted in this rapidly changing health-care environment that includes unbelievable technological advances.

Thank you.

CONTRIBUTORS

Michele M. August-Brady, DNSc, RN
Associate Professor of Nursing
Moravian College, Nursing Department
Bethlehem, Pennsylvania

Vera Brancato, EdD, RN, BC
Professor and Director
Center for Enhancement of Teaching
Kutztown University
Kutztown, Pennsylvania

Peggy L. Chinn, PhD, RN, FAAN
Professor Emerita
University of Connecticut School of Nursing
Storrs, Connecticut

Lucille A. Joel, EdD, RN, FAAN
Professor, College of Nursing
Rutgers—The State University of New Jersey
Newark, New Jersey

Susan Leddy, PhD, RN
Professor Emerita
Widener University
Chester, Pennsylvania

Deborah C. Messecar, PhD, RN, CNS
Associate Professor
Oregon Health & Science University
School of Nursing
Portland, Oregon

Barbara A. Moyer, EdD, RN
Assistant Professor of Nursing
DeSales University
Center Valley, Pennsylvania

Robert G. Mulligan, MA, MEd
Doctoral Student
Neumann College
Aston, Pennsylvania

Judy Irene Murphy, PhD, RN, CNE
Associate Professor
Massachusetts College of Pharmacy and
    Health Services
Boston, Massachusetts

Marilyn E. Parker, PhD, RN
Professor and Director
College of Nursing
Florida Atlantic University
Boca Raton, Florida

Mary E. Partusch, PhD, RN
Professor of Nursing
Nebraska Methodist College
Omaha, Nebraska

Mary Anne Rizzolo, EdD, RN, FAAN
Senior Director, Professional Development
National League for Nursing
New York, New York

Pamela Roberts, MSN, RN
Nursing Lab Manager
Department of Nursing
Montgomery County Community College
Blue Bell, Pennsylvania

Savina O. Schoenhofer, PhD, RN
Professor, Department of Graduate Nursing
Alcorn State University
Natchez, Mississippi

Susan M. P. Scholtz, DNSc, RN
Associate Professor of Nursing
Moravian College, Nursing Department
Bethlehem, Pennsylvania

Joan Stanley, PhD, CRNP, FAAN
Senior Director, Education Policy
American Association of Colleges of Nursing
Washington, DC

Marilyn Stoner, PhD, RN
Associate Professor of Nursing
California State University
San Bernardino, California

Theresa M. Valiga, EdD, RN, FAAN
Chief Program Officer
National League for Nursing
New York, New York

Ruth Wittmann-Price, DNSc, RN, CNE
Assistant Professor, Nursing & Health
DeSales University
Center Valley, Pennsylvania

Mary-Anne Andrusyszyn, RN, EdD
Associate Professor
Counsellor and President Elect, Iota Omicron
    Chapter, STTI
Faculty of Health Sciences, School of
    Nursing
The University of Western Ontario
London, Canada

Julia Aucoin, DNS, RN, BC
Assistant Professor
University of North Carolina
Greensboro, North Carolina

Joan Garity, EdD, RN
Associate Professor
University of Massachusetts
Boston, Massachusetts

Gretchen Heery, APRN, BC
Adjunct Faculty
Cedar Crest College
Allentown, Pennsylvania

Kathleen G. Hoover, PhD, RN
St. Louis University
St. Louis, Missouri

Rose Kearney-Nunnery, PhD, RN
Vice President of Academic Affairs
Technical College of the Low Country
Beaufort, South Carolina

Carol T. Kostovich, PhD, RN
Associate Professor, School of Nursing
Saint Xavier University
Chicago, Illinois

Laurie V. Nagelsmith, MS, RN
Clinical Nurse Specialist
Director, Baccalaureate Nursing Program
Excelsior College
Albany, New York

**Karin J. Opacich, PhD, MHPE, OTR/L,
    FAOTA**
Project EXPORT Director and
Assistant Director, National Center for Rural
    Health Professions
University of Illinois-Rockford
and
Curriculum Consultant
Opacich Consultative Services
Rockford, Illinois

Carole Anne Pepa, PhD, RN
Associate Professor
College of Nursing
Valparaiso University
Valparaiso, Indiana

Laurel Pierangli, MS, RN
University of Scranton
Scranton, Pennsylvania

Marydelle Polk, PhD, ARNP-BC
Coordinator, PHC-MSN Program
Florida Gulf Coast University
Fort Myers, Florida

**Mary Carol G. Pomatto,
    MS, EdD, ARNP-CNS**
Professor and
Chair Department of Nursing
Pittsburg State University
Pittsburg, Kansas

Susan Poslusny, PhD, RN
Associate Professor & Chair
DePaul University Department of Nursing
Chicago, Illinois

Carmen Roche, BScT, MScT
Professor
McMaster-Mohawk-Conestoga Collaborative
    BScN Program
Hamilton, Ontario

Savina O. Schoenhofer, PhD, RN
Professor of Graduate Nursing
Alcorn State University
Alcorn, Mississippi

Rosalee J. Seymour, EdD, RN
Associate Professor
East Tennessee State University
Johnson City, Tennessee

Nancy Sharts-Hopko, PhD, RN, FAAN
Director, Doctoral Program
Villanova University
Philadelphia, Pennsylvania

M. Elaine Tagliareni, RN, PhD
Director, Nursing Program
Community College of Philadelphia
Philadelphia, Pennsylvania

Janis Waite, RN, MSN, EdD
Associate Professor
Saint Francis Medical Center College of
  Nursing
Peoria, Illinois

Nan Russell Yancey, RN, PhD
Professor
Director of Graduate Studies
College of Nursing and Health Professions
Lewis University
Romeoville, Illinois

ACKNOWLEDGMENTS

The writing of this textbook has been an important undertaking. We value the contributions of the chapter authors who helped shape and define this new textbook on Nursing Education. These chapters represent an enormous amount of work and thought. We believe that this blend of philosophy and application will enhance the knowledge of educators who are dedicated to teaching the next generation of nursing educators. As you reflect on the names of the contributors, you will see outstanding experts in the world of nursing education from Dr. Chinn who presents a wonderful way to develop your own nursing philosophy to Dr. Valiga, Dr. Rizzolo, and Dr. Stanley who explain the future implications of nursing education. You will see other innovative nurse educators, namely, Dr. August-Brady, Dr. Brancato, and Dr. Scholtz who are role models for excellence in education and research in our immediate circle of colleagues. Robert Mulligan is not only a wonderful educator and "tells you how it is in managing a classroom" but a great friend of nursing as well. Dr. Parker, Dr. Schoenhofer, and Dr. Messecar have presented a wonderful foundation for the science and art of nursing education; whereas, Dr. Leddy, Dr. Stoner, Dr. Joel, Dr. Partusch, and Pamela Roberts highlight important application methodologies that help in facilitating the instruction, supervision, and evaluation of novice nursing educators. Finally, Dr. Murphy takes you on a journey from novice to expert, using a variety of visionary strategies.

We also gratefully acknowledge the support of the editors and publishers for their expertise in helping to format and polish this work, from Joanne DaCunha who tried to keep us on target (which was quite a task at times) to Caryn Abramowitz whose gracious manner and efficient style kept things moving along very smoothly as the various chapter versions hit our desks.

Finally, we want to dedicate this book to our future nursing educators who will be our nursing mentors for the next generation of nursing students. Nursing education is indeed an art and a science that encompasses the three very important domains of nursing: education, clinical practice, and research. We are grateful to have had this opportunity to collectively and collaboratively influence the domain of nursing education.

Thank you.

CONTENTS

NURSING EDUCATION: FOUNDATIONS FOR PRACTICE EXCELLENCE

Chapter Outline

1

FOUNDATIONS FOR NURSING EDUCATION

Marilyn E. Parker
Savina O. Schoenhofer

Learning Outcomes

On completion of this chapter, the reader will be able to:

• Explain the characteristics of nursing as a discipline.
• Discuss why nursing is considered a practiced discipline.
• Identify the patterns of knowing.
• Trace the evolution of the philosophy and practice of nursing education methods.

Key Terms

Concepts
Environment
Epistemology
Ethical
Grand nursing theory
Health
Learned profession
Metaparadigm
Ontology
Person
Personal
Sociopolitical

The focus of this chapter is to discuss nursing education in relation to the discipline of nursing and to understand the how and why of the evolution of nursing education in the manner that we know it today. Teaching methods for nursing education do not exist in a vacuum. It is important that future, novice, and seasoned nurse educators make a clear connection between the nature of nursing as a discipline and the ways of teaching selected and invented for nursing education. In teaching nursing, faculty never teach a "piece" of value or information in isolation—when teaching that "piece," we are always teaching it as a meaningful aspect of the discipline, and thus we are teaching the discipline.

The basic premise of this chapter is that teaching methods must be tailored to the nature of nursing as a discipline. Part of the decision-making about selection of teaching methods involves an understanding of the content of nursing knowledge, the structure of that content, and the values and beliefs that underlie the nature of the discipline. In this chapter, we intend to prepare the reader to think broadly, critically, and specifically about the possible use of the methods described in this book. We take the view that methods don't work except when people can work them effectively. Part of effectively choosing, modifying, and inventing methods for nursing education involves a deep and clear understanding of nursing as a discipline, and an equally clear and deep understanding of nursing education as the vehicle for facilitating knowledge and understanding of the discipline. With an appropriate knowledge and understanding of the discipline, nurses can design effective nursing care and thus actualize the highest purpose of the discipline of nursing.

The chapter focuses on the broad context of nursing as a discipline of knowledge. Included in the discussion will be philosophical foundations and practical implications for choosing/inventing teaching methods that work for nursing education. Philosophical and theoretical foundations offer coherent and enduring values to guide choice of method. Practical implications provide the link between nursing as a discipline and nursing as a profession. Classic scholars have expressed this link in terms like "practice discipline" (Dickoff, James, & Wiedenbach, 1968) and **"learned profession"** (Rogers, 1970).

Nursing as a Discipline

It is important for the nurse educator to conceptualize nursing as a discipline. First we will examine the idea of disciplines, as articulated initially by King and Brownell (1976). We will then discuss nursing as a learned profession, a discipline that has a direct and immediate practice imperative, and relate that idea to nursing education. It is necessary to examine the issue of what is to be taught, as a precursor to questions of how to teach and how to facilitate learning.

Characteristics of Disciplines

Classic education theorists, King and Brownell (1976), developed a descriptive set of characteristics of disciplines as a foundation for their treatment of curriculum issues. These characteristics were intended to be generic descriptors of all disciplines:

- Community of scholars
- Focused on a unique social need
- Specialized network
- Specific knowledge and skill
- Contains a value system
- Has an established instructive community

The key to the nature and uniqueness of any discipline is the unique focus and perspective it takes on human concerns. Each discipline illuminates an aspect of what it means to be human and to live in the world. A description of these characteristics and the importance of each to nursing is found in Parker (2006).

The most fundamental of those characteristics is that a discipline addresses an explicit unique social need. This tells us that each discipline offers a unique way of viewing human concerns and, in fact, each discipline is unique. King and Brownell (1976) described disciplines as *communities of scholars* voluntarily working together around a *focused and unique social need or concern.* A discipline *imaginatively* creates and uses *specialized networks, methods, and materials* designed to produce and employ *specific knowledge and skills* in response to that focused and unique concern. A discipline has a *value system* and is organized as an *instructive community.* Each discipline illuminates an aspect of what it means to be human and to live in the world.

New disciplines emerge in two ways. One way for a discipline to develop is when a more focused perspective is taken by a critical mass of members of an existing discipline—a new discipline can emerge, such as the practice discipline of physical therapy. This discipline emerged as knowledge of anatomy, physiology, and physics were used in developed scholarship and practice focused on prevention and healing of physical **health** disorders. Such a new discipline would be created from a body of research, scholarship, and theories as well as from new or unique contributions to society that have been distinguished from those related to existing disciplines.

The second manner in which a discipline develops is from the intersecting margins of two or more disciplines. In this manner, a new discipline may emerge whose focus is constructed from specialized aspects of several parent disciplines. A discipline such as biochemistry is an example of a new discipline derived from the expanse of biology and chemistry.

These same processes can produce subdisciplines and specializations within a discipline, that is, minor, specialized focal interests that retain a clear link to the focus of the broader discipline, such as physical therapy being practiced in different settings to include acute care, rehabilitation, and athletics.

These processes of discipline development have contributed to the expansion of the formal knowledge and practice of nursing, and concomitantly added clarity to the central focus of the discipline and service of nursing. These processes have also led to specialization within the discipline of nursing practice.

The Nature of Nursing as a Practiced Discipline, a Learned Profession

Nursing practice is both the source and goal of nursing knowledge. The scholarship, research, theories, and education of nursing are grounded in the practice of the discipline of nursing. Selecting and creating effective nursing education methods relies on an understanding that the content of nursing encompasses the goals and methods of nursing practice and the integral connections of practice with distinctive practice-related knowledge. The use of a nursing-practice situation is a teaching method that draws on expert knowing of the teacher and stimulates creative and thoughtful learning. Study of the complexity and beauty of nursing practice gives substance and meaning to the idea of a practiced discipline, a learned profession.

Nursing as a practiced discipline and learned profession takes a unique focus on what it means to be human. Nursing is a discipline that is often grouped with several disciplines categorized as human service or health-related disciplines, such as social work, medicine, and physical therapy. The interests and responsibilities of nursing as a distinct discipline within a group of disciplines are necessarily different from, though connected to, those of the other related disciplines.

For example, social work, medicine, physical therapy, and nursing are connected through their concern for the health and well-being of persons by practices to promote health and prevent disease. If there were no unique knowledge constructed from nursing's perspective and contributed to the larger knowledge base, there would be no need for a discipline called nursing among the health and human service disciplines. Without a unique body of nursing knowledge, there is no basis for a claim for a unique service or practice. In other words, it is nursing's unique knowledge base that warrants a unique service or practice called professional nursing.

One more link in this logical sequence brings us to the major purpose for nursing education and, thus, the central principle for designing curricula, whether at the program level or at the level of the single lesson. That purpose is to assist persons desiring to enter into the professional role of nursing to develop knowledge and understanding of nursing as a basis from which to design, offer, and evaluate nursing care. Teachers of nursing can best facilitate learning by using distinctive knowledge of the discipline and practice of nursing for each learning experience while being open to and encouraging new ways of thinking, knowing, and being in nursing. This analysis makes evident the principle that selection and use of teaching methodologies for nursing education must be tailored to the unique focus and purpose of the discipline of nursing.

In the field of education, it is a well accepted tenet that instruction be tailored to the content and to the learner. Putting these three ideas together (discipline, content, learner) helps us understand that any teaching method used to educate for nursing must be in concert with the uniqueness of the nursing discipline and that students of nursing require educational strategies that maximize the development of the values, knowledge, and skills that make up the body of nursing knowledge.

Nursing's Unique Focus

To arrive at a clear articulation of the content of the discipline, we now ask: What is the unique focus taken by nursing on human service/human health concerns? To answer this question, scholars have taken several approaches. One approach has been to articulate various conceptual systems descriptive of nursing as a unique discipline and profession, systems often-called grand nursing theories. The other approach has been to discern the universal unifying **concepts** addressed by the discipline; nursing's **metaparadigm** is one name given to this approach.

Grand Nursing Theory

Beginning in the 1960s and continuing through the remainder of the 20th century, formal systems of nursing value, thought, and action were developed by a number of nursing scholars. The impetus for theoretical development of the discipline was supported by the National League for Nursing (NLN) in recognition of the need for clarity about the discipline in curriculum development efforts. These formal systems—variously called **grand nursing theories,** conceptual models, conceptual frameworks, and nursing philosophical frameworks—express explicit conceptualizations of nursing as a discipline and professional practice. Some examples of the grand nursing theories or frameworks include but are not limited to Orem's Self-Care Deficit Nursing Theory, Rogers' Science of Unitary Human Beings, Parse's Human Becoming School of Thought, and Boykin and Schoenhofer's Theory of Nursing As Caring. The content of each of the comprehensive integrated systematic views of nursing (the grand nursing theories) consists of three interrelated systems: a system of concepts and relationships among and between the concepts, an undergirding value system, and a language system that expresses a unique and organized perspective of the discipline.

To illustrate, these interrelated systems will be briefly described in relation to the theory of Nursing As Caring. The conceptual system dimension of the theory of Nursing As Caring can be expressed in its statement of focus of the discipline of nursing: *nursing is nurturing persons living caring and growing in caring* (Boykin & Schoenhofer, 2001, p. 1). This statement contains the central organizing concepts (**person** and caring) in relationship, and is further amplified by the concepts of *knowing person as caring, call for nursing, nursing response, nursing situation, caring between*, and *enhancing personhood* (p. 1). The value system undergirding the nursing as caring theory is expressed in the statements: *persons are caring by virtue of their humanness* (p. 1) and *personhood is enhanced through participating in nurturing relationships with caring others* (p. 1). The language system is the vehicle that makes the value-oriented conceptual system accessible for use. The language system of the nursing as caring theory is everyday language enhanced by a language of caring that draws on Mayeroff's (1991) caring ingredients and Roach's (1992) 5 Cs of caring.

At the heart of each of the grand nursing theories is a clear and explicit statement of the unique focus of the discipline. The full conceptual or philosophical theory is an elaboration that brings that unique focus into integrated practical significance for use in direct practice, and in teaching, administration, and scholarship. Controversy about the use of these grand nursing theories continues among nurse educators. At one extreme of the controversy is the position that unless a curriculum is grounded in and structured by one of the explicit grand nursing theories, there is no clear coherent guide to the nature and content of the discipline. At the other extreme is the argument that the pursuit of knowledge ought to be unbounded and that whatever nursing faculty teach is by definition nursing knowledge.

Universal Unifying Concepts

As part of the NLN conceptual framework movement in the 1970s, the idea of major encompassing concepts was introduced. Grand theories contain the major concepts accepted as essential in the discipline of nursing. Yura and Torres (1975), for example, wrote about person, **environment,** health, and nursing. Fawcett's (1978) study of a range of nursing literature led to the wide acceptance of what she identified as nursing's metaparadigm concepts and stimulated further proposals for naming those concepts. For example, Kim (1987) articulated four domains of nursing as the concepts relevant to the discipline: client, client-nurse encounters, practice, and environment. Newman, Simes and Corcoran-Perry (1991) proposed an integrated statement of nursing focus, intended to encompass and transcend other efforts at grand theory and specification of metaparadigm concepts: "nursing is the study of caring in the human health experience" (p. 3). These and other various sets of metaparadigm concepts have been used by nurse educators in several ways, as broad and complete or partial conceptual frameworks and curriculum organizers, and as detailed concepts that structure specific knowledge content.

Some nursing curricula employ neither grand nursing theories nor sets of universal unifying nursing paradigmatic concepts, but rather the curriculum framework is imported from other disciplines, such as biology, anthropology, and psychology. Some faculties may take the position that there is no unique body of nursing knowledge but that nursing is the skilled application of various other fields of knowledge in practical situations that occur in settings of nursing practice. This view was much more prevalent prior to the NLN conceptual framework initiative of the late 1960s and early 1970s, before widespread dissemination of the concept of nursing as a practice discipline (for example, see Dickoff, James, & Wiedenbach, 1968) and a learned profession (see Rogers, 1964).

Foundations of Curriculum Design for Nursing

Although this text centers on the creative use of teaching methods that work in nursing education, educators understand that methods do not exist apart from a framework of values, beliefs, and ideas. The foundation of curriculum design for nursing education resides in an explicit expression of the values, beliefs, and focal ideas of the discipline of nursing, which give direction to the specification of programmatic content, structure, materials, and methods. Whether the curriculum framework and design of programs of nursing education take their focus from a highly systematized extant general theory of nursing or from a more fluid, less systematized conception of nursing's metaparadigm, the focus of the program must be on the discipline of nursing. It is this broad framework and programmatic design that ultimately determines the appropriateness of specific teaching methods to advance knowledge for nursing.

Essential Ways of Knowing Nursing

It is crucial that nurse educators understand that multiple ways of knowing are needed and even essential in education for nursing practice. (Please refer to Chapter 3 for further explanation of ways of knowing.) Because of the nature of nursing as moral and practical in purpose and holistic in scope, ways of knowing and pathways to knowledge must be multidimensional. Historically, nursing was taught and learned largely as artful applications of traditional practices. In the middle of the 20th century, the concept of nursing as science gained acceptance, primarily among students and faculties in programs of graduate and doctoral education. The work of Dickoff, James, and Wiedenbach (1968), the Nursing Development Conference Group (1973), and others provided ideas and language that encouraged further development in what might be termed the epistemological dimensions of nursing.

Publication of Carper's (1979) scholarship on patterns of knowing essential for nursing ushered in a sea change in the way scholars and educators approached inquiry. Historically incompatible patterns of knowing in nursing that underpinned the two sides of the art/science argument were brought together in Carper's thesis that knowing in nursing required four patterns or pathways. Not only empirical and **ethical** knowing, but also **personal** and aesthetic knowing—all four combined—are legitimate and even essential ways of knowing for nursing. Two additional patterns have been added to the literature—**sociopolitical** (White, 1995) and unknowing (Munhall, 1983). The work of Chinn and Kramer (2003) has significantly elaborated on the depth and scope of Carper's initial explication by using the patterns of knowing to structure nursing knowledge. Possibilities for the creation and selection of nursing education methods are greatly expanded when nurse educators have a detailed understanding of the idea of multiple patterns of knowing and particularly the idea that knowing in nursing requires all patterns and ways of knowing identified by Carper and others. Understanding the complexity of nursing practice has given rise to the various ways of knowing nursing that appear in the literature. Teaching nursing using perspectives of these multiple ways of knowing assists students to comprehend the scope and depth of nursing knowledge and its use in practice.

Tracing the History of Nursing Education Methods: Philosophy and Practice

We will now briefly trace the evolution of the philosophy and practice of nursing education methods. A sense of history is important to creating and selecting effective nursing education methods.

The ongoing interplay of **ontology** and **epistemology** has influenced the history of nursing education methods. This interplay of ontology and epistemology is a process that constantly evolves in the pursuit of understanding human existence and knowledge. This larger philosophical sphere of human studies influences all disciplines, including nursing. Nursing as a service deals with people and, as such, incorporates the metaphysical studies of why people exist and in what condition and how human beings gain knowledge and interact with the environment. The history of methods of teaching/learning closely parallels the evolution of the idea of nursing as a practiced discipline and the ways of knowing are considered important to this evolutionary history.

The apprenticeship model was prevalent in the early days of nursing education. Until the 1970s, the education for nursing was widely termed "training." In fact, there was little thought given to education for nursing. By the 1950s and 1960s, behavioral psychology had permeated education, including nursing education. The introduction of this learning theory was an ideal philosophy and practice for what was considered "nurse's training." Approaches to training that had been fine-tuned for military and industrial needs in an earlier decade resonated with nurse educators, bringing a sense of systematization and professionalism to nursing education. The model of curriculum development set forth by Tyler (1969) was attractive to nursing educators, as well as others in the field of education, due to its orderly, scientific approach to the structure of curricula. Although a thorough discussion of the behavioral Tylerian model of curriculum is beyond the scope of this chapter, Bevis (1989) has presented an excellent analysis of the impact of the Tylerian model in nursing education. The Tylerian model has been one of the dominant models used in nursing education for several decades and is based primarily on the logic of deduction and empirical knowledge. In the Tylerian framework of education, which is still used by some educators today to varying degrees, objectives are stated and education is presented to meet the objectives rather than the unique learning needs of the student (Bevis, 1989).

As the behavioral curriculum was becoming status quo in schools of nursing, new and competing psychological and educational theories of teaching/learning were being introduced. Humanistic and emancipatory theories of curriculum, widely influential in nursing, included those of Rogers, Green, and Freire. Carl Rogers' humanistic psychology was founded on principles antithetical to those of behaviorism. The Rogerian (1970) theory emphasized freedom and creativity, rather than strict prescription to achieve specified end-products sought in behaviorism. Many schools of nursing, particularly those mounting baccalaureate and higher degree programs, adopted humanistic psychology tenets in the curriculum. As humanism was infiltrating all corners of nursing education, two new philosophies were being introduced into nursing education. The aesthetic and emancipatory pedagogy articulated by Greene (1978) resonated with an emerging interest in caring as a basic value and substantive concept in nursing (Watson, 1989). In the same era, the emancipatory empowerment approach in community development espoused by Freire (1988) gained visibility in nursing education. Both of these theories promoted the learning environment as a nonauthoritarian domain in which both teacher and students were equal, reflective learners. Knowles' theory of adult learning (1970) also influenced the shift in higher education in the last quarter of the 20th century. Many principles of andragogy or adult learning embraced a more emancipatory educational philosophy, which views the student as an active participant in learning rather than a recipient of education. This broad evolutionary trend in nursing education was also influencing education programs of many other disciplines and professions. Similar issues were being addressed in the fields of education and other social sciences.

The work of leading scholars in nursing education clearly reflects the zeitgeist of freedom and creativity prevalent in education and the larger social environment. As in earlier eras, the NLN committed its institutional resources to the dissemination of new education philosophies and practices throughout the arena of nursing education. Two areas of scholarship exercise considerable influence on nursing education philosophy and practice in the last decade of the 20th century and into the 21st. The work of Bevis and Watson (1989) addressing the caring curriculum as consonant with fundamental values of nursing as a discipline and profession is illustrative of one stream of influence. In addition, an important influence is the philosophy and practice of narrative pedagogy, initiated by Diekelmann (Diekelmann & Diekelmann, 2000).

Nursing educators have shown that the use of narratives, which allow students to incorporate lived experiences and a discussion of these experiences into the learning environment, informs nursing practice. Narrative pedagogy arises out of the common lived experiences of students, teachers, and clinicians in nursing education. It is a sharing and interpreting of the narratives that is important. This new phenomenological pedagogy is identified through interpretive research in nursing education.

Summary

In this chapter, we have focused on the idea of nursing as a discipline practiced as a learned profession and its relevance to the creation and selection of nursing education methods. Methods are embodied expressions of ideas and values important to an enterprise. In the nursing education enterprise, it is important that choice of teaching/learning method be grounded in the nature of nursing as understood in the distinctive focus of nursing, the values and interrelated concepts and practice methods that define the discipline. Accepting the role of nurse educator implies a commitment to inquiry into the very nature of the discipline. The methodological choices nurse educators make for facilitating learning in nursing directly express a view of nursing, either reflectively or unreflectively. Nurse educators recognize their responsibility for role modeling. What we are advocating in this chapter is the value of modeling in nursing education practice a clear conception of nursing as a discipline and learned profession. Choice of teaching method is a significant component of the lessons nurse educators teach—it is important that these choices reflect a conception of nursing as a discipline, a learned profession.

R e f e r e n c e s

Bevis, E. O. (1989). Illuminating the issues: Probing the past, a history of nursing curriculum development—the past shapes the present. In E. O. Bevis, & J. Watson, *Toward a caring curriculum: A new pedagogy for nursing* (pp. 13–35). New York: National League for Nursing.

Bevis, E. O., & Watson, J. (1989). *Toward a caring curriculum: A new pedagogy for nursing.* New York: National League for Nursing.

Boykin, A., & Schoenhofer, S. O. (2001). *Nursing as caring: A model for transforming practice.* Sudbury, MA: Jones & Bartlett.

Carper, B. A. (1979). Fundamental patterns of knowing in nursing. *Advanced Nursing Science, 1*(1), 13–23.

Chinn, P. L., & Kramer, M. K. (2003). *Integrated knowledge development in nursing.* (6th ed.). St. Louis: Mosby.

Dickoff, J., James, P., & Wiedenbach, E. (1968). Theory in a practice discipline. Part I. Practice oriented theory. *Nursing Research, 17*, 415–435.

Diekelmann, N., & Diekelmann, J. (2000). Learning ethics in nursing and genetics: Narrative pedagogy and the grounding of values. *Journal of Pediatric Nursing, 15*, 226–231.

Diekelmann, N., Schuster, R., & Nosek, C. (1998). Creating new pedagogies at the millennium: The common experiences of using distance education technologies. University of Wisconsin-Madison Teachers. Retrieved January 1, 2007. **http://www.uwc.edu/cio/diekelmann.htm**

Fawcett, J. (1984). The metaparadigm of nursing. Current status and future refinements. *Journal of Nursing Scholarship, 16*, 84–87.

Fawcett, J. (1978). The "what" of theory development. In *Theory development: What, why, how?* (NLN Pub. No. 15-1708.) New York: National League for Nursing.

Freire, P. (1988). *Pedagogy of the oppressed.* New York: Continuum Publishing Co.

Greene, M. (1978). *Landscapes of learning.* New York: Teachers' College Press, Columbia University.

Kim, H. S. (1987). Structuring the nursing knowledge system: A typology of four domains. *Scholarly Inquiry for Nursing Practice: An International Journal, 1*(1), 99–110.

King, A. R., & Brownell, J. A. (1976). *The curriculum and the disciplines of knowledge.* Huntington, NY: Robert E. Krieger Pub. Co.

Knowles, M. S. (1970). *The modern practice of adult education. Andragogy versus pedagogy.* Englewood Cliffs, NJ: Prentice Hall/Cambridge.

Mayeroff, M. (1991). *On caring.* New York: Harper & Row.

Munhall, P. (1983). Unknowing: Towards another pattern of knowing in nursing. *Nursing Outlook, 41,* 125–128.

Newman, M., Simes A., & Corcoran-Perry, S. (1991). The focus of the discipline of nursing. *Advances in Nursing Science, 14*(1), 1–6.

Nursing Development Conference Group. (1973). *Concept formalization in nursing: Process and product.* Boston: Little, Brown.

Parker, M. E. (2006). *Nursing theories and nursing practice* (2nd ed.). Philadelphia: F A Davis.

Roach, S. M. (1992). *The human act of caring.* Ottawa: Canadian Hospital Association.

Rogers, M. E. (1964). *Reveille in nursing.* Philadelphia: FA Davis Co.

Rogers, M. E. (1970). *An introduction to the theoretical basis for nursing.* Philadelphia: FA Davis.

Tyler, R. W. (1969). *Basic principles of curriculum and instruction.* Chicago: The University of Chicago Press.

Watson, J. (1989). *A new paradigm of curriculum development.* In Bevis, E. O., & Watson, J., *Toward a caring curriculum: A new pedagogy for nursing* (pp. 37–49). New York: National League for Nursing.

White, J. (1995). Patterns of knowing: Review, critique and update. *Advanced Nursing Science, 17*(4), 73–86.

Yura, H., & Torres, G. (1975). Today's conceptual framework within baccalaureate nursing programs. In *Faculty-curriculum development, Part III: Conceptual framework –Its meaning and function* (NLN Pub No. 15-1558) (pp. 17–25). New York: National League for Nursing.

REVIEW QUESTIONS

- What are the basic characteristics of nursing that makes it a practice discipline?
- What is the unique focus taken by nursing on human service or health concerns?
- Does nursing have a unique body of knowledge or is it the application of various other fields of knowledge in a practice setting?
- Is nursing an art or a science?

CRITICAL THINKING EXERCISES

▶ Identify how you would implement the Carper's patterns of knowing using a nursing theorist found on the Internet nursing Web page.

▶ Develop a nursing map for the discipline of nursing.

▶ Interview a nursing professor and describe how the program implemented a nursing theorist.

▶ How do you see the patterns of knowing (Carper, 1979) implemented in your practice?

▶ What are the future implications for educators in nursing as the curricula change?

Diekelmann, N., Schuster, R., & Nosek, C. (1998). Creating new pedagogies at the millennium: The common experiences of using distance education technologies. University of Wisconsin-Madison Teachers. Retrieved January 1–19, 2007. http://www.uwc.edu/cio/diekelmann.htm

Diekelmann found in studying her teaching practices that narratives reveal human meanings and concerns, moral issues, and the practical know-how embedded in concrete teaching episodes. Dialoguing about a particular incident about teaching can in itself reflect understanding and therefore teach. Diekelmann proposes that teachers know much more than they can ever say about teaching. The precepts offered by a pedagogical theory inevitably fall short in prescribing teaching practices, because the theory must be filled out, or challenged by the particular teacher, with particular students, and particular subject matter. This kind of practical pedagogical knowledge development can occur through discussion and interpretation of narrative accounts of particular teaching incidents (p. 322).

Tourville, C., & Ingalis, K. (2003). The living tree of nursing theories. *Nursing Forum 38*(3) 21–30, 36.

Three behavioral theories have been used to develop major nursing theories: interactive, systems, and developmental. The purpose of this article is to provide a symbolic image as a framework for nurses to visualize the multiple nursing theories starting with the first nurse theorist, Florence Nightingale. The article concludes that the Living Tree helps organize various nursing theories so a nurse can apply the theories to practice.

Chapter Outline

PHILOSOPHICAL FOUNDATIONS FOR EXCELLENCE IN TEACHING

2

Peggy L. Chinn

Learning Outcomes

On completion of this chapter, the reader will be able to:

- Understand the different philosophies of nursing education.
- Articulate underpinning assumptions of philosophies.
- Critique the philosophy contained in a school of nursing mission statement.
- Describe the components of Carpers' ways of knowing.
- Provide examples of Noddings' four major processes that are essential to a caring education.
- Practice methodologies that enhance dialogue.

Key Terms

Aesthetics	Natural environment
Andragogy	Pedagogy
Caring	Personal knowing
Confirmation	Praxis
Creativity in practice	Reflective practice
Culture	Responsibility
Empirics	Rights
Ethics	Socioeconomic
Integrity	Sociopolitical knowing
Justice	Wholeness
Modeling	

Excellent teaching is based on deliberately selected values and ideas. Excellent teaching is **praxis**—thoughtful reflection and action that occur in synchrony, in the direction of transforming the world (Chinn, 2004b). Praxis is a circular, ongoing process in which you examine the underlying ideas you wish to put into practice, form your approach in the classroom and put it into practice, examine what actually happened in light of your ideas, refine your ideas and adjust your practice, then move through the cycle again. What you seek for yourself and your students becomes the same as what you do as a teacher.

Even if you assume that you do not have a philosophy of education, as a teacher, your actions are formed by assumptions about what education should be, how you should act as a teacher, and what is important in your teaching. Some of these hidden philosophies are sound; others you will want to discard or revise once you examine the ideas that give shape to your actions. In some cases, you will start out with something that is going on in the classroom that is dissatisfying, and will discover that the root of the problem involves a value or a fundamental belief that you do not share. This process of exploring the meaning of what you practice in the classroom is the start of forming your own deliberately chosen philosophy of teaching.

Who You Are and How You Teach

This chapter provides an overview of how philosophies influence nursing education, and the philosophical perspectives on which nursing knowledge and theory rest. Philosophies clarify the values and assumptions that underlie how we view the world and, in turn, how we interact (see Box 2–1 and Table 2–1). Theories, which are based on underlying philosophies or assumptions, provide a more structured explanation of the dynamics that come together to form experience. Philosophies address questions like "Why is this important?" and "What does this mean?" Theories address questions like "How does this happen?" This chapter focuses on underlying philosophical ideas that are fundamental to the discipline of nursing, both in theory and in practice. To begin exploring philosophies for nursing education, consider the statements in Box 2–1 about students and teachers. As you read each statement, revise it as needed to reflect your own personal belief.

Box 2–1 Ideas Underlying Who You Are and How You Teach

Students are a blank slate, and it is the teacher's responsibility to teach them what they need to know.

Students will try to get away with the least amount of effort, and it is up to the teacher to motivate them to make the effort needed to learn.

Students will cheat whenever they can, and it is up to the teacher to prevent cheating.

Students generally try their best, and what the teacher needs to do is provide them with good opportunities to learn.

Students learn best when they perceive a need to know something, and the teacher's job is to help them understand the reasons for learning what they are required to learn.

Students are motivated to earn good grades, not necessarily to learn, so it is the teacher's responsibility to redirect the focus on learning.

Students only retain what they will use, so the teacher must design the teaching plan based on what they will probably use in the clinical area.

TABLE 2–1 Philosophy and Education Continuum Chart

Modernity <———————————————————————————————————> Post Modernity

Traditional and Conservative <—————————> Contemporary and Liberal

Authoritarian (convergent) <—————————> (divergent) Nonauthoritarian

	Idealism	Realism	Pragmatism	Existentialism
General or World Philosophies	Ideas are the only true reality, the only thing worth knowing. Focus: *Mind*	Reality exists independent of human mind. World of physical objects ultimate reality. Focus: *Body*	Universe is dynamic, evolving. Purpose of thought is action. Truth is relative. Focus: *Experience*	Reality is subjective, within the individual. Individual rather than external standards. Focus: *Freedom*
Originator(s)	Plato, Socrates	Aristotle	Pierce, Dewey	Sartre, Kierkegaard
Curricular Emphasis	Subject matter of mind: literature, history, philosophy, religion.	Subject matter of physical world: science, math.	Subject matter of social experience. Creation of new social order.	Subject matter of personal choice.
Teaching Method	Teach for handling ideas: lecture, discussion.	Teach for mastery of facts and basic skills: demonstration, recitation.	Problem solving; Project method.	Individual as entity within social context.
Character Development	Imitating examples, heroes.	Training in rules of conduct.	Making group decisions in light of consequences.	Individual responsibility for decisions and preferences.
Related Educational Philosophies	**Perennialism:** Focus: Teach ideas that are everlasting. Seek enduring truths, which are constant, not changing, through great literature, art, philosophy, religion.	**Essentialism:** Focus: Teach the common core, "the basics" of information and skills (cultural heritage) needed for citizenship. (Curriculum can change slowly.)	**Progressivism:** Focus: Ideas should be tested by active experimentation. Learning rooted in questions of learners in interaction with others. Experience and student centered.	**Reconstructionism/ Critical Theory:** Focus: Critical pedagogy. Analysis of world events, controversial issues, and diversity to provide vision for better world and social change.

(table continued on page 18)

TABLE 2–1 Philosophy and Education Continuum Chart (continued)

Key Proponents	Robert Hutchins Jacque Maritain Mortimer Adler Allan Bloom	William Bagley Arthur Bestor E. D. Hirsch Chester Finn Diane Ravitch Theodore Sizer	John Dewey William Kilpatrick	George Counts J. Habermas Ivan Illich Henry Giroux Paulo Freire
Related Theories of Learning (Psychological Orientations)	**Information Processing:** The mind makes meaning through symbol-processing structures of a fixed body of knowledge. Describes how information is received, processed, stored, and retrieved from the mind.	**Behaviorism:** Behavior shaped by design and determined by forces in environment. Learning occurs as result of reinforcing responses to stimuli. **Social Learning** Learning by observing and imitating others.	**Cognitivism/ Constructivism:** Learner actively constructs own understandings of reality through interaction with environment and reflection on actions. Student-centered learning around conflicts to present knowing structures.	**Humanism:** Personal freedom, choice, responsibility. Achievement motivation towards highest levels. Control of own destiny. Child centered. Interaction with others.
Key Proponents	R. M. Gagne E. Gagne Robert Sternberg J.R. Anderson	Ivan Pavlov John Watson B.F. Skinner E.L. Thorndike Albert Bandura	Jean Piaget U. Bronfenbrenner Jerome Bruner Lev Vygotsky	J.J. Rousseau A. Maslow C. Rogers A. Combs R. May

Permission obtained from Dr. LeeNora M. Cohen, OSU–School of Education, August, 2006.

Each of these statements reflects a particular philosophy of education, and there are theories of learning and education that are grounded in one or more of these statements. If these statements are taken as a literal description of all students and teachers, clearly they are overgeneralizations. As theoretical propositions, they reflect a relationship between two or more concepts that might be accurate to reality, but that are open to empiric testing and ultimate revision based on the empiric evidence.

The critical thinking statements about philosophy reflect underlying beliefs about human nature and the **responsibility** of teachers, and they guide how teachers plan and implement their teaching practices. Consider phrases such as "students are a blank slate," or "students learn best when ..." These types of statements, followed by statements that prescribe a particular teacher responsibility, are grounded in a patriarchal philosophical assumption of a subordinate student and a dominant teacher who knows better than the student. They also reflect a pedagogical approach to education, or one that is grounded in assumptions about learners who like children, lack experience and knowledge. Phrases that focus on students as agents, such as "students learn best when they perceive a need to know ..." reflect **andragogy,** an approach to education that is grounded in the assumption that learners are mature and capable of actively participating in the learning experience.

Some equate **pedagogy** to educational approaches for children and andragogy to educational approaches for adults (Knowles, Holton, & Swanson, 2005). It may be more effective to identify these terms not with age or developmental state, but rather with the assumed needs of the learner. If adults are new to a field of learning, they may initially lack the ability to participate actively in the learning experience and will benefit from a teaching approach that assumes their need for a great deal of guidance and direction in the learning process (pedagogy). As mature learners, bright school-agers, many teens, and most adults, gain early experience with the material, and quickly progress toward the ability to co-create the learning experience, at which time the teaching approach can shift to encourage their active participation (andragogy).

A phrase such as "students retain only what they will use" is grounded in a pragmatic philosophy, or a general world view that assigns the most value or worth to that which is useful, or functional. A phrase such as "students are motivated to earn good grades" reflects a teleological philosophy, meaning that actions are directed by the purpose they serve, rather than by their causes. The phrase "students will cheat whenever they can" reflects an underlying philosophy of inherent evil in all people, whereas the phrase "students generally try their best" reflects an underlying philosophy of inherent good in all people.

Clearly, some of these philosophical positions are incompatible with one another. It is illogical to hold simultaneously the opposing beliefs that all people are inherently good, and that all people are inherently bad. In most of the previous examples in which students are assumed to be evil or bad, however, the teacher is implicitly assumed to be good, well-intended, or at least well motivated. This kind of philosophy reflecting a struggle between good and evil is common in cultures that are founded on a Judeo-Christian philosophy in which the struggle between good and evil originated at the time of creation. In contrast, it is also possible to assume that such a struggle does not exist and that people can be capable of evil but generally reach for a higher good (Noddings, 1989).

It is no easy task to sort out one's own personal philosophy, and most people have inconsistencies and contradictions in their values and views that are difficult to address. Every nurse educator has a personal history grounded in **culture,** religion, and social and political traditions that have become engrained in our thinking certain world views, some of which we struggle to change or overcome, and some of which we hold dear. To begin to form and subsequently to

> What are the fundamental ideas from general philosophies and theories that form nursing as a discipline?
> What are specific examples of educational philosophy that other nurse educators have articulated?
> What is one's own practice as a teacher? (Shellenbarger, Palmer, Labant, & Kuzneski, 2005).

examine one's own philosophy of nursing education, it is necessary to reflect actively on the questions in Box 2–2.

Patterns of Knowing or Fundamental Ideas That Form Nursing as a Discipline

The following sections provide ideas about each of the three areas of reflection enumerated in Box 2–2, emphasizing issues to consider as you engage in your own reflection.

Barbara Carper (1978) examined early nursing texts for their philosophical perspectives and identified four fundamental patterns of knowing that underpin nursing knowledge. The four patterns are:

- **Empirics,** the science of nursing
- **Ethics,** the moral component of nursing knowledge
- **Personal knowing,** the inner experience of nursing
- **Aesthetics,** the art of nursing

These four patterns of knowing have become widely accepted as underlying nursing knowledge and practice. White (1995) proposed a fifth pattern:

- **Sociopolitical knowing,** the context of nursing

At least several, sometimes all, of these five patterns of knowing are typically reflected in nursing school philosophies in some manner. This fact indicates that as a principle, nursing faculty tend to acknowledge fundamental patterns of knowing in their course content and activities. Consider the philosophy of the program in which you currently teach. If your program does not have a philosophy, find one from another program, or see for example (Mission and Philosophy, School of Nursing University of Connecticut, 2004). As you read any curriculum philosophy document, you can examine it in light of each of the fundamental patterns of knowing. If you find that any of the patterns are simply not reflected, then you can conclude that an essential component of nursing knowledge is likely to be neglected in the courses that are taught. Or, if you find one or more of the patterns to be overly predominant, then the other patterns are likely to be neglected in the course content. As you examine your chosen document, consider the following.

Empirics

Empirics is typically the dominant pattern of knowing in nursing curricula. As you examine your school's philosophy, consider to what extent empirics is emphasized, and make a note of your observation. When focusing on empirics, the philosophy will contain phrases that refer to: nursing theory and theory from other disciplines, the sciences in general, and medicine.

Theory is generally taken to mean scientific theory that explains human experiences that can be measured or accessed through the physical senses. Experiences that are not strictly physical, or that are hard to observe, such as hope or grief, for example, are addressed in empiric theory in ways that point to observable dimensions of the experience, such as posture or motions, verbal or facial expressions, or sequences of behavior. These kinds of theories typically constitute what nursing philosophies refer to as the foundation for nursing practice.

The "Sciences" in General

Many nursing philosophies specifically state that nursing is based on the more general physical and human sciences. Rarely, a philosophy will also mention the arts and humanities as a foundation for nursing practice.

Medicine

Medicine is generally assumed to mean a practice based on scientific theory that addresses pathophysiology and pathopsychology. Many nursing philosophies include medical science as a foundation for nursing practice. If you do not find this in the philosophy you are examining, make a special note of this omission. Later, when you examine the course content, you may find a stunning disconnect—a large emphasis on medical theory in the actual course content outlines.

Ethics

Ethical considerations usually appear in a school's statement of philosophy. As you examine your philosophy, consider which of the following dimensions of ethical knowing are included: **rights** and **justice,** responsibility, **integrity** and ethical comportment, and **caring** as a moral imperative.

Rights and Justice

Nursing philosophies often include a statement that acknowledges the right of all people to health or health care. Or, you may see statements concerning what people deserve in terms of respect, regardless of various personal dimensions, such as **socioeconomic** status, race, religious belief, and so forth.

Responsibility

Many nursing philosophies address the responsibilities of the nurse, dimensions of professionalism, obligations to serve, and accountability for one's own practice. Advocacy for the rights of patients is a common ethical dimension for nursing.

Integrity and Ethical Comportment

Statements that refer to the nurse's obligation to act with integrity and within the cultural expectations of morality are usually not specific to a particular moral or ethical standard, but refer more generally to conduct that meets general ethical standards, such as honesty, truth-telling, abiding by legal requirements of practice, and so forth.

Caring as a Moral Imperative

The moral obligation to care is often subtle. It is assumed in statements that refer to the nurses' obligation to care for people regardless of race or creed, for example. There is a slight but important difference in a statement that says a nurse is obligated to have compassion and respect for others, and one that states that a nurse is obligated to care for others in all circumstances. Occasionally, you will find statements in nursing philosophies that indicate that a nurse is not obligated to care for a person when, for example, the nurse's religious beliefs conflict with the care that is required.

Personal Knowing

Personal knowing is not often included as an explicit part of a school's philosophy. Personal knowing is the inner experience of becoming a whole and genuine self. Personal knowing is essential for engaging in a caring and healing encounter with another. Statements that refer to the nature of the nurse as a human being and as one in relation to others imply beliefs related to personal knowing. Elements of a philosophy that reflect personal knowing include: **reflective practice,** therapeutic use of self, and the unique nature of human beings.

Reflective Practice
Statements that refer to the development of expertise in nursing infer a kind of practice that develops through personal reflection on one's own practice, resulting in gaining personal insight, meaning, and growth arising from the practice itself (Schön, 1987).

Therapeutic Use of Self, or Self-in-Relation
In principle, many nursing philosophies explicitly state, or tacitly assume that a large component of nursing involves the therapeutic use of self, or the nurse's ability to enter into a dynamic human relationship with others that is directed toward caring and healing.

Unique Nature of Human Beings
Many nursing philosophies hold the tenet that human beings are unique and individual. This statement is usually in a context that also addresses respect for the uniqueness of the other person, often without specific reference to the idea that the nurse is also a unique individual. Any general statement about the uniqueness of individuals also implies that in order to know and understand another's uniqueness, one must know the self.

Aesthetics

Aesthetics is closely related to personal knowing in that both are concerned with a dimension of uniqueness. Aesthetics, however, concerns the ability to discern the deeper meaning of a situation, and the creative ability to respond to a situation in its **wholeness.** It is the ability of the nurse to bring forth something that is possible in a situation, and that without the nurse would not be possible. Philosophical statements that reflect aesthetic knowing include: **creativity in practice** and the transformative nature of nursing.

Creativity in Practice
Creativity and the art of nursing practice is not typically included in the philosophies of schools of nursing, but there may be statements that could link to this important component of nursing. Even the premise that each person is unique implies that an element of creativity is necessary in an interaction that occurs between two or more people. Statements that refer to the importance of culture imply the ability to discern cultural meanings and to be responsive to different cultures.

Transformative Nature of Nursing Practice
When nursing is viewed as a practice that has its own foundation and purpose, and not one that is dependent upon the practice of medicine, then nursing acquires agency as a practice that can transform reality, or bring forth changes toward health, healing, and wellness. Philosophical statements that refer to a purpose of nursing, such as achieving high-level wellness, peaceful death, or healing and well-being, imply that the nurse has the ability to engage in a kind of creative practice that is responsive to what is, but that moves experience toward a new and different reality.

Sociopolitical Knowing

Sociopolitical knowing concerns context and environment. Most philosophies of Schools of Nursing include statements that acknowledge the importance of one's context as inherently significant to health and well-being. Statements that relate to sociopolitical knowing include: culture, family and community; **natural environment**; socioeconomic aspects of health; and governmental, organizational, and political structures.

Culture, Family and Community

These aspects of a person's context are generally regarded as inherent in the idea of "wholism," which assumes that a person cannot exist in individual isolation, but as one who develops within, and participates in developing, a meaningful social network.

Natural Environment

Although generally it is assumed that the natural environment plays an important role in health, it is usually neglected as a component within philosophies of nursing education (Kleffel, 1991). Examine your philosophy for statements that point to the importance of a clean and healthy environment, which are supported by a sociopolitical will to protect and nurture the physical environment.

Socioeconomic Aspects of Health

Like the natural environment, socioeconomic factors are generally understood as related to health and well-being, but explicit reference to socioeconomics is rare. Your philosophy might address this aspect of health indirectly, for example in acknowledging the right of individuals to receive care regardless of socioeconomic status. Missing in this kind of reference is the idea that a nurse might have a role to play in changing the contexts in which socioeconomic factors are a detriment to human health and well-being.

Governmental, Organizational, and Political Structures

Political structures are closely related to culture and community, but they are not the same thing, and these structures are at the heart of determining health-care rights, services, quality of care, and opportunity for participation in decision-making. Examine your philosophy for elements that refer to the nurse's role as an advocate, or that position the nurse as an agent in determining the quality of care, as a leader and change-maker, or as an active participant in the community. Also look for statements that position all people as creators, participants, and decision-makers in their own health care. Although many of these statements do not explicitly address organizational and political structures, they set the stage for active participation and influence in such structures.

Common Assumptions in Nursing Theory

There are several important texts that summarize the elements of major nursing theories known as grand theory (Chinn & Kramer, 2004; Fawcett, 1993; Meleis, 1991). These theories address the general, broad nature of nursing, setting forth ideas about the fundamental goals and purposes of nursing, and explanations of the fundamental dynamics that occur in a nurse-patient interaction to achieve these broad goals. There are also many middle-range theories published in journal articles and summarized in texts (Smith & Liehr, 2003). Middle-range theories focus on specific human health experiences that occur commonly in nursing practice, such as uncertainty in illness, family stress, and unpleasant symptoms. Middle-range theory provides a comprehensive description of the specific experience, explanations of the dynamics that occur as the experience unfolds, and either explicit or implied explanations concerning the dynamics in the nurse-patient interaction related to the experience. Similarly, situation-specific theories address specific nursing phenomena, but also incorporate specific contexts and are readily applicable to practice (Im & Meleis, 1999).

Whether a nursing theory is considered a grand theory, a middle-range theory, or a situation-specific theory, there are common fundamental tenets or assumptions upon which they are based that characterize theory as nursing theory (Chinn, 1989). These assumptions provide the framework or the foundation for nursing as a discipline, and underpin what and how we teach in nursing. The assumptions that characterize a nursing perspective in theory should also appear in a nursing education philosophy, either explicitly or impliedly. Examine the major assumptions of the nursing theory guiding your own educational institution may be an enlightening exercise. Look for the following major assumptions of nursing theory in your school philosophy.

Health is Wholeness

There is an abiding and consistent theme running throughout nursing literature that identifies health in its fullest, whole dimension as the fundamental goal of nursing. Health is defined in various ways and specific dimensions or aspects of health vary from theory to theory. But fundamentally, health is conceptualized as a dynamic experience that embraces all aspects of human existence.

The Primacy of Human Uniqueness and Subjectivity

Nursing theories consistently point to the person's unique perceptions and experience as the starting point from which to understand human health experience. Although theories, by definition, draw general conclusions about the nature of a phenomenon, nursing theories provide conceptual space for experience to be interpreted and understood in the context of the individual's unique experience. Subjectivity is typically understood to be developed within a relational, social, and cultural context, but even given certain general understandings about culture, nursing's focus consistently seeks to understand a person's uniqueness within their context.

Caring and Supportive Relationship

Not all nursing theories specify caring per se as the central concept, but nursing theories consistently espouse nurturing, growth-producing, healing relational contexts or interactions that support movement toward health and wellness. Some theories include or focus on the specific nature of the relationship between nurse and patient or family. Others focus on the significant relationships of family, community, society, or environment that influence the evolution of a specific health experience.

Putting It All Together

By examining your school's philosophy, you can compare it to what you personally believe, and the ways in which you view the world, yourself, and others with whom you interact. You now have a start toward developing your own personal philosophy, which incorporates the essential tenets of nursing's fundamental patterns of knowing in nursing and assumptions that are consistent with theoretical nursing perspectives. You may also have a start toward developing a theory of nursing education. Your philosophy will consist of those statements that you take as givens, as assumptions that you take to be constant and enduring. A theory of education includes descriptions and explanations that you think represent your experience as accurately as possible, but that you are also aware may not yet be the best or most accurate explanations. Theoretical ideas are built from your philosophy, but theories reside in the empiric realm; they are ideas about reality that are subject to empiric examination and change. As an example, a philosophy might have a strong component that views the nurse as an advocate for patient rights (ethical knowing). A related theory might address the kind of organizational structure that is proposed to provide a strong environment in which nurse advocacy results in a higher quality of care. This theory would provide the structure from which to design research exploring the characteristics of the organizational structure, resulting in evidence demonstrating the extent to which this structure actually results in a high quality of care and positive patient outcomes.

Noddings' (1995) philosophy of caring education illustrates a well-developed educational philosophy (Chinn, 1999). Noddings' philosophy is significant for nursing education because it embraces the fundamental perspective of caring relationship that underlies nursing theory. This is a key element that must characterize nursing education if we are to know what we do, and do what we know. If we seek to teach students how to engage in caring and supportive relationships in order to promote growth, health, and healing, then as teachers we are compelled to teach in ways that demonstrate exactly this kind of relationship. If we do not do so, we are essentially sending the message "do as I say, not as I do."

The next section of this chapter summarizes key elements of Noddings' philosophy, along with implications for teaching practices that arise from each philosophical element. The final section of this chapter will then provide suggestions for reflecting on your teaching practices. These two sections, taken together, lead you through praxis—reflection on what you know (what you value and what you believe to be true, right, and good in education) and what you do (as reflected in your teaching practices). The outcome, hopefully, will be a thoughtful statement of your personal philosophy of nursing education, and a foundation from which to affirm, change, or develop teaching practices that are consistent with your philosophy.

Noddings' Philosophy of Caring Education

There are four major processes or principles that Noddings specifies as essential to caring education: **modeling,** dialogue, practice, and **confirmation.** Each of these processes leads directly to teaching practices that demonstrate beliefs and values of caring education. The practices that are suggested for each of Noddings' principles are drawn from *Peace and Power* guidelines for group process (Chinn, 2004b; Falk-Rafael, Anderson, Chinn, & Rubotzky, 2004).

Modeling

Modeling is showing in action and interaction what it means to care. Caring in teaching, as in all caring relationships, does not mean "anything goes." Rather, it means that you care about yourself as a nurse educator; you take your role as teacher seriously; you are clear about what is required to be a nurse; and you are clear about professional and personal standards of nursing. At the same time, you care deeply about each student, and are committed to creating the best possible learning environment for everyone. Specific actions that model what it means to care as a teacher are listed in Box 2–3.

Dialogue

Dialogue underpins all interactions between and among students and teachers. It is an interactive exchange that brings to conscious awareness what everyone is doing, and more importantly, why. Everyone in the group is brought into the discussions with equal opportunity to participate and enter into the dialogue. The teacher creates a context for dialogue that is reflective, so that every

Provide clear standards for achievement, and keep your promise to abide by these standards.
Demystify all aspects of the learning experience so that students are not left to guess or figure it out on their own.
Be open about your own philosophy, goals, and values for the learning experience.
Be responsive to all concerns that are expressed about the experience of learning.
Be flexible (consistent, not rigid); assure fundamental quality of achievement while encouraging creativity and individuality for each student's experience.
Make all learning resources equally available to everyone, including the resources that you draw on as the teacher.
Encourage everyone to do their best, and assist each student in deciding what his or her best performance can be realistically.
Give specific feedback that not only points out what needs to change or improve, but what students can do to move toward the standard of achievement that you have provided.
Eliminate vague value terms in providing feedback (good, poor, satisfactory, etc.) and use instead specific descriptions of what you see in the student's performance in relation to the learning goals you have provided ("Your answer to Ms. Jones showed an accurate understanding of her concerns.").
Build in options for learning experiences that students can create and ground in what is most meaningful to them.

learning experience becomes a "text"—a focus for reflection that brings forth awareness of the meaning of each learning experience. Specific actions that promote caring dialogue are listed in Box 2–4.

Practice in Caring

Practice in caring is the practice of cooperation and sharing. The dominant practices of patriarchal education view cooperation and sharing as "cheating." In the context of caring education, cooperation and sharing are valued as critical learning tools for not only gaining knowledge and understanding, but also for developing valuable human interaction skills that serve communities and societies well. Concerns for each student's individual achievement are addressed within a context of cooperation and sharing in ways that call forth individual responsibility, and each individual's best performance. Specific actions that promote practice in caring are listed here:

Box 2–4 Specific Actions That Promote Caring Dialogue

Include early and ongoing discussion in the group that brings to the group everyone's intentions, hopes, and dreams for the learning experience; discuss individual differences and how these can be integrated into the experience of the whole.
Encourage negotiation so that everyone's concerns are addressed to the extent possible.
Let go of the idea that you alone as teacher have to address each concern; encourage and draw on everyone's ideas for addressing individual concerns.
Use time at the end of each learning experience for each student to share his reflection on the learning experience, and use these reflections as a foundation for the next experience.
Create a context for discussion so that every voice is heard and respected.

- Engage broad audiences: instead of being the only person to see and evaluate a student's work, encourage students to share their work openly and invite everyone's feedback.
- Provide guidelines for everyone to use in providing constructive criticism of one another's work.
- Build in opportunities for students to receive feedback on their constructive criticism skills.
- Encourage presentations of student work both in and outside of class (to clients, or groups of nurses in the community, for example), and draw on the feedback they receive from these groups.
- Build in opportunities for students to share with the group resources and information that they discover outside of class.

Confirmation

Confirmation is the practice of affirming and encouraging the best for all. As the teacher, you have the responsibility to identify basic standards of achievement that are grounded in professional standards of nursing care, and that provide for students explicit descriptions of the basic performance expectations required for the particular learning experience. At the same time, within a caring context your responsibility is to learn and know students as individuals, and encourage them to reach the professional standards in ways that express their own desires, expectations, and highest good. Each student's achievement must meet the expectations of the student as well as those of the teacher. When a student cannot meet these expectations, the teacher responds with compassion and understanding and shifts the focus for interacting with the student in the direction of assisting the student to find a path that better suits her abilities or needs at this moment in time. Since confirmation in most educational contexts also involves grading, there are immense challenges in maintaining a focus on caring practices, but it is possible to do so (Chinn, 2004a). Practices that demonstrate the principle of confirmation are listed in Box 2–5.

Box 2–5 Specific Actions That Promote Practice in Caring

Build in opportunities for students to receive ample formative feedback, where they can make mistakes without being "graded," and use feedback to refine their achievement.

Clearly and specifically describe ways for students to demonstrate what they have accomplished in relation to each expectation for the learning experience.

Abandon single expectations for all; build in ways to acknowledge that a student has met fundamental standards of achievement, and when they have excelled in some dimension of achievement.

Create a learning context in which constructive criticism is invited and welcomed.

Use student portfolios as a means for students to demonstrate what they have accomplished, and to begin building a professional résumé.

Encourage students to use the criteria for achievement to assess their own work, and to share their self-assessment as part of their portfolio.

Provide opportunities for the group to celebrate one another's contributions to the learning experience, and of one another's achievements.

Use criterion-based assessment; criteria for achievement flow from the expectations for learning but express in concrete terms what the student needs to demonstrate in order to meet the criteria for achievement.

Conceptually define grades, rather than defining grades on an arbitrary scale of numbers. Example: "C" = meeting basic standards of care, "B" = meeting basic standards as well as influencing the continuity of care that meets basic standards, "A" = in addition, critiques existing standards of care and proposes a new standard.

Reflective Practice

This process of examining your philosophy and your course materials will become an on-going one. The other critical component in your praxis of teaching will be to make space to reflect critically at the end of each course, going over what you intended to happen, and what actually happened. Use the student evaluations as one component that influences your reflection. Be open and receptive to student comments, while also valuing your own insights and inner knowing of the circumstances within which the student perspective developed. If at all possible, engage in discussion with students about their experience several weeks after the experience, when insights and understandings about what they learned and how they learned will be interpreted from a different (and possibly better informed) perspective. Share your perspectives on the experience with the students and invite their reaction to any changes you are considering.

Another often neglected source for critical reflection is that of faculty colleagues. When you invite their feedback, be aware of their own philosophy and perspectives concerning nursing education. You will benefit from learning the perceptions of those who do not share your values, but you will be particularly interested in the feedback of those who do share your values. Feedback coming from each of these perspectives will help you continue to refine both your values and beliefs, and your practices as a teacher.

It may seem that these reflective processes are too time-consuming for an already overworked nurse educator. Indeed, engaging in this kind of reflective practice places a real demand on your time, energy, and emotional/intellectual capacities. However, what you will gain is immense. You will acquire a renewed and renewable sense of satisfaction in your teaching. You will reach a point when you avoid, and even eliminate, some of the most distressing and time-consuming demands of teaching—the demands coming from students who are floundering, dissatisfied, distressed, anxious, and uncertain. Your level of preparation for each new course will improve, and your well-developed course materials will provide a sound framework that makes it possible to get right to the heart of teaching and learning.

Summary

This process of examining your philosophy and your course materials will become an on-going process. The other critical component in your praxis of teaching will be to make space to reflect critically at the end of each course, going over what you intended to happen, and what actually happened. Use the student evaluations as one component that influences your reflection. Be open and receptive to student comments, while also valuing your own insights and inner knowing of the circumstances within which the student perspective developed. If at all possible, engage in discussion with students about their experience several weeks after the experience, when insights and understandings about what they learned and how they learned will be interpreted from a different (and possibly better informed) perspective. Share your perspectives on the experience with the students and invite their reaction to any changes you are considering.

Another often neglected source for critical reflection is that of faculty colleagues. When you invite their feedback, be aware of their own philosophy and perspectives concerning nursing education. You will benefit from learning the perceptions of those who do not share your values, but you will be particularly interested in the feedback of those who do share your values. Feedback coming from each of these perspectives will help you to continue to refine both your values and beliefs, and your practices as a teacher.

It may seem that these reflective processes are too time-consuming for an already overworked nurse educator. Indeed, engaging in this kind of reflective practice places a real demand on your time, energy, and emotional/intellectual capacities. But what you will gain is immense. You will acquire a renewed and renewable sense of satisfaction in your teaching. You will reach a point when you avoid, and even eliminate, some of the most distressing and time-consuming demands of teaching—the demands coming from students who are floundering, dissatisfied, distressed, anxious, and uncertain. Your level of preparation for each new course will improve, and your well-developed course materials will provide a sound framework that makes it possible to get right to the heart of teaching and learning.

Carper, B. A. (1978). Fundamental patterns of knowing in nursing. *Advances In Nursing Science, 1*(1), 13–23.

Chinn, P. L. (1989). Nursing patterns of knowing and feminist thought. *Nursing and Health Care, 10*(2), 71–75.

Chinn, P. L. (1999). A philosophy of nursing education. Retrieved October 22, 2005, from **http://ans-info.net/Caring%20curriculum_files/frame.htm**

Chinn, P. L. (2004a). A praxis for grading. In M. H. Oermann & K. T. Heinrich (Eds.), *Annual review of nursing education* (Vol. 2, pp. 89–109). New York: Springer Publishing.

Chinn, P. L. (2004b). *Peace & power: Creative leadership for building communities* (6th ed.). Boston: Jones & Bartlett.

Chinn, P. L., & Kramer, M. (2004). *Integrated knowledge development in nursing* (6th ed.). St Louis: Mosby.

Falk-Rafael, A. R., Anderson, M. A., Chinn, P. L., & Rubotzky, A. M. (2004). Peace and power as a critical feminist framework for nursing education. In M. H. Oermann & K. T. Heinrich (Eds.), *Annual review of nursing education* (Vol. 2, pp. 217–235). New York: Springer Publishing.

Fawcett, J. (1993). *Analysis and evaluation of conceptual models of nursing* (3rd ed.). Philadelphia: FA Davis Co.

Im, E.-O., & Meleis, A. I. (1999). Situation-specific theories: Philosophical roots, properties, and approach. *Advances in Nursing Science, 22*(2), 11–24.

Kleffel, D. (1991). Rethinking the environment as a domain of nursing knowledge. *Advances in Nursing Science, 14*(1), 40–51.

Knowles, M. S. I., Holton, E. F., & Swanson, R. A. (2005). *The adult learner: The definitive classic in adult education and human resource development* (6th ed.). Burlington, MA: Elsevier.

Meleis, A. I. (1991). *Theoretical nursing: Development & progress* (4th ed.). Philadelphia: J.B. Lippincott.

Mission and Philosophy, School of Nursing University of Connecticut [Electronic (2004). Version]. Retrieved October 22, 2005 from **http://web1.uits.uconn.edu/nursing/Mission.html.**

Noddings, N. (1989). *Women and evil.* Berkeley, CA: University of California Press.

Noddings, N. (1995). *Philosophy of education.* Boulder, CO: Westview Press.

Schön, D. A. (1987). *Educating the reflective practitioner.* San Francisco: Jossey-Bass Publishers.

Shellenbarger, T., Palmer, E. A., Labant, A. L., & Kuzneski, J. L. (2005). Use of faculty reflection to improve teaching. In M. H. Oermann & K. T. Heinrich (Eds.), *Annual review of nursing education* (Vol. 3, pp. 343–357). New York: Springer Publishing.

Smith, M. J., & Liehr, P. (2003). *Middle range theory for nursing:* Springer Publishing.

White, J. (1995). Patterns of knowing: Review, critique, and update. *Advances in Nursing Science, 17*(4), 73–86.

REVIEW QUESTIONS

- Consider the philosophy of the program in which you currently teach. Identify the patterns of knowing: empirics, ethics, personal knowing, aesthetics, and sociopolitical knowing. Develop a grid to determine if the patterns are equally distributed throughout the philosophy. If a pattern is not found in the philosophy, provide suggestions for integration within the document.
- Because the personal knowing pattern is often not included in a school's philosophy, identify statements that reflect on this pattern, focusing on reflective practice, therapeutic use of self, and the unique nature of human beings.
- Reflect on your own practice. Provide examples of how you engaged in caring and supportive relationships. Explain how you may be able to model these behaviors for students in a clinical setting.
- Review the four major processes that Noddings specifies as essential to caring education: modeling, dialogue, practice, and confirmation. Develop case studies and ask students to determine which of the processes are exemplified in them.

CRITICAL THINKING EXERCISES

Having reached this point in this chapter, you are now ready to reflect on your own practice as a teacher. If you have not already done so, make a list (or a narrative) describing the values, beliefs, and ideas that you hold dear as a teacher. Reflect on your statements in light of the nursing patterns of knowing and the fundamental assumptions common to nursing theories. Next, select a course syllabus that you have used, or one that you are developing. Examine your syllabus in light of the values and beliefs that you have outlined, and begin to make revisions, additions, or deletions to bring your course materials into alignment with your values.

ANNOTATED RESEARCH SUMMARY

Coyle-Rogers, P., & Cramer, M. (2005). The phenomenon of caring: The perspectives of nurse educators. *Journal for Nurses in Staff Development, 21*(4), 160–170.

This research uses a phenomenological approach and uncovered themes related to the perception of nurse educators' role in caring. The themes discovered were intuitive discovery, supportive guidance, respect, promoting independence, and shared success. Discussion of the themes indicated potential outcome divergence.

Also noted were differences in what students/orientees and nurse educators believe to be caring behaviors related to independence and rescue strategies. Nursing educators, regardless of employment situation, are encouraged to use these findings to understand their role perceptions by students and orientees.

Chapter Outline

THE ART AND SCIENCE OF NURSING EDUCATION

3

Deborah C. Messecar

Learning Outcomes

On the completion of this chapter, the reader will be able to:

- Describe the history of nursing science.
- Understand the ways of knowing that can affect student learning.
- Identify appropriate nursing process language.
- Discriminate between different teaching methodologies.
- Analyze evidence-based practice and its use for nursing education.
- Describe the assets and deficits of different teaching methodologies.

Key Terms

Conceptual mapping
Evidence-based practice
NIC/NOC/NANDA
Problem-based learning (PBL)
Questioning
Science of nursing
Storytelling

The body of knowledge that serves as the rationale for nursing practice defines how it is that nurses know and understand their world. Carper's (1978) article on the fundamental patterns of knowing in nursing specifies the important dimensions upon which nursing knowledge can be characterized. There are four main kinds of knowledge in nursing:

- Empirics: knowledge that or "factual knowledge"
- Aesthetics: knowledge how or "practical knowledge"
- Personal knowledge: knowledge of people, places, and things, or "knowledge by acquaintance"
- Ethics: knowledge of what ought to be done, or "moral knowledge"

Understanding these patterns of knowledge is critical for any faculty members engaged in teaching and mastering nursing. By examining the kinds of knowing that provide the discipline with its particular perspectives and significance, the instructor gains an increased awareness of the complexity and diversity of nursing knowledge. Although each type of knowledge is considered necessary for achieving mastery in nursing, none of them alone should be considered sufficient. This chapter will cover the essential patterns of knowing in nursing and will illustrate how these patterns inform clinical judgment. A brief history of the **science of nursing** education will be presented along with a summary of selected current research and initiatives in nursing education and how they apply to fundamental patterns of knowing in nursing.

Carper's Ways of Knowing

Four fundamental patterns of knowing in nursing were originally identified by Carper in 1978 from an analysis of the conceptual and syntactical structure of nursing knowledge. The four patterns include: empirical, aesthetic, personal, and ethical knowledge.

Empirics, the Science of Nursing

Empirics, or the science of nursing, is the pattern of knowing that is focused upon the description, classification, and explanation of phenomena that are perceptible by direct observation or experience. In other words, empirics is the factual knowledge of the discipline. It is consciously accessible and acquired by observation, inspection, and deductive reasoning (Stein, Corte, Colling, & Whall, 1998). Empiric (or semantic) knowledge is a product of formal educational experiences like reading a professional journal or accessing a textbook (Stein et al. 1998). Empirical knowledge is based on factual descriptions of persons, places, or situations that can be verified by others.

Empiric knowledge or "knowing that" is the category of knowledge that comes to mind when we think about knowledge acquired in the classroom that is derived from research in basic and nursing sciences. In Benner's early work describing the transition from novice to expert nurse, this is the theoretical type of knowledge that drives nursing action (Benner, 1983, 1984). If empiric knowledge was sufficient to guide nursing practice, students could simply memorize procedures from a manual of nursing practice; no clinical application would be required to attain competence. As an illustration, take the example of the nurse doing a simple procedure like a catheter insertion. The procedure manual tells you what supplies to collect, how to proceed step-by-step, and identifies conditions or problems that require special attention. But when the process of inserting a Foley catheter is complicated by the real life contingency—like a patient who has benign prostatic hypertrophy, a condition not necessarily described in the manual—theoretical or empiric knowledge alone may not be sufficient.

Aesthetics, the Art of Nursing

Aesthetics, or the art of nursing, is the type of knowledge underlying the performance of nursing practice, or "knowing how." Aesthetic knowledge lies beneath the skillful performance of the manual and technical procedures in nursing, as well as the ability to grasp the significance of a patient's behavior immediately and respond insightfully to it. Learning the art of nursing requires students to master the ability to put together disparate facts and details about a patient's behavior into a holistic understanding of what is significant in that behavior. Through empathy, the nurse gains understanding of the patient's felt experience and therefore has a larger repertoire of choices in designing and providing nursing care that is effective and satisfying. Because this way of knowing is not based on empirical knowledge or that which can be directly observed, the validity of this type of knowledge is only apparent once the nurse has managed to produce care that is helpful and beneficial. Aesthetic knowledge is action-oriented and includes both the manual/technical skills of the profession as well as the intellectual skill necessary for grasping a situation, making a care plan, and then intervening in a clinical encounter (Stein et al. 1998).

Aesthetic knowledge is more complex than empirical knowledge and requires both motor skills and strategies and rules to make sense of information. This practical knowledge is what Benner has also described as "knowing how" and is absolutely essential for making astute judgments. Practical knowledge is gained through experience, which is not acquired through the mere passage of time, but only when one's frame of reference about what can be expected is somehow altered or challenged in an actual, real-life situation (Benner, 1984). The complex acquisition of skills sometimes escapes our capacity to describe even simple activities theoretically (Kuhn, 1970; Polanyi, 1958). As a result, some practical knowledge will not be easily reduced to step-by-step explanation.

For example, when an experienced nurse encounters a crisis situation, such as a patient presenting in an emergency room with a rapidly dropping blood pressure, the knowledge needed is readily solicited. To the outside observer, the nurse is able to respond almost intuitively, based on an immediate grasp of the clinical situation, and just seems to know what to do. The beginning nurse however, will respond slowly, trying to reason things through based on theoretical knowledge as he struggles to figure out which particular aspect of factual knowledge applies. It is through application that the nurse begins to develop practical knowledge that refines and extends the theoretical base of practice. Hence, the means of acquiring "hands-on" knowledge include not only laboratory sessions and bedside experiences, but also observation of experts' problem solving in selected situations as in clinical rounds or seminars. Reflection on practice is key for developing this type of practical knowledge (Tanner, 2006).

Personal Knowing in Nursing

Personal knowing in nursing assumes that gaining self-awareness is a vital aspect of professional development. Personal knowing in nursing is defined as that knowledge of self that supports a therapeutic interpersonal process between the nurse and the patient. Personal knowledge is acquired through interactions, relationships, and transactions among individuals. Personal knowledge is based on the existentialist view that people are continuously evolving over time. In the existentialist view, being cannot be made a subject of objective enquiry, it is revealed to the individual by reflection on his own unique concrete existence in time and space. Hence, each self-aware individual comes to understand their own existence in terms of their experience of themselves and their situation.

The recognition of other individuals and communication with them is a criterion of authentic existence. To be authentic, one must preserve one's own individual personal identity, while allowing others to have the freedom to make their own choices as they also constantly engage in the process of becoming. By having an authentic personal relationship with the patient, the nurse is able to help the patient achieve higher levels of individual well-being that would be impossible without this therapeutic use of self.

This form of knowledge in nursing is perhaps the most difficult to master and teach, but yet is the most essential knowledge for understanding the meaning of health for the patient. Personal knowledge is acquired gradually through interaction between the nurse and the patient and is the product of personal experience in practice (Stein et al., 1998). Writing about feelings is one way to facilitate personal knowing.

According to Higgins (1996), journal writing can be used as a mode of thinking about practice with nursing students. Capacchione's (1989) journal method is unique because it develops both sides of the brain: the rational, verbal left hemisphere and the artistic, intuitive right hemisphere. Drawing is a right brain function. With this technique, students learn to have faith and hope in themselves and can learn to inspire it in others.

Ethics, the Moral Knowledge in Nursing

Ethics or the moral knowledge in nursing is focused on making decisions on right and wrong action in the context of the care and treatment of patients. It involves the struggle to identify what ought to be done in situations of ambiguity or uncertainty. Knowledge of ethical codes alone will not be sufficient to provide the nurse with answers to moral questions in nursing. Students come to the clinical situation with their own fundamental disposition toward what is good and right, and often these values remain unspoken, and unrecognized—even though they may profoundly influence what students notice in a given situation, the options they may consider taking, and what they ultimately decide to do (Tanner, 2006). Allowing students to tell their stories reinforces their humanistic values. For example, Higgins (1996) had first-year students come together for a seminar, which began with introductions and asking each student to share the stories that led to them choosing nursing as a career. The purpose of this exercise was to build upon the caring values that the students brought to nursing. Subsequent sessions built upon this work. By examining the values by which students decide what is morally right, they gain greater awareness of what is involved in making moral choices and being responsible for the choices made.

Carper's model of the ways of knowing in nursing not only highlights the importance and centrality of empirical, factual, and theoretically derived knowledge, but recognizes the equally essential knowledge gained through clinical practice. This is because both personal and aesthetic knowledge are postulated to come from experience that is more than the mastery of a list of technical skills (Stein, Corte, Colling, & Whall, 1998). Strict dedication to content coverage needs to be replaced with development of flexible skill sets that can be used across settings (Tanner, 2002, 2004). Faculty should alter what and how they teach accordingly.

The next section of this chapter will trace the evolution of how the empirical science of nursing has been organized and described for the novice nurse. The history of going from use of the nursing process, to a proliferation of classification schemes, and on to **evidence-based practice** developed around practice guidelines and critical pathways will be described.

Following this description of processes, taxonomies, and evidence-based protocols, the chapter reviews current research and initiatives that communicate the contextual, interpretive, and interpersonal knowledge deemed important in Carper's ways of knowing in nursing.

Science of Nursing Education

By examining some of the roots of the nursing process, the scientific basis of nursing actions, and its limitations in describing nursing practice knowledge will become clearer.

History

In the early 1960s a model called "The Nursing Process" was developed by Orlando (Orlando, 1961). The idea is that the patient must be the central character; nursing care needs to be directed at improving outcomes for the patient. The model emphasizes that nursing actions are directed toward some goal, and are deliberative. There are five steps of the model:

• Assessment
• Diagnosis
• Planning
• Implementation
• Evaluation

In this model, clinical judgment is viewed as a linear problem-solving activity, which the nurse uses to identify nursing interventions directed toward the resolution of diagnosed problems. By using this model, greater emphasis was placed on nursing care planning. In 1971, the concept of nursing diagnosis developed as a statement describing the phenomenon, and which nurses independently diagnose and treat. A major national effort to develop taxonomy of nursing diagnoses began. The organization that started this process was formed in 1982, as the **North American Nursing Diagnosis Association (NANDA)** and has been responsible for linking the use of standardized languages with the nursing process.

Benefits and Limitations of the Nursing Process

The nursing process model corrects the perception that nurses only follow doctor's orders, or practice according to a set of rigid protocols, rather through an analysis of what the patient needs and responding to that need. By emphasizing application of empiric knowledge to problems in practice, the nursing process model has had a profound influence on the development of nursing as a discipline, and on the improvement of patient care. It has had broad utility in nursing education because it reminds students of the value of comprehensive assessment, and thorough understanding of problems before taking action. In addition, the nursing process emphasizes the need to be thoughtful, deliberative, and systematic in making nursing decisions. As a framework for practice, the nursing process reminds nurses of the value of nursing care planning and mutual goal setting with the patient and the importance of science in decision-making (Tanner, 2006). Several aspects of the nursing process are problematic, however. First, the nursing process, when employed by the novice nurse, can overplay the importance of empiric knowledge over personal and aesthetic knowledge (Henderson, 1982, 1987). The value of other ways of knowing that expert nurses use, such as intuition (Benner & Tanner, 1987; Jacavone & Dostal, 1992; Pyles & Stern, 1983; Rew, 1988; Schraeder & Fischer, 1987), may be ignored. The nursing process' seemingly linear approach to problem solving, as usually documented in a student care plan, also does not reflect the sometimes serendipitous (Corcoran, 1986), or heuristic (short-cut) methods of conclusion drawing on which experienced nurses rely (O'Neill, 1995; Tanner, Padrick, Westfall, & Putzier, 1987; Westfall, Tanner, Putzier, & Padrick, 1986). The assumption of objectivity in the model is also problematic, as it ignores the value of personal knowledge embodied by the term "knowing the patient" (Jenks, 1993; Jenny & Logan, 1992; MacLeod, 1993; Radwin, 1995; Tanner, Benner, Chesla, & Gordon, 1993). The model also presupposes that the patient is the passive recipient of nursing actions that the nurse then evaluates from her perspective as effective or not effective. As a result, students may not identify a potential ethical issue until after it is clear that the care plan goals are at odds with the patient and family's desires. Although the model has been used extensively to teach beginning nursing students the care planning process, numerous studies have shown that it fails to describe adequately the processes of nursing judgment used by expert nurses (Benner, Chesla, & Gordon, 1993; Fonteyn, 1994; Tanner, 1998; Timpka & Arborelius, 1990; Westfall, Tanner, Putzier, & Padrick, 1986).The nursing process and the writing of care plans can sometimes focus students too heavily on the mastery of content, in lieu of critical thinking (Porter-O'Grady, 2001).

Nursing Process, Nursing Standardized Languages, and Evidence-Based Nursing

While the nursing process may be helpful to a novice nurse in developing an initial plan of care for a patient, it has been difficult for students to capture the detailed judgments and decisions that expert nurses make. Thus, supplements to describing nursing action have formed. The original impetus to develop a standard vocabulary for describing health-care phenomena in nursing was to facilitate more widespread use of computers in documentation of care (Werley, Devine, Zorn, Ryan, & Westra, 1991). A standard vocabulary permits the coding of nursing information so that data are available, reliable, valid, and comparable across settings. More importantly, use of a standard vocabulary as opposed to free text notes, ensures that information regarding categories of nursing diagnoses, interventions, and outcomes are easily retrievable and trackable across settings. In order to have the capacity to track a nurse's contribution to these outcomes, a standard vocabulary for nursing is essential. These context-free elements of the process, organized into taxonomic structures for diagnosing, treating, and organizing nursing care are based upon research evidence that can be used to direct nurses' clinical decision-making (Jadad, Haynes, Hunt, & Browman, 2000; McCloskey & Bulechek, 2000).

NMDS

To respond to the need for developing a standard vocabulary, a minimum set of nursing essential core data was developed to allow for grouping and comparison of nursing data collected across various populations, settings, geographic locations, and time. The Nursing Minimum Data Set (NMDS) is a minimum set of items of information with uniform definitions and categories concerning the specific dimension of nursing. The NMDS includes three broad categories of elements: (1) nursing care, (2) patient or client demographics, and (3) service elements. Elements that also are included in the Uniform Hospital Discharge Data Set (UHDD) are indicated by an asterisk (University of Iowa Nursing Informatics, 2006) in Box 3–1.

The nursing care elements of the NMDS include nursing diagnosis, nursing intervention, nursing outcome, and intensity of nursing care. The NMDS provides access to nursing core data while also meeting the information needs of multiple data users in the health-care system. Its primary contribution to practice is that it provides data for quality improvement and trend tracking. NMDS contribution to education comes from facilitating awareness in students of the necessity

Box 3–1

39

Science of Nursing Education

Nursing Care Elements

1. Nursing Diagnosis
2. Nursing Intervention
3. Nursing Outcome
4. Intensity of Nursing Care

Patient or Client Demographic Elements

*5. Personal Identification
*6. Date of Birth
*7. Sex
*8. Race and Ethnicity
*9. Residence

Service Elements

*10. Unique Facility or Service Agency Number
*11. Unique Health Record Number or Patient or Client
 12. Unique Number of Principle Registered Nurse Provider
*13. Episode Admission or Encounter Date
*14. Discharge or Termination Date
*15. Disposition of Patient or Client
*16. Expected Payer for Most or This Bill (Anticipated Financial Guarantor for Services)

*Also included in the Uniform Hospital Discharge Data Set (UHDDS).

to document care appropriately using the nursing process model, and ensuring integration of information management in the undergraduate and graduate curricula.

Unfortunately, no single classification system for the NMDS nursing elements is widely and universally accepted. A number of competing systems have emerged. Classification schemes for nursing diagnosis, interventions, and outcomes of care include: (1) the North American Nursing Diagnosis Association (NANDA, 1992); (2) the Omaha Community Health Problem and Intervention Classification System (Martin & Scheet, 1992); (3) the Nursing Interventions Classification (McCloskey & Bulechek, 1992); and (4) the Nursing Outcomes Classification (Johnson & Maas, 1997). These four classification systems were recognized by the American Nurses Association Steering Committee on Databases to Support Clinical Nursing Practice as usable for documenting nursing practice (McCormick et al., 1994).

NANDA

The focus of this classification scheme is on the NMDS nursing element diagnosis. Of the four classification schemes, NANDA has the longest history. In the 1970s, the association was formed to develop labels for nursing diagnosis. At present, more than 167 diagnosis labels have been developed. An organizing framework of nine general patterns was developed in 1991. Diagnoses are arranged alphabetically in the taxonomy and are coded using the International Classification of Disease (ICD) framework (NANDA International, 2005). New terminology is included via a systematic and rigorous process. The labels are easy to use clinically. NANDA bridges the gap between theory and clinical practice to help apply nursing diagnosis concepts to patients (Lunney, 2005). A nursing diagnosis helps the nursing student to organize his assessment information into a coherent pattern described by the diagnosis taxonomy. The taxonomy is research-based; hence the student's clinical judgment about the patient's responses to actual or potential health problems or life processes are linked to empirically validated concepts.

Omaha Classification System (OCS)

The Visiting Nurses Association of Omaha developed the Omaha Classification Scheme for nurses in community and public health service. The project was supported with a contract from the Division of Nursing, PHS, US DHHS (McCormick et al., 1994). The Omaha system was designed to provide a framework for integrating a clinical practice and documentation system (Martin, Leak, & Aden, 1992). The problem classification scheme has four domains: (1) environmental (e.g., sanitation); (2) psychosocial (e.g., caretaking); (3) physiological (e.g., circulation); and (4) health-related behaviors. The classification scheme includes a rating scale for outcomes that uses a numeric measurement to evaluate changes in the client's knowledge and behavior status in relation to specified health-related problems and selected time frames (Martin, Scheet, and Stegman, 1993). The intervention scheme is divided into four broad areas: health teaching, treatment and procedures, case management, and surveillance. Because this system was developed for community health, most of the users are practicing in that setting. In a survey conducted from 2001 to 2005, approximately 75% of home care and public health organizations reported using Omaha System software (Martin, 2005). The OMAHA classification system has been linked to the NANDA and other classification systems.

The Nursing Interventions Classification (NIC)

Researchers at the University of Iowa developed the **Nursing Interventions Classifications (NIC)** with a grant from the National Center for Nursing Research. The authors used a national Delphi survey of masters-prepared nurses to generate the original list of 336 specific interventions (Moorehead, McCloskey, & Bulechek, 1993). Currently, the NIC contains more than 514 research-based, standardized clinical interventions grouped into seven categories: (1) basic physiological, (2) complex physiological, (3) behavioral, (4) safety, (5) family, (6) health system, and (7) community (Dochterman & Bulechek 2004; McCloskey & Bulechek, 2000). The NIC has been validated by a sample of 121 nurses from the Midwest Nursing Research Society. NIC's creators used input from this survey to revise the original taxonomy. NIC is continuously updated and has an ongoing process for feedback and review (McCloskey & Bulechek, 2000). NIC is designed to be used by all nursing specialties in any setting. It can also be used by other providers to document their interventions (Dochterman & Bulechek, 2004). NIC is included as one data set that will meet the uniform guidelines for information system vendors in the American Nurses Association's Nursing Information and Data Set Evaluation Center (NIDSEC). The NIDSEC was established by the American Nurses Association (ANA) to review, evaluate against defined criteria, and recognize information systems from developers and manufacturers that support documentation of nursing care within automated Nursing Information Systems (NIS) or within Computer-based Patient Record systems (CPR).

The Nursing Outcomes Classification (NOC)

In order to complete the requirements for documentation of a nursing clinical encounter, researchers from the NIC team realized the necessity of a system to classify patient outcomes. Johnson and Maas published the **Nursing Outcomes Classification (NOC)** in 1997. The 330 outcomes can be used across episodes of care and in various settings. The outcomes have been linked to NANDA International diagnoses, Gordon's functional patterns, the Taxonomy of Nursing Practice, the Omaha Classification System, resident admission protocols used in nursing homes, the OASIS System used in home care, and NIC interventions. Although the classification system is mostly individually focused (311 of the 330 outcomes are at the individual level), the outcomes can be aggregated to provide some measure of community and family outcomes and an additional 10 family and nine community level outcomes have been developed (Iowa Outcomes Project, Johnson, Maas, & Moorhead, 2000).

Before the development of the classification taxonomies, there was no systematic way to document nursing actions in a common language that novice nurses could use as a guide to the wide array of possible diagnoses, interventions, and outcomes. Although nursing diagnoses have been a part of the organization of most major care planning textbooks since NANDA's inception, there has been no easy way to link nursing diagnosis and intervention with the patient's signs and symptoms, demographic characteristics, medical diagnoses, and therapies. The NIC/NOC system can be used by the nursing instructor to facilitate teaching beginning nurses how to assess a patient and then link that assessment to a list of potential interventions and hoped-for outcomes (McCloskey & Bulechek, 2000). Because the lists are not proscriptive, the student nurse, along with the instructor, must exercise clinical judgment when selecting the intervention. The classifications cannot replace nursing judgment, nor are they absolutely necessary for nursing decision-making to take place, they simply provide one possible systematic way to document and communicate about nursing actions.

Each of the databases has different advantages for different users. The NANDA diagnosis classification scheme is probably the most widely recognized method for categorizing nursing diagnoses. This scheme, however, does not offer a taxonomy for interventions and outcomes. The OCS is a more complete classification system because it does include taxonomies for diagnoses, interventions, and outcomes, but it has not changed substantially since the original work. The NIC/NOC, unlike the systems derived in community health settings, was designed to be universally applicable in any care environment. The NIC/NOC employed panels of nurse experts to develop its taxonomy. The NIC/NOC have evolved after several stages of development and validation. Only NANDA, NIC, and NOC have ongoing research efforts to keep them current (Dochterman & Bulechek, 2004). The three systems have now been integrated since the formation of the NIC/NOC/NANDA (NNN) Taxonomy of Nursing Practice.

Evidenced-Based Practice

In nursing education, students and faculty daily confront questions about assessment, treatment, prevention, and cost-effectiveness of care. In evidence-based practice, the best available evidence, moderated by patient circumstances and preferences, is applied to improve the quality of clinical judgments and facilitate cost-effective health care. If clinical research is to improve clinical care, it must be relevant, of high quality, and accessible. The research should provide evidence of efficacy, effectiveness, and cost-effectiveness for typical inpatient and outpatient practice settings (Haynes, 1999) (Box 3–2).

Box 3-2 Determining Quality of Research

Three basic questions are used to evaluate a study critically (University of Alberta, 2006):
• What are the results?
• Are the results of the study valid?
• Can the results be applied to my patient?

Barriers to Evidence-Based Care

Evidence-based health care promotes the collection, interpretation, and integration of valid, important, and applicable patient-reported, clinician-observed, and research-derived evidence. Yet in medicine, only about half the therapeutic interventions used in inpatient (Nordin-Johansson & Asplund, 2000; Suarez-Varela, Llopis-Gonzalez, Bell, Tallon-Guerola, Perez-Benajas, & Carrion-Carrion, 1999) and outpatient (Ellis, Mulligan, Rowe, and Sackett, 1995) care in internal and family medicine are supported in the research literature with evidence of efficacy. The other half of the interventions either has not been studied or has only equivocal supportive evidence. Several problems exist with using the research literature for evidence-based practice in both nursing and medicine.

First, only a small fraction of the total research literature includes the efficacy studies of clinical practice that form the basis for evidence-based medicine (Haynes, 1993). This clinical research literature has been beset for decades with study design and reporting problems (Fletcher & Fletcher, 1979; Schor & Karten, 1966)—problems that still exist in the recent randomized trial (Moher, Jadad et al., 1995), systematic review (Moher, Cook et al., 1999; Sacks, Reitman, Pagano, & Kupelnick, 1996) and guidelines (Shaneyfelt, Mayo-Smith, & Rothwangl, 1999) literature. In the past, it was not surprising that most clinicians considered the research literature to be unmanageable because of its volume (Williamson, German, Weiss, Skinner, & Bowes, 1989) and of limited applicability to clinical practice because they would not be able to access it quickly enough to consider it on a busy clinical practice (Greer, 1988; McAlister, Graham, Karr, & Laupacis, 1999).

Moreover, the Internet and other sources of research evidence have increased exponentially. But the skills to retrieve and critically appraise this information are not easy to develop. Evidence-based practice is a way of thinking that requires discipline and practice to assess, "Where is the evidence for this?" and to weigh it against the validity and reliability of daily practice activities. Systems that provide both patients and clinicians with valid, applicable, and useful information may result in care decisions that are more concordant with current recommendations, are better tailored to individual patients, and ultimately are associated with improved clinical outcomes. Although the Internet and other sources of research evidence have provided patients with many more options for obtaining health information, they have also increased the potential for patients to misinterpret or become misinformed about research results (Jadad, Haynes, Hunt, & Browman, 2000; Kaplan & Brennan, 2001). As a result, patients are now less dependent on clinicians, including nurses, for information, but still trust clinicians the most for help with selecting, appraising, and applying a profusion of information to health decisions (Harris Interactive, 2000). Hence, in spite of the difficulties, nurses will have to be able to access and use this kind of information.

Furthermore, we know from Carper's model that nursing is much more than empiric–knowledge-based practice (Higgins, 1998). The art of nursing also needs to be studied to validate its contributions to quality care. In the future, qualitative nursing research will add essential components to nursing knowledge. Research on expert practice suggests that clinical judgment looks more like engaged practical reasoning, with the clinician being attuned to subtle changes in the patient's clinical state, attending to salient information, and understanding and responding to patient's issues and concerns often without any conscious deliberation at all (Tanner, Benner, Chesla, & Gordon, 1993). As a result, nursing research using qualitative methods is very suitable for developing the holistic knowledge of the discipline of nursing that expert practice requires.

What is the True Nature of Evidence-Based Practice and Clinical Judgment?

Clinical judgment is more than a disengaged, analytical, and objective process directed toward resolution of problems and/or achievement of clearly defined ends. Clinical judgment is defined as an interpretation or conclusion about a patient's needs, concerns, or health problem and the decision to take action (or not), and to use or modify standard approaches, or to improvise new ones as deemed appropriate by the patient's response (Tanner, 1998). Clinical judgment requires empiric, aesthetic, ethical, and practical knowledge that is abstract, able to be generalized, and applicable in many situations. Nursing knowledge may be derived from empiric science and theory, but it grows with experience as scientific abstractions are filled out in practice. The less commonly recognized practical, aesthetic, and ethical types of knowledge are often tacit and are an important factor in aiding clinicians to be able to recognize clinical states instantaneously. An additional component of these types of nursing knowledge is the importance of knowing the individual patient and being able to draw upon this understanding to predict and anticipate individual patient responses. Clinical judgment requires a disposition for critical thinking. An instructor can further develop the student's critical thinking skills by integrating all four types of knowledge into the planned learning activities for the students.

Building Clinical Judgment Through Evidence-Based Practice

Acquiring the skills to make expert clinical judgments is an extraordinarily complex process. In this process, the faculty role changes from acting as the deliverer of content, to being the facilitator of learning and the designer of clinical learning experiences to develop clinical reasoning (Tanner, 2002). Clinical reasoning is defined as the process by which nurses and other clinicians make their judgments, and includes the deliberate process of generating alternatives, weighing them against the evidence, and choosing the most appropriate course of action. Clinical reasoning implies that conditions of uncertainty are what prompt the seeking, appraising, and implementation of new knowledge by clinicians. The openness to accept that there may be different, and possibly more effective methods of care than those that are currently employed acts as the impetus to weighing evidence against expectation, norm, or standard. A modified concept of evidence-based practice acknowledges the many types of nursing knowledge. See Box 3–3.

By building the student's skills in information accessing and processing, students become independent in their ability to identify and answer their evidence-related practice questions. By adding an emphasis on Carper's ways of knowing, instructors can help students develop their per-

---

Box 3–3 Framing Questions Using Evidence-Based Practice Approaches and Carper's Ways of Knowing (John, 1995).

Empirics

What knowledge did or should have informed me?

Aesthetics

Why did I respond as I did? And what were the consequences of that for the learner? Others? Myself?

Personal

How did I feel in this situation? And what internal factors were influencing me?

Ethics

How did my actions match my beliefs? And what factors made me act in an incongruent way?

sonal, aesthetic, and ethical knowledge. The heavy emphasis in most programs on critical thinking skills attests to the complexities of the modern health-care environment and the need for nurses to be able to make sound clinical decisions based on relevant and current evidence (Ferguson, & Day, 2005). Several innovative pedagogical strategies have been developed to enhance nursing student's critical thinking ability. **Problem-based learning, conceptual mapping, storytelling,** and **questioning** are among some of the most promising innovations developed (Billings & Halstead, 1998).

Current Research and Initiatives

Several innovative teaching strategies have been proposed to integrate the various forms of nursing knowledge, with a more broadly defined evidence-based approach to educating nursing students.

Problem-Based Learning

Problem-based learning (PBL) encourages students to identify their own gaps in knowledge. It is a process-driven method for learning, which has as its goal self-directed information retrieval, and utilization of that information to solve clinical problems. Students direct their own learning, and critique the adequacy of their mastery of needed knowledge. PBL is a method of active, student-centered and student-driven, collaborative, inquiry-based learning. PBL involves student learning that is organized around self-directed work, which makes students responsible for their learning regarding a particular "problem" or question (Siu, Laschinger, & Vingilis, 2005). PBL moves the educator away from expert lecturer to being a facilitator of small groups and individual self-directed, active learning. In a study comparing PBL with conventional lecture approaches, the PBL students rated themselves higher on a measure of clinical problem-solving ability (Siu et al., 2005). Key in this approach is the development of nurses who master the ability to engage in their own learning. Education in the 21st century requires the development of nursing students as effective problem solvers. Students are bombarded with a vast amount of information from multiple and diverse sources. These sources need to be reflective of both the art and science of the profession (Jacobs, Rosenfeld, & Haber, 2003). PBL pedagogy, in combination with evidence-based practice, is an approach that has been used at University of South Carolina–College of Nursing (Anderson, 2000). Students are confronted with a case study designed to help them master environmental nursing content. The students work in pairs and seek out an actual or potential environmental health hazard in their community. In the course, students explore the impact of hazard exposure on community health, examine principles of risk perception and risk communication, explore environmental health resources, and experience community involvement. In this approach, students acquire the clinical knowledge and decision-making skills to provide evidence-based care to vulnerable patients experiencing environmental health hazards.

Conceptual Mapping

Conceptual mapping depicts concepts and the relationship of concepts visually and can be used to help students develop and reinforce their mastery of content. A concept map helps the student integrate new knowledge with old by creating a knowledge graph that depicts networks of concepts. Nodes represent concepts and links represent the relations between concepts. The labeled links explain the relationship between the nodes. The arrow describes the direction of the relationship, and can be uni-directional or bi-directional. Concept maps help students develop understanding of nursing knowledge, explore new information and relationships, access prior knowledge, and gather new knowledge and information.

Concept mapping has been proposed as an alternative to having students create the traditional nursing care plan (Ignatiavicius, 2004). The concept map helps the student demonstrate synthesis with a minimum of writing compared with the usual care plan approach of integrating knowledge. This advantage can be enhanced further by the instructor questioning the student about the rationale for the relationships depicted in the map (Billings & Halstead, 2004). Disadvantages include the difficulty in interpretation of student maps, which may be time-consuming to read and interpret.

Storytelling

The use of storytelling as a pedagogy has been described and recommended by Severtsen and Evans (2000). Storytelling can be empowering for the nurse and the patient. Storytelling prompts nursing students to grow developmentally by accessing their intuitive awareness and helping them to gain self-awareness (Koithan, 1994). The use of storytelling in clinical education involves four principles: guiding, respecting, bearing witness, and community-centered practice. In guiding, students were asked to tell a short story at the beginning of each session about how their week had gone. By using this process, the faculty members were able to help the students get to know each other through listening and telling their stories. In respecting, thinking with stories (treating the story as a whole entity) not about the stories (reducing them to content that we analyze) was emphasized to help students learn how to respect and empower their student colleague storytellers in the classroom. Often, students were sharing clinical encounters. By practicing bearing witness, the students learn the therapeutic value of listening and bearing witness to a patient's story. This often comes as a surprise to novice clinicians who have an expectation that they must always intervene to relieve suffering. With the above practiced skills, the students developed community-centered practices that represented the caring values the faculty members were trying to instill.

Questioning

As in many other professions, one strategy for developing critical thinking skills involves questioning. Questions help the novice nurse (or novice professional in many domains) learn how to transfer theoretical knowledge into applied knowledge experience (Chase, 1983; Infante 1981; Klassens, 1988; McCue, 1981). The use of questions to facilitate clinical learning has been documented previously (Craig & Page, 1981; Scholdra & Quiring, 1973). Sellappah, Hussey, Blackmore, and McMurray (1998), in their study of the content of clinical instructors' questions, found that most of the clinical teachers they followed and observed asked low-level knowledge questions in a disorganized and scattered fashion. Low-level questions focused on basic knowledge and comprehension, such as "What is a normal ph?" A high-level analysis, synthesis, or evaluation question, however, prompts critical thinking on the part of the student. An example of a high-level question might be: "If they reverse the narcotic what will happen to the patient?" The researchers concluded that clinical instructors have to be taught the skill of questioning, and how to use questioning strategy effectively. The findings of studies have indicated that clinical teachers' ability to ask high-level questions improved significantly after receiving instructions about the use of questioning strategies (Craig & Page, 1981). Therefore, more attention needs to be given to developing clinical teachers' effective use of questioning strategies.

Technology and Innovation in Nursing Education

Teaching technologies are undergoing rapid change. In the not too distant past, rapid adoption of new technologies, without adequate planning for or understanding of key pedagogical implications, occurred. In spite of these initial difficulties, the self-directed learning encouraged by these technologies has been shown to be equivalent or superior to more traditional methods (Armstrong & Frueh, 2003). This section of the chapter presents information about the use of some of the more common technologies (Internet, CD-ROM, and Simulation) and their usefulness as tools to facilitate self-directed learning.

Problems with Technology Mediated Teaching

Technology problems with course delivery, and a drop in student satisfaction with Web-based versus traditional delivery have been reported by multiple nurse educators (Billings, 2000; Cragg, 1994a; Cragg, 1994b; DeBourgh, 2003; Ryan, Carlton, & Ali, 1999; Yucha & Princen, 2000). The inconsistency of basic Internet skills among students, and the lack of standardization of Web browsers, platforms, and computers among groups of students cause dissatisfaction with course delivery (DeBourgh, 2003). Reports of student dissatisfaction with the visual appeal and interface design of course Web sites have been common (DeBourgh, 2003; Rouse, 1999). Interface design relates to the way in which screen elements are used to navigate the application and provide access to the media contained within (Ribbons, 1998). In addition, unstable or poorly performing Internet course software substantially undermines student satisfaction with Web-based course delivery (Ayoub, Vanderboom, Knight, Walsh, Briggs, & Grekin, 1998; Block, Pollock, & Hutton, 1999; DeBourgh, 2003; Milstead & Nelson, 1998).

Advantages of Technology Mediated Reaching Approaches

Internet-based learning takes place in a virtual classroom. Access to a computer theoretically gives students the opportunity to learn anyplace, anytime, anywhere. This flexibility mitigates some of the educational barriers to learning for nurses and nursing students in the clinical setting, such as irregular work schedules (McAlpine, Lockerbie, Ramsay, & Beaman, 2002) or limited time (Reinert & Fryback, 1997). Test results from Internet-based courses have shown similar or higher-than-average scores when compared with those of traditional classroom courses (Andrusyszyn, Iwasiw, & Goldenberg,1999; Billings, Skiba, & Connors, 2005). Some findings have indicated that Internet-based group discussions were deeper and more diverse than equivalent classroom-based interactions, with outcomes equaling or exceeding those of classroom courses (Billings, Skiba, & Connors, 2005; Cravener, 1999; Ryan, Carlton, & Ali, 1999). Indications are that Internet-based courses can actually enhance student participation, with greater numbers of students conversing (Bangert, 2005). One difference between classroom-based learning and Internet-based learning is that students do not need to compete to be recognized or heard; instead, students have time to think more deeply about the quality of their responses. According to Billings and Rowles (2001), dialogue, discussion, writing assignments, mini-lectures (i.e., the length of one typed page), games, and critical thinking exercises work well in online environments because all participants in the online learning community must participate, whereas in traditional classrooms, participants can be more passive learners.

Use of Multimedia and Simulation

Multimedia CD-ROMs can compensate for or avoid problems encountered in Web-based delivery due to Internet service provider (ISP) problems, insufficient home Internet infrastructure, or Web-courseware failures. In addition, CD-ROMs require less technical know-how for students to use. This decreases the amount of time students would ordinarily spend acquiring new computer skills rather than focusing on course content (Cravener, 1999; Geibert, 2000; Leasure, Davis, & Thievon,

2000). Active learning combined with prompt feedback that helps learners decide what material they know and what they do not know are key features of CD-ROM learning (Jeffries, 2000). CD-ROM development projects, however, have been plagued by student complaints that they would have liked more detailed coverage of additional topics (Marshall & van Soeren, 2000). Other educators who have piloted or tested CD-ROM development recommend that CD-ROM instruction not be used alone, but rather as a supplement to other types of instruction providing more faculty-student interaction (Bauer, Geront, & Huynh, 2001; Jeffries, 2000; Madorin & Iwasiw, 1999; Wells et al., 2003).

Simulations can be used to create learning experiences and will help reinforce content and increase learner self-efficacy to manage responses to a clinical practice situation. See Chapter 9 on learning laboratories. Simulations can include the use of mannequins, as in cardiopulmonary resuscitation practice, sequences of skills with models such as an intravenous practice arm; human simulation using play acting, and very high-tech interactive patient simulators (Billings & Halstead, 2005). In active simulation, the instructor acts as a role model and coach. During student-directed practice sessions, the traditional role of the instructor can be supplanted with a technology-mediated self-directed learning approach. The ability to alter the simulation activities so that they just barely exceed the current knowledge and abilities of the student, makes simulation particularly effective as a tailored teaching strategy (Lupien & George-Gay, 2001).

Summary

Understanding the types of knowledge as described by Carper is important in comprehending some of the essential foundational knowledge acquisitions needed in the teaching learning process for nursing education. The history of the science of nursing also adds insight to the vast realm of knowledge needed to synthesize the art and science of nursing. The nursing process is used to assist in organizing the scientific data and has paved the way for evidence-based educational practices. Other organizational strategies such as NIC and NOC have also added to the knowledge base of nursing science and provided a common language for better communication and interpretation. Teaching methodologies must move beyond factual information and promote critical-thinking for the role of the nurse in this complex and technologically enhanced healthcare system.

R e f e r e n c e s

Andrusyszyn, M., Iwasiw, C., & Goldenberg, D. Computer conferencing in graduate nursing education: Perceptions of students and faculty. *Journal of Continuing Education in Nursing, 36*(9), 272–278.

Anderson, J. (2000). *Environmental health nursing project on small group/problem based teaching resources* from website at **http://www.aoec.org/CEEM/methods/southcarolina2.html**

Armstrong, M., & Frueh, S. (Eds.). (2003). *Telecommunications for nurses: Providing successful distance education and telehealth* (2nd ed.). New York: Springer.

Ayoub, J. L., Vanderboom, C., Knight, M., Walsh, K., Briggs, R., & Grekin, K. (1998). A study of the effectiveness of an interactive computer classroom. *Computers in Nursing, 16*(6), 333–338.

Bangert, A. W. (2005). The seven principles of effective teaching: a framework for designing, delivering, and evaluating an Internet-based assessment course for nurse educators. *Nurse Educator, 30*(5), 221–225.

Bauer, M., Geront, M., & Huynh, M. (2001). Teaching blood pressure measurement: CD-ROM versus conventional classroom instruction. *Journal of Nursing Education, 40*, 138–141.

Benner, P. (1983). Uncovering the knowledge embedded in clinical practice. *Image: The Journal of Nursing Scholarship, 15*(2), 36–41.

Benner, P. (1984). *From novice to expert: Excellence and power in clinical nursing practice.* Menlo Park, CA: Addison-Wesley.

Benner, P., & Tanner, C. (1987). Clinical judgment: How expert nurses use intuition. *American Journal of Nursing, 87*(1), 23–31.

Billings, D. M. (2000). A framework for assessing outcomes and practices in web-based courses in nursing. *Journal of Nursing Education, 39*(2), 60–67.

Billings, D. M., & Halstead, J. A. (1998). *Teaching in nursing: A guide for faculty.* Philadelphia: WB Saunders.

Billings, D. M., & Halstead, J. A. (2004). *Teaching in nursing: A guide for faculty.* Philadelphia: Saunders.

Billings, D. M., & Rowles, C. (2001). Development of continuing nursing education offerings for the World Wide Web. *Journal of Continuing Education in Nursing,32*(3), 107.

Billings, D. M., Skiba, D. J., & Connors, H. R. (2005). Best practices in Web-based courses: Generational differences across undergraduate and graduate nursing students. *Journal of Professional Nursing; 21*(2), 126–133.

Block, D. E., Pollock, T. J., & Hutton, S. J. (1999). Technoglitches in distance education. *Computers in Nursing, 17*(5), 232–234.

Capacchione, L. (1989). *The creative journal for children: A guide for parents, teachers and counselors.* Boston: Shambhala Publications.

Carper B.A. (1978). Fundamental patterns of knowing in nursing. *Advances in Nursing Science, 1*(1), 13–23.

Chase B. M. (1983). Clinical experience made easy. *Journal of Nursing Education, 22*(8), 347–348.

Cragg, C. E. (1994a). Distance learning through computer conferences. *Nurse Educator, 9*(2), 10–14.

Cragg, C. E. (1994b). Nurses' experiences of a post-RN course by computer mediated conferencing: Friendly users. *Computers in Nursing, 12*(5), 221–226.

Craig J. L., & Page, G. (1981). The questioning skill of nursing instructors. *Journal of Nursing Education, 20*(5), 18–23.

Cravener, P. A. (1999). Faculty experiences with providing online courses thorns among the roses. *Computers in Nursing, 17*(1), 42–47.

DeBourgh, G. A. (2003). Predictors of student satisfaction in distance-delivered graduate nursing courses: what matters most? *Journal of Professional Nursing, 19,* 149–163.

Dochterman, J., & Bulechek, G. (Eds.). (2004). *Nursing interventions classification (NIC)* (4th ed.). St. Louis: Mosby.

Dochterman, J. M., & Jones, D. (2003). *Unifying nursing languages: The harmonization of NANDA, NIC, and NOC.* Washington, DC: American Nurses Publishing.

Ellis, J., Mulligan, I., Rowe, J., & Sackett, D. L. (1995). Inpatient general medicine is evidence based. A-Team, Nuffield Department of Clinical Medicine. *Lancet, 346*(8972):407–410.

Ferguson, L., & Day, R. (2005). Evidence-based nursing education: Myth or reality. *Journal Nursing Education, 44*(3), 107–115.

Fletcher, R. H., Fletcher, S. W. (1979). Clinical research in general medical journals: A 30-year perspective. *New England Journal of Medicine, 301*(4),180–183.

Fonteyn, M. E., & Cooper, L. F. (1994). The written nursing process: Is it still useful to nursing education. *Journal of Advanced Nursing, 19*(2), 315–319.

Geibert, R. C. (2000). Integrating Web-based instruction into a graduate nursing program taught via video-conferencing challenges and solutions. *Computers in Nursing, 18*(1), 26–34.

Graveley, E., & Fullerton, J. T. (1998). Incorporating electronic-based and computer-based strategies: Graduate nursing courses in administration. *Journal of Nursing Education, 37,* 186–188.

Greer, A. L. (1988). The state of the art vs. the state of the science: The diffusion of new medical technologies into practice. *International Journal of Technology Assessment in Health Care, 4*(1):5–26.

Harris Interactive. Ethics and the Internet: Consumers vs. Webmasters, Internet Healthcare Coalition, and National Mental Health Association. Oct 5, 2000.

Haynes, B. (1999). Can it work? Does it work? Is it worth it? The testing of healthcare interventions is evolving [editorial]. *British Medical Journal, 319*(7211), 652–653.

Haynes, R. B. (1993). Where's the meat in clinical journals [editorial]? *ACP Journal Club,* Nov–Dec, A16.

Henderson, V. (1982). Is the study of history rewarding for nurses? *Society for Nursing History Gazette, 2*(1),1–2.

Henderson, V. (1987). The nursing process in perspective. *Journal of Advanced Nursing, 12*(6), 657–658.

Higgins, P. (1996). Caring as therapeutic in nursing education. *Journal of Nursing Education, 35,* 134–136.

Higgins, P. (1998). Response to "A Theoretical Analysis of Carper's Ways of Knowing Using a Model of Social Cognition." *Scholarly Inquiry for Nursing Practice: An International Journal, 12,* 61–64.

Infante, M. S. (1981). *The clinical laboratory in nursing education* (2nd ed.). New York: John Wiley.

Iowa Outcomes Project, Johnson, M., Maas, M, & Moorhead, S. (Eds.). (2000). *Nursing outcomes classification (NOC)* (2nd ed.). St. Louis: Mosby.

Jacavone, J., & Dostal, J. (1992). A descriptive study of nursing judgment in the assessment and management of cardiac pain. *Advances in Nursing Science, 15*(1), 54–63.

Jacobs, S. K., Rosenfeld, P., & Haber, J. (2003). Information literacy as the foundation for evidence-based practice in graduating nursing education: A curriculum-integrated approach. *Journal of Professional Nursing, 19*(5), 320–328.

Jadad, A. R., Haynes, R. B., Hunt, D., & Browman, G. P. (2000). The Internet and evidence-based decision-making: A needed synergy for efficient knowledge management in health care. *CMAJ: Canadian Medical Association Journal, 162*(3), 362–365.

Jeffries, P. D. (2000). Development and test of a model for designing interactive CD-ROMs for teaching nursing skills. *Computers in Nursing, 18*(3), 118–124.

Jenks, J. M. (1993). The pattern of personal knowing in nurse decision making. *Journal of Nursing Education, 32,* 399–405.

Jenny, J. J., & Logan, J. (1992). Knowing the patient: One aspect of clinical knowledge. *Image: The Journal of Nursing Scholarship, 24,* 254–258.

John, C. (1995). Framing learning through reflection within Carper's fundamental ways of knowing in nursing. *Journal of Advanced Nursing, 22(2),* 226–234.

Johnson, M., & Maas, M. (1997). *Nursing outcomes classification (NOC).* St Louis: Mosby.

Kaplan, B., & Brennan, P. F. (2001). Consumer informatics supporting patients as co-producers of quality. *Journal of the American Medical Informatics Association, 8,* 309–316.

Klassens, E. L. (1988). Improving teaching for thinking. *Nurse Educator, 13*(6), 15–19.

Koithan, M. (1994). The seeing self: Photography and storytelling as a health promotion methodology. In P. Chinn & J. Watson, (Eds.), *Art and aesthetics in nursing* (pp. 247–261). New York: National League for Nursing Press.

Kuhn, T. (1970). *The structure of scientific revolutions* (2nd ed.). University of Chicago Press.

Leasure, R. A., Davis, L., & Thievon, S. L. (2000). Comparison of student outcomes and preferences in a traditional vs. World Wide Web-based baccalaureate nursing research course. *Journal of Nursing Education, 39,* 149–154.

Lunney, M. (2005). *Critical thinking & nursing diagnoses: case studies & analyses.* North American Nursing Diagnosis Association.

MacLeod, M. (1993). On knowing the patient: Experiences of nurses undertaking care. In A. Radley (Ed.), *Worlds of illness: Biographical and cultural perspectives on health and disease* (pp. 38–56). London: Routledge.

Madorin, S., & Iwasiw, C. (1999). The effects of computer-assisted instruction on the self-efficacy of baccalaureate nursing students. *Journal of Nursing Education, 38,* 282–285.

Marshall, M. J., & van Soeren, M. H. (2000). Development and evaluation of a pathophysiology CD-ROM for nurse practitioner distance education. *Computers in Nursing, 18*(2), 87–92.

Martin, K., Leak, G., & Aden, C. (1992). The Omaha System: A research-based model for decision making. *Journal of Nursing Administration, 11,* 47–52.

Martin, K., & Scheet, N. (1992). *The Omaha system: Applications for community health nursing.* Philadelphia: W. B. Saunders.

Martin, K., Scheet, N., & Stegman, M. (1993). *American journal of public health, 83,* 1730–1734.

Martin, K. S. (2005). *The Omaha system: A key to practice, documentation, and information management* (2nd ed.). St. Louis: Elsevier.

McAlister, F. A., Graham, I., Karr, G. W., & Laupacis, A. (1999). Evidence-based medicine and the practicing clinician. *Journal of General Internal Medicine, 14*(4), 236–242.

McAlpine, H., Lockerbie, L., Ramsay, D., & Beaman, S. (2002). Evaluating a Web-based graduate level nursing ethics course: Thumbs up or thumbs down? *Journal of Continuing Education in Nursing, 33*(1), 12–18.

McCloskey, J., & Bulchek, G. (1992). *Nursing interventions classifications (NIC).* St. Louis: C. V. Mosby Year Book.

McCloskey, J., & Bulechek, G. (2000). *Nursing interventions classifications (NIC)* (3rd ed.). St. Louis: C. V. Mosby Year Book.

McCormick, K., Lang, N., Zielstorff, R., Milholland, D., Saba, V., & Jacox, A. (1994). Toward standard classification schemes for nursing language: Recommendations of the American Nurses Association Steering Committee on Databases to Support Clinical Nursing Practice. *Journal of the American Medical Informatics Association, 1*, 421–427.

McCue, H. (1981). Clinical teaching and the nursing process—implication for nurse teacher education. *The Australian Nurses' Journal 10*(7), 36–37.

Milstead, J. A., & Nelson, R. (1998). Preparation for an online asynchronous university doctoral course: Lessons learned. *Computers in Nursing, 16*(5), 247–258.

Moher, D., Cook, D. J., Eastwood, S., Olkin, I., Rennie, D., & Stroup, D. F. (1999). Improving the quality of reports of meta-analyses of randomised controlled trials: The QUOROM statement—Quality of Reporting of Meta-analyses. *Lancet, 354*(9193):1896–1900.

Moher, D., Jadad, A. R., Nichol, G., Penman, M., Tugwell, P., & Walsh, S. (1995). Assessing the quality of randomized controlled trials: an annotated bibliography of scales and checklists. *Controlled Clinical Trials, 16*(1):62–73.

Moorehead, S. A., McCloskey, J., & Bulechek, G. (1993). Nursing Interventions Classification: A comparison with the Omaha System and the Home Health Care Classification. *Journal of Nursing Administration, 23*, 23–29.

NANDA International. (2005). *NANDA's Nursing diagnoses: Definitions and classifications 2005–2006.*

Nordin-Johansson, A., & Asplund, K. (2000). Randomized controlled trials and consensus as a basis for interventions in internal medicine. *Journal of Internal Medicine, 247*(1):94–104.

North American Nursing Diagnosis Association. (1992). *NANDA nursing diagnosis: Definitions and classifications.* Philadelphia: NANDA.

O'Neill, E. S. (1995). Heuristics reasoning in diagnostic judgment. *Journal of Professional Nursing, 11*(4), 239–245.

Orlando, I. J. (1961). *The dynamic nurse-patient relationship, function, process and principles.* New York: G. P. Putnam.

Polanyi, M. (1958). *Personal knowledge.* London: Routledge and Kegan Paul.

Pyles, S. H., & Stern, P. N. (1983). Discovery of nursing gestalt in critical care nursing: The importance of the gray gorilla syndrome. *Image: The Journal of Nursing Scholarship, 15*(2), 51–57.

Radwin, L. E. (1995). Conceptualizations of decision making in nursing: Analytic models and "knowing the patient". *Nursing Diagnosis, 6*(1), 16–22.

Reinert, B. R., & Fryback, P. B. (1997). Distance learning and nursing education. *Journal of Nursing Education, 36*(9), 421–427.

Rew, L. (1988). Intuition in decision making. *Image: The Journal of Nursing Scholarship, 20*(3), 150–154.

Ribbons, R. M. (1998). Guidelines for developing interactive multimedia: Applications in nurse education. *Computers in Nursing, 16*(2), 109–114.

Rouse, D. P. (1999). Creating an interactive multimedia computer-assisted instruction program. *Computers in Nursing, 17*(4), 171–176.

Ryan, M., Carlton, K. H., & Ali, S. (1999). Evaluation of traditional classroom teaching methods versus course delivery via the World Wide Web. *Journal of Nursing Education, 38*, 272–277.

Sacks, H. S., Reitman, D., Pagano, D., & Kupelnick, B. (1996). Meta-analysis: An update. *Mt Sinai Journal of Medicine, 63*(3–4):216–224.

Scholdra, J. D., & Quiring, J. D. (1973). The level of questions posed by nursing educators. *Journal of Nursing Education, 12*(3), 15–20.

Schor, S., & Karten, I. (1966). Statistical evaluation of medical journal manuscripts. *JAMA, 195*(13): 1123–1128.

Schraeder, B. D., & Fischer, D. K. (1987). Using intuitive knowledge in the neonatal intensive care nursery. *Holistic Nursing Practice, 1*, 45–51.

Sellappah, S., Hussey, T., Blackmore, A. M., & McMurray, A. (1998). The use of questioning strategies by clinical teachers. *Journal of Advanced Nursing, 28*(1), 142–148.

Severtsen, B. M., & Evans, B. C. (2000). Education for caring practice. *Nursing and Health Care Perspectives. 21*(4), 172–177.

Shaneyfelt, T. M., Mayo-Smith, M. F., & Rothwangl, J. (1999). Are guidelines following guidelines? The methodological quality of clinical practice guidelines in the peer-reviewed medical literature. *JAMA, 281*(20):1900–1905.

Siu, H. M., Laschinger, H. K. S., & Vingilis, E. (2005). The effect of problem-based learning on nursing students' perceptions of empowerment. *Journal of Nursing Education, 44*(10), 459–469.

Stein, K. F., Corte, C., Colling, K. B., & Whall, A. (1998). A theoretical analysis of Carper's Ways of Knowing using a model of social cognition. *Scholarly Inquiry for Nursing Practice: An International Journal, 12*, 43–60.

Suarez-Varela, M. M., Llopis-Gonzalez, A., Bell, J., Tallon-Guerola, M., Perez-Benajas, A., & Carrion-Carrion, C. (1999). Evidence-based general practice. *European Journal of Epidemiology, 15*(9):815–819.

Tanner, C. (1998). State of the science: Clinical judgment and evidence-based practice: Conclusions and controversies. *Communicating Nursing Research, 31*, 14–26.

Tanner, C. (2002). Clinical education, circa 2010. *Journal of Nursing Education, 41*(2), 51–52.

Tanner, C. (2004). The meaning of curriculum: Content to be covered or stories to be heard? *Journal of Nursing Education, 43*(1), 3–4.

Tanner, C. (2006). Thinking like a nurse: A research-based model of clinical judgment in nursing. *Journal of Nursing Eduction, 45*(6), 204–211.

Tanner, C.A., Benner, P., Chesla, C., & Gordon, D. R. (1993). The phenomenology of knowing the patient. *Image: The Journal of Nursing Scholarship, 25*, 273–280.

Tanner, C. A., Padrick, K. P., Westfall, U. A., & Putzier, D. J. (1987). Diagnostic reasoning strategies of nurses and nursing students. *Nursing Research, 36*(6), 358–363.

Timpka, T., & Arborelius, E. (1990). The primary-care nurse's dilemmas: A study of knowledge use and need during telephone consultations. *Journal of Advanced Nursing, 15*, 1457–1465.

University of Alberta (accessed 2006). Catwalk: Critically appraised topic: **http://www.library.ualberta.ca/subject/healthsciences/catwalk/evaluate/index.cfm**

University of Iowa Nursing Informatics. (accessed February 2006). Brief Synopsis of the Nursing Minimum Data Set (NMDS) taken from: **http://www.nursing.uiowa.edu/NI/collabs_files/Synopsis%20NMDS%20Nov%202003.pdf**

Wells, M. J., Wilkie, D. J., Brown, M., Corless, I. B., Farber, S. J., Judge, M. K. M., & Shannon, S. E. (2003). Technology survey of nursing programs: Implications for electronic end-of-life teaching tool development. *CIN: Computers, Informatics, Nursing, 21*(1): 29–36.

Werley, H., Devine, E., Zorn, C., Ryan, P., & Westra, B. (1991). The Nursing Minimum Data Set: Abstraction tool for standardized, comparable, essential data. *American Journal of Public Health, 81*, 421–426.

Westfall, U. E., Tanner, C. A., Putzier, D. J., & Padrick, K. P. (1986). Activating clinical inferences. A component of diagnostic reasoning in nursing. *Research in Nursing and Health, 9*, 269–277.

Williamson, J. W., German, P. S., Weiss, R., Skinner, E. A., & Bowes, F. D. (1989). Health science information management and continuing education of physicians: A survey of U.S. primary care practitioners and their opinion leaders. *Annals of Internal Medicine, 110*(2):151–160.

Yucha, C., & Princen, T. (2000). Insights learned from teaching pathophysiology on the World Wide Web. *Journal of Nursing Education, 39*, 68–72.

Review Questions

- How are Carper's four ways of knowing elicited by specific types of questions?
- What was the purpose of NANDA in relation to nursing knowledge development?
- What are the expectations and patient considerations of evidence-based practice in nursing?
- How does the role of technology impact knowledge development in nursing?

Critical Thinking Exercises

A clinical group of undergraduate fundamental nursing students are learning the nursing process and applying it to a client with anemia. During post-conference they bring in research articles that support specific interventions. They develop a group concept map about the client and develop three nursing diagnoses with appropriate NANDA language. The research articles they have retrieved support dietary iron intake and blood replacement but the students' assessment reveals that the client is a vegetarian and is of a culture and religion that does not accept blood products. How would you guide their knowledge development in this clinical scenario in the context of Carper's ways of knowing?

Annotated Research Summary

McGrath D. & Higgins A. (2006). Implementing and evaluating reflective practice group sessions. *Nurse Education in Practice, 6*(3), 175–181

McGrath and Higgins (2006) studied the introduction of reflection as a way of knowing with a group of diploma nursing students. Reflection was being studied as one mechanism to develop thoughtful practitioners within the technologically enhanced environment of health care. Implementation of reflective session strategies along with traditional lecture over the course of a year showed an increase in critical thinking in this study.

Stockhausen, L. (2006). Métier artistry: Revealing reflection-in-action in everyday practice. *Nurse Education Today, 26*(1), 54–62.

Stockhausen (2006) studied artistry in practice in the clinical setting through a well developed ethnographic study. She describes a new concept reflection-in-action (termed Métier Artistry) that experienced nurses use when caring for clients with student nurses. This educational discovery assisted learning in the clinical area and the author encourages its use as a method that shows great potential for clinical education. Examples are provided in the article.

Ruth-Sahd, L. A., & Hendy, H. M. (2005). Predictors of novice nurses' use of intuition to guide patient care decisions. *Journal of Nursing Education, 44*(10), 450–458.

Ruth-Sahd (2005) studied intuition in novice nurses (N = 323) as a way of knowing. Intuition was evaluated by an 18-item subscale identified by Miller from the Miller Intuitiveness Instrument. The results showed that older, more life experienced students with previous hospitalizations and more social support were more apt to use intuition as a way of knowing.

Little, M. (2006). Personal knowing through performance and feedback workshops. *Journal of Nursing Education, 45*(3), 131–135.

Newly graduated RNs are expected to be competent health educators for individuals, groups, and communities. To prepare for this complex role, nursing students need time to focus on developing basic teaching skills and self-confidence in a nonthreatening learning environment. Of primary importance to novice teachers' development is taking the time to identify and appreciate the personal dimensions that are an integral part of the health educator role. Carper identified personal knowing as one of the four ways of knowing in nursing. This article describes an innovative praxis strategy that used videotaped performances, learner feedback, and self-reflection to encourage personal knowing in relation to the experience of nursing students learning to teach groups of clients.

Chapter Outline

4

Nursing as a Career

Michelle August-Brady

Learning Outcomes

On the completion of this chapter, the reader will be able to:

- Comprehend the severity of the nursing faculty shortage.
- Articulate current qualifications for the role of nurse educator.
- Describe essential components of the nursing faculty role in the 21st century.
- Appraise current challenges in nursing education.

Key Terms

Authentic student-teacher relationship
Evidence-based practice
Learning
Nursing education research

D o you have a passion for advancing the quality of nursing practice? Do you have a passion for teaching and **learning**? Are you interested in pedagogical research? If you have answered yes to these questions, you already possess the characteristics that motivate the majority of nurse educators and you may want to consider a career in nursing education. The purpose of this chapter is to discuss the future of nursing education as a career, qualifications for the role of nurse educators, current challenges in nursing education, and possible resources to support such a career path.

Dwindling Supply and Increasing Demand

Perhaps there is no better time to talk about forging a career in nursing education than now. Over the past several years, much attention has been placed on recruitment and retention strategies as a result of the continuing nursing shortage. Less attention has been placed on the nursing faculty shortage, yet this problem has been brewing ever so quietly for several years. The nursing faculty shortage became more visible with the success of recruitment strategies to nursing, when the demand for nursing faculty rose. There can be little fruitful discussion of nursing education as a career without reference to the current reality of faculty shortage.

There is ample evidence of the decreasing supply and increasing demand for nursing faculty. According to the American Association of Colleges of Nursing's (AACN) *Survey on Vacant Faculty Positions* (AACN, 2005), a national nursing faculty vacancy rate of 8.5% exists, which increased from a vacancy rate of 8.1% in 2004. Tens of thousands of prospective nursing students are denied entrance into nursing programs because of dwindling faculty resources. A dwindling supply and increasing demand for nursing faculty in turn perpetuates the nursing shortage. This vacancy rate is likely to increase in the foreseeable future for the following reasons. First, nursing faculty retirements are expected in large numbers over the next decade because of the exodus of baby boomers. The National League for Nursing (NLN) projects that "75% of the current faculty population is expected to retire by 2019" (2004, p. 5). Second, there has been a declining rate at which graduate nursing students are choosing a career in nursing education (NLN, 2004). AACN's introduction of the clinical nurse leader (CNL) and the doctorate of nursing practice (DNP) degree programs is not likely to contribute faculty supply, and some fear that it may worsen supply issues. For example, prospective candidates may decide on earning a practice-based doctorate as opposed to a traditional research-based doctorate. Individuals who have earned practice-based doctorates will possess expertise more congruent with practice environments, and will not be grounded in theoretical and research knowledge needed for a career in academe. Moreover, the development of the CNL and DNP curricula require additional investments of faculty time and resources that may augment current resource challenges.

A myriad of other factors exist that influence the current nursing faculty shortage. Salary is a consideration in that clinical positions offer significantly higher salaries than academic positions, due to the relatively fixed budget constraints of academic institutions (AACN, 2003). Students with graduate degrees in nursing have more career options within and outside the profession. In nursing, advanced practice nurses may choose clinical positions that are congruent with their values and skills, and offer more compensation than nursing education. In the corporate environment, opportunities are available for nurses with advanced degrees in pharmaceutical research and sales, insurance industries, publishing companies, and entrepreneurial and other options. These options generally offer higher compensation packages than those available in academe.

Although public perception of nurses remains high, the general public does not have clear ideas about what nurses do and nurses have remained relatively silent in educating them about the work of nursing (Buresh & Gordon, 2000). In the media, nurses are often portrayed in an anti-intellectual context and nurses are viewed as less knowledgeable members of the health-care team. Nurse educators often find themselves in similar circumstances. A chemistry professor would rarely be asked what her doctoral degree was in, but nursing professors are frequently asked this question, which signals outdated perceptions on the part of the general public.

The fact that there already is a national nursing faculty shortage should not paralyze individuals from considering nursing education as a career. In fact, our current reality opens the door for thoughtful and innovative discussion that is likely to produce more promising models for the education of nursing students in the 21st century. Research is an integral part of that discussion as nurse educators are challenged to examine best practices in nursing education. For example, nurse educators have traditionally held clinical practice with students as sacred learning time. Yet, one may question whether faculty to student ratios of 1:12 or more result in effective clinical learning. Are there more effective ways of promoting clinical judgment in students? This is but one area in need of research in nursing education, there are many others.

Qualifications

In order to teach nursing, one must be a registered nurse who has received advanced educational preparation in a clinical specialty. A masters degree in nursing is required to teach in a 2- or 4-year program. Most 4-year colleges or universities require a doctoral degree for tenure track positions, however.

Due to greater recognition of the nursing faculty shortage, schools of nursing have become more interested in developing nursing education program tracks or post–masters certificates in nursing education for those individuals who have previously earned a masters degree in nursing. Many of these programs are available in an accelerated fashion, online, or are blended offerings, thereby appealing to a variety of students.

Because these programs are targeted for the working nurse, courses are often offered on a specific schedule to enhance planning, or courses are offered through distance education, thereby saving travel time. Nursing education programs offer greater flexibility today than in the past. For example, students seeking to earn a post–masters certificate in nursing education may often use those earned credits toward a doctoral degree in the future, rather than duplicating required courses.

Graduate course work in educational and learning theory is needed to provide the additional grounding in the area of best practices with regard to teaching and learning. In order to facilitate learning and intellectual curiosity in students, nurse educators must be fully knowledgeable in the area of educational theory and educational psychology while engaging in practices that facilitate self-reflection in one's own practice. Educators must understand the process of learning so that teaching strategies are used to engage students actively in their own learning. Expressive and/or reflective journaling before and after clinical experiences are powerful means of encouraging students to think about their anxieties, assumptions, and decision-making related to patient care. By reflecting on one's work, nurse educators continually challenge themselves to improve teaching practices that promote learning while also role modeling the importance of self-reflection as a lifelong learning strategy for students. Case studies, simulated learning, and problem-based learning are other strategies that require students to assume a more active role in their learning. The nurse of the future needs to be educated as a thinker and not just a doer, so strategies that encourage critical reflection or thoughtful analysis of one's practice must be emphasized and modeled.

Role of the Nurse Educator in the 21st Century

There are many national reports indicating the need for change in health care and in the education of health-care professionals in particular. In its report entitled *Crossing the Quality Chasm: A New Health System for the 21st Century*, the Institute of Medicine (IOM, 2001) acknowledges that the education of health professionals is in need of major change and asserts that the clinical education of health professionals is outdated and not responsive to the present or future needs in health care. As its guiding vision, the IOM (2003) makes the recommendation that health professionals should be educated to deliver patient-centered care within an interdisciplinary team that emphasizes evidence-based practice, quality improvement approaches, and informatics. Furthermore, the IOM (2003) recommends that all health professionals should have core competencies that are shared across disciplines in order to improve the quality of patient care. This backdrop of needed change will serve as the starting point for discussions regarding essential attributes needed in nursing education. Emphasis on student learning, promotion of evidence-based practice, and development of **authentic student-teacher relationships** are those attributes that are foundational to effective teaching.

Emphasis on Student Learning

Over the past decade, American higher education has shifted from a teacher-centered to a student-centered approach (Barr & Tagg, 1995). Such changes are aimed at the development of intellectual inquiry and the promotion of critical thinking, attributes necessary to solve problems in a world characterized by escalating ambiguity and complexity. Understanding and facilitating student learning must be a priority for the nurse educator of the 21st century. In a world where information increases exponentially, "covering content" needs to be replaced with teaching students how to learn both effectively and efficiently. In order to do this, educators need to understand how learning occurs and how to create learning environments in which students become active participants in learning. In **nursing education research,** there always has been a greater focus on the outcomes of learning, rather than on understanding the processes involved in learning (Tanner, 2001). But research aimed at understanding how students learn may result in the development of best practices in teaching. For example, there is some empirical support for the use of concept mapping as a strategy that promotes critical thinking (August-Brady, 2005; Daley, Shaw, Balistrieri, Glasenapp, & Piacentine, 1999). More educational research is needed to establish a strong evidence base in teaching and learning.

In order to facilitate learning, nurse educators must be cognizant of a variety of factors that students bring to the learning setting. Individual student characteristics, such as culture, age, gender, previous educational or life experiences, and socioeconomic factors, influence how they learn. Demographic changes in the student population also require that educators fully understand generational differences in teaching and learning. For example, a typical classroom may consist of second-degree students or second-career students (Boomers), returning or transfer students who may be in their mid 20s and 30s (Genexers) or students who attend college immediately after graduating from high school (Millennials). The nurse educator of the future needs to be sensitive to a growing array of factors that influence how one learns and must use a variety of pedagogical approaches that meet the needs of this diverse population of student learners. Skillful assessment of student learning outcomes is also needed in order to evaluate how students learn and the degree to which teaching strategies encourage meaningful learning.

Nursing education offers many opportunities for individuals to use their creativity and innovative thinking as they design curricula that prepare nursing students for the complexities of the contemporary health-care environment. Fitzpatrick (2005) suggests that what has been done in nursing education is based on past practices and tradition and not based on research. A recent survey of nursing students suggests that the content demands of the nursing curricula are so great that little time is left for students to assimilate that content into useful clinical knowledge (Norman, Buerhaus, Donelan, McCloskey, & Dittus, 2005). Del Bueno (2005) supports the assertion that content-laden nursing education curricula may be the root cause of students not being able to translate knowledge learned in the classroom into clinical judgment needed in practice. Novice nurses are less aware of their thinking and learning processes when compared with experienced nurses (Daley, 1999) and one may question whether the educational programs emphasizing content mastery have allowed students time to process learning. Nurse educators will be challenged to develop newer models of teaching if students are to learn how to be thoughtful, reflective practitioners. This is an area of much needed research in nursing education.

Promotion of Evidence-Based Practice

The primary focus of health-care institutions today is on the provision of quality care within a cost-effective framework. This emphasis on outcomes has led to a national movement requiring evidence-based care. Much work remains to be done, however. Pravikoff, Tanner and Pierce (2005) conducted a survey to determine the readiness of U.S. nurses for **evidence-based practice** and found that respondents reported a lack of value for research in practice. The value of research to practice may not have been highlighted in these respondents' educational programs.

The movement toward evidence-based practice requires that educators and practitioners engage in collaborative research. The formation of partnerships between academic institutions and health-care institutions provides opportunities for research and improved practice. Such endeavors offer exciting opportunities for educators to work with practitioners through research projects designed to assess the evidence base for quality nursing interventions. The nurse educator of the future must form collaborative relationships not only with practicing nurses but also with other members of the health-care team. Fluidity must characterize disciplinary boundaries as all team members seek to provide quality outcomes for health care. With patient-centered care as its focus, nursing and medicine, for example, need to collaborate in clinical studies in order to improve outcomes of care. Most importantly, nurse educators must role model this behavior for students so that students learn that practice and research coexist and cannot be seen as separate entities.

The nurse educator of the future needs to design learning opportunities that are grounded in nursing practice in which students critically evaluate practice from a process and outcome perspectives. For example, undergraduate students need to experience the process of research that is linked to clinical practice in order to appreciate its central role in shaping practice (August-Brady, 2005). In this way, research becomes meaningfully grounded in practice rather than a theoretical topic unrelated to the practice setting. Evidence-based practice is here to stay and discussions centering on nursing education and nursing practice must be strongly grounded in nursing research.

Emphasis on Authentic Student-Teacher Relationships

Historically, teachers derive much satisfaction from working with students. Nurse educators often have a passion for teaching students and are privileged to be able to influence the professional and personal development of students. Hence, most educators stay in nursing education because of the rewards involved in seeing students learn and grow into their nursing identity.

There is mounting evidence to suggest that a thoughtful student-teacher relationship is essential for students to develop and grow. A move from a behaviorist approach to the humanistic approach in nursing education began in the late 1980s with the landmark work of Bevis and Watson (1989). The traditional behaviorist model viewed students as empty vesicles who were eager to receive knowledge transmitted from the teacher. The humanistic approach recognizes that students have their own experiences that enrich learning while also viewing the student as a participant in learning. Since that time, others have carefully examined the centrality of the student-teacher connection in promoting learning. Gillespie (2002) found that a connected student-teacher relationship allowed students to focus on not only learning, the development of clinical judgment, communication and organizational abilities, and the ability to synthesize and use nursing knowledge, but also fostered the development of students' professional identity. Diekelmann (2001) suggests "knowing and connecting" and "creating places: keeping open a future of possibilities" as central experiences for teachers and learners (p. 57). Connecting with students and knowing them as individuals is central to effective teaching and learning.

What does this mounting evidence on student-centered approaches to teaching and learning suggest to aspiring nurse educators? The current research suggests that learning and student development are promoted through strategies aimed at getting to know students and connecting to students through more thoughtful, concerted means. Gillespie (2005) asserts that a connected student-teacher relationship is characterized by the teacher nursing with students so that students "experience self-confirmation of their existing capacities and, prompted by the example of the clinical teacher, become aware of potential capacities" (p. 215). When investigating student perceptions of effective and ineffective clinical instructors, Tang, Chou, and Chiang (2005) found that students perceived that the most effective clinical instructors were those having strong interpersonal relationships with students and rated "solves problems with students" as the highest-rated item within that category (p. 190). This would suggest that working together with students and role modeling professional behaviors are powerful determinants of effective teaching.

The nurse educator of the future will need to establish authentic relationships with students grounded in mutual trust and respect so that students gain the self-confidence to achieve their potential. The humanistic paradigm offers opportunities to relate to students as mentors and role models rather than primarily as evaluators. Such an approach is necessary in order to educate a student population that is far more heterogeneous than in past decades.

Challenges for the Nurse Educator in the 21st Century

One of the biggest challenges facing nurse educators today is the need to establish an independent evidence base in nursing education. Research in nursing education has been relatively devalued in terms of funding (Diekelmann & Ironside, 2002). Innovative studies that are conducted often consist of small samples and narrow settings, and often are not replicated. As a result, there is little development of the science of nursing education. Compounding the funding issues, some doctoral programs in nursing have not officially recognized nursing education as a developing science, and limit doctoral dissertations to clinical practice areas. This prevents students from engaging in scholarly investigations in nursing education and limits the growth of the science of nursing education.

There have been many changes in nursing education in recent years. Changes in student populations, educational delivery methods, diversity in practice settings, technological advances in health care, and new modes of curriculum delivery have altered the landscape of nursing education (Ferguson & Day, 2005). The challenge for nurse educators is to engage in research aimed at determining the effectiveness of nursing education. Without a science base underlying teaching, educators may be inclined to use more traditional approaches to teaching. Such approaches are based on past experiences and tradition. Fitzpatrick (2005) encourages nursing faculty "to put aside traditional tools of teaching and learning and to listen to students stories about how to make nursing education more meaningful to their lives as professional nurses" (p. 205).

How students learn, for example, is an area that merits careful examination. There has been much attention in nursing education on outcomes of learning, specifically critical thinking abilities. Nursing education has long recognized that curricula are content laden and that the approach to education needs to change (Bevis & Watson, 1989; Peters, 2000). As information continues to multiply exponentially, students are challenged to make use of efficient and effective means of learning. The learning process to date has been largely unexamined with teaching strategies implemented on unexamined assumptions about student learning (August-Brady, 2005). Research aimed at examining the process of learning may lead to more effective teaching practices and more capable nursing graduates. A strong proponent for the science of nursing education, the National League for Nursing, advocates for the value of pedagogical research and the provision of financial resources for pedagogical research (NLN, 2005).

Another challenge facing nursing education, as mentioned earlier, is the national shortage of faculty, a situation that is likely to worsen before it improves. The average age of a nursing professor with a doctoral degree is 56 years. According to the National League for Nursing (Valiga, 2004) approximately 75% of the current nursing faculty population is expected to retire by 2015. Compared to other disciplines, it takes nursing faculty two times longer to complete graduate education culminating in a doctoral degree. This is primarily because nurses accrue several years in practice before pursuing graduate study, practice full-time, and often juggle multiple roles while attending graduate school.

Given that it currently takes approximately 16 years for nursing faculty to complete graduate education, the prospects of increasing faculty supply any time soon are not promising (Valiga, 2004). Because of this grim reality, new models for educating nursing faculty need consideration. Accelerated programs have started to appear, offering prospective faculty a fast track in graduate courses. Care must be taken so that prospective faculty are offered courses in educational theory and are provided with immersion experiences in classroom and clinical instruction in order to prepare graduate students adequately for the teaching role.

Recruitment and retention efforts currently directed toward the nursing shortage need to include recognition of the faculty shortage. State and federal monies are becoming more available for nurses who plan to pursue nursing education. Although funding is needed to attract prospective faculty, additional efforts are needed to retain nursing faculty. In addition to common responsibilities shared by all faculty, the nursing faculty has additional responsibilities, including the expectation to maintain clinical practice expertise, clinical instruction of increasing numbers of students caring for highly acute and complex patients with accompanying responsibilities, and hours spent in developing positive collaborative relationships with clinical agencies. An expectation to "do it all" adds an additional burden that does not seem to exist in other disciplines (Rudy, 2001). Such additional responsibilities need to be factored into the workload of nursing faculty and those responsibilities need to be recognized, valued, and compensated as they would be in a corporate environment. Individuals enter nursing education for a variety of reasons, including but not limited to, shaping the profession, being intellectually stimulated, and working in an autonomous role with an expected degree of flexibility. According to data from the NLN (2004), individuals leave academe because of the heavy workload and poor salaries when compared with the corporate environment.

Strong orientation programs are needed to assist in the development and retention of junior faculty members as they learn to navigate through academe. Senior faculty members may provide invaluable resources for junior faculty members in terms of informal or formal mentoring. Continued professional development in nursing education is needed by most junior faculty members. Fortunately, many such opportunities exist in nursing in terms of conferences or more formal means. The Education Scholar Program endorsed by AACN is a Web-based program aimed at the promotion of teaching and professional scholarship primarily for educators in the health professions (www.educationscholar.org). The National League for Nursing offers a certification in nursing education, which formally recognizes the specialized knowledge of nurse educators. Certification in nursing education, as in other areas of nursing practice, communicates to others that the highest standards of excellence are being met.

There is a need for a serious national debate regarding credentialing in nursing education. In order to teach nursing in accredited nursing programs, one must have earned a masters degree in nursing. Traditionally, nurses enter graduate programs after establishing themselves as practitioners, which results in nursing faculty entering academe much later when compared with other disciplines. This translates into fewer productive years as a teacher. Concerned about the faculty shortage crisis, AACN (2003) questions whether a baccalaureate degree in nursing should be prerequisite to a masters degree in nursing. It is conceivable that students with undergraduate degrees in disciplines other than nursing may offer a broader and potentially richer perspective to nursing. These are interesting, provocative questions and, in the absence of empirical evidence, worth serious deliberation.

Resources

Due to the recognized nurse faculty shortage, a variety of resources are now available for individuals interested in learning more about nursing education as a career. The American Nurses Association (ANA) has clearly articulated its vision of nursing education in the future and calls for the attraction of nurse faculty early in their careers. Information about nursing education as a career may be found on a variety of nursing Web sites, including the American Nurses Association, the National League for Nursing, and the American Association of Colleges of Nursing.

Professional nursing organizations such as the National League for Nursing have supported the movement to increase nursing education's evidence base by developing Nursing Education Research Grants. Through such grants, educators are encouraged to develop and test innovative models of education.

Increasingly, monies are becoming available for nurses seeking to enter graduate education with the goal of pursuing a faculty role. Loan forgiveness programs are available that considerably reduce the cost of graduate study. Most loan forgiveness programs require that the recipient teach in an accredited school of nursing for a prescribed period of time. Scholarships are also available for prospective nursing faculty.

Summary

This chapter highlighted some of the essential components of newly envisioned nursing education and some of the challenges that nursing education faces. This is a pivotal time to consider nursing education as a career for several reasons. Nurse educators are challenged to use their creativity as they develop innovative models of education that are responsive to the current and future demands of a complex health-care environment. Given that pedagogical research is beginning to be recognized and valued, nursing education would benefit from research related to teaching and learning, the design of flexible models of education, and the evaluation of related outcomes. The advancement of the science of nursing education presents yet another opportunity for nursing faculty members to forge their collective efforts in shaping the direction of professional nursing.

References

American Association of Colleges of Nursing. (2003). Faculty shortages in baccalaureate and graduate nursing programs: Scope of the problem and strategies for expanding the supply. Washington, DC: AACN.

American Association of Colleges of Nursing. (2005). Special survey of AACN membership on vacant faculty positions. Washington, DC: AACN.

August-Brady, M. (2005). The effect of a metacognitive intervention on approach to and self-regulation of learning in baccalaureate nursing students. *Journal of Nursing Education, 44,* 297–304.

August-Brady, M. (2005). Teaching undergraduate research from a process perspective. *Journal of Nursing Education, 44,* 519–521.

Barr, R., & Tagg, J. (1995). From teaching to learning – A new paradigm for undergraduate education. *Change, 27*(6), 13–26.

Bevis, E., & Watson, J. (1989*). Toward a caring curriculum: A new pedagogy for nursing.* New York: National League for Nursing.

Buresh, B., & Gordon, S. (2000*). From silence to voice.* Ithaca, NY: Cornell University Press.

Daley, B. (1999). Novice to expert: An exploration of how professionals learn. *Adult Education Quarterly, 49*(4), 133–148.

Daley, B., Shaw, C., Balistrieri, T., Glasenapp, K., & Piacentine, L. (1999). Concept maps: A strategy to teach and evaluate critical thinking. *Journal of Nursing Education, 38,* 42–47.

Del Bueno, D. (2005). A crisis in critical thinking. *Nursing Education Perspectives, 26,* 278–282.

Diekelmann, N. (2001). Narrative pedagogy: Heideggerian hermeneutical analyses of lived experiences of students, teachers, and clinicians. *Advances in Nursing Science, 23,* 53–71.

Diekelmann, N., & Ironside, P. (2002). Developing a science of nursing education: Innovation with research. *Journal of Nursing Education, 41,* 379–380.

Ferguson, L., & Day, R. (2005). Evidence-based nursing education: Myth or reality? *Journal of Nursing Education, 44,* 107–115.

Fitzpatrick, J. (2005). Can we "escape fire" in nursing education? *Nursing Education Perspectives, 26,* 205.

Gillespie, M. (2002). Student-teacher connection in clinical nursing education. *Journal of Advanced Nursing, 37,* 566–576.

Gillespie, M. (2005). Student-teacher connection: A place of possibility. *Journal of Advanced Nursing, 52,* 211–219.

Institute of Medicine. (2001). *Crossing the quality chasm: A new health system for the 21st century.* Washington, DC: National Academy Press.

Institute of Medicine. (2003). *Health professions education: A bridge to quality.* Washington, DC: National Academy Press.

National League for Nursing. (2004). Report on the national study of faculty role satisfaction. New York: National League for Nursing.

National League for Nursing. (2005). *Transforming nursing education.* New York: National League for Nursing.

Norman, L., Buerhaus, P., Donelan, K., McClosky, B., & Dittus, R. (2005). Nursing students assess nursing education. *Journal of Professional Nursing, 21,* 150–158.

Peters, M. (2000). Does constructivist epistemology have a place in nursing education? *Journal of Nursing Education, 39,* 166–172.

Pravikoff, D. S., Tanner, A. B., & Pierce, S. T. (2005). Readiness of U.S. nurses for evidence-based practice: Many don't understand or value research and have had little or no training to help them find evidence on which to base their practice. *American Journal of Nursing, 105*(9), 40–52.

Rudy, E. (2001). Supportive work environments for nursing faculty. *AACN Clinical Issues, 12*(3), 401–410.

Tang, F., Chou, S., & Chiang, H. (2005). Students' perceptions of effective and ineffective clinical instructors. *Journal of Nursing Education, 44,* 187–192.

Tanner, C. (2001). Measurement and evaluation in nursing education. *Journal of Nursing Education, 40,* 3–4.

Valiga, T. (2004). *Nursing education shortage: A national perspective.* Paper presented at the Congressional Briefing presented by the A. N. S. R. Alliance. Washington, DC.

REVIEW QUESTIONS

- What are reasons for the decreased supply of nursing faculty educators today?
- According to the Institute of Medicine report (2001), what changes need to occur in the education process for future nursing faculty?
- Your chairperson in nursing has decided that the department will institute a humanistic faculty-student approach throughout its curriculum. Identify strategies to help in this paradigm change.
- Your department of nursing is approached by the nursing administration from a large teaching medical center. The administration is interested in forming a partnership between the university and center for evidence-based practice research. Explain why this type of collaboration will be beneficial for both parties. Identify a variety of topics that could be addressed using evidenced-based research.

CRITICAL THINKING EXERCISE

As the chairperson of a nursing department, you are responsible for developing an advertisement for a full-time faculty position at your program. What attributes will you identify as essential for this faculty position?

ANNOTATED RESEARCH SUMMARY

Peters, M. A., & Boylston, M. (2006). Mentoring adjunct faculty: Innovative solutions. *Nurse Educator 31*(2), 61–64.

Rising enrollments in schools of nursing have increased the demand for qualified nursing faculty. In the midst of a nurse faculty shortage, many academic institutions are relying on adjunct faculty to fill the gap. The increasing number of adjunct faculty and their need for orientation to the faculty role presents a challenge to schools and departments of nursing. The authors discuss innovative solutions to these challenges.

Schaefer, K. M., & Zygmont, D. (2003). Analyzing the teaching style of nursing faculty: Does it promote a student-centered or teacher-centered learning environment? *Nursing Education Perspectives 24*(5), 239–245.

The purposes of this study were to (a) describe the predominant teaching style of a group of nursing faculty members, either as teacher-centered or student-centered; and (b) to compare teaching style to the instructional methods the faculty members used in the courses they taught and to their stated philosophies of teaching/learning. Findings indicate that the participants were more teacher-centered than student-centered; their written philosophies supported the teacher-centered approach. However, evidence that faculty used student-centered language, often in a teacher-centered context, indicates that participants in the study may recognize the need for a student-centered environment but may have difficulty with implementation. Recommendations for faculty members and administrators are offered.

Kopp, E. M., & Hinkle, J. L. (2006). Understanding mentoring relationships. *Journal of Neuroscience Nursing 38*(2), 126–131.

This article explains how mentoring may be used as a growth-and-development strategy for the recruitment and retention of nursing. It examines and discusses mentoring from both a conventional and contemporary perspective and addresses the new paradigm now evident in nursing.

Chapter Outline

CURRICULUM DEVELOPMENT

Susan Leddy

5

Learning Outcomes

On completion of this chapter, the reader will be able to:

- Describe the processes of curriculum development.
- Appreciate the communication processes that can affect curriculum development.
- Analyze the elements that influence determination of program outcomes.
- Utilize information about students in implementing curriculum change.
- Participate in curriculum development through an understanding of the curriculum process.

Key Terms

Active learning
Behaviorist model
Curriculum
Curriculum development
Epistemological model
Faculty philosophy
Framework
Level objectives
Matrix

Negative synergy
Nursing theorist model
Passive learning
Philosophy
Practice protocols
Process
Skills
Values

Curriculum is the totality of formal and informal content that imparts the **skills,** attitudes, and **values** considered important in achieving specific educational goals. A curriculum needs to be flexible in order to accommodate changes in the environment that influence the content of the curriculum. For example, the use of Web-based technology is an area of competence that many faculty need to address. Eventually, an accumulation of many small modifications upsets curricular integrity, and the entire curriculum has to be re-conceptualized and revised. All curriculum decisions should be made based on a review of the total curriculum.

The concept of curriculum (in contrast to an accumulation of disparate courses) developed in the mid-1800s. In 1892, a college preparation curriculum in Chicago labeled various course subjects, specified content for each course at each level, and ordered a sequence of courses. From the 1920s, a technical approach to creating curricula was in practice, reaching an apex in nursing with the influential models developed by Tyler (1950) and Taba (1962). Steps in the technical approach to **curriculum development** include (1) define the goals; purposes, or objectives; (2) define experiences or activities related to the goals; (3) organize the experiences and activities; and (4) evaluate the goals.

In 1998, Wiggins and McTighe changed the order of the stages to what has been called a backward design. The steps in this design include: (1) identify the desired results; (2) determine the acceptable evidence; and (3) plan teaching experiences and instruction based on standards, as opposed to a curriculum based on activities. For example, a faculty member may decide that students need experiences with clients who have teaching needs, rather than simply assigning students to a clinical setting every week for 16 hours. This method starts from the end—the desired results based on goals or standards—and then derives the curriculum from performance, or the evidence of learning called for by the standard (Wiggins & McTighe, 1998). In a study designed to compare results from a backward designed curriculum with those from a traditional curriculum, students from the backward designed curriculum outperformed traditional students in meeting outcome goals (Kelting-Gibson, 2005). This chapter espouses a hybrid approach: it starts the curriculum development **process** with identification of desired outcomes, and continues by designing activities to achieve those outcomes. First, it is important to have an overview of the stages of curriculum development.

Overview of the Stages of Curriculum Development

"Curriculum development is a deliberate process, not an event, that takes concentrated time, effort and faculty commitment" (Dillard & Laidig, 1998, p. 78). The process consists of a series of systematic, logical, dynamic, spiraled, and progressive stages (Torres & Stanton, 1982) that can be time-consuming and labor-intensive (Hull, St. Romain, Alexander, Schaff, & Jones, 2001). The stages of the curriculum development process as described in this chapter are as follows:

1. Identify the characteristics desired of the graduate of the program. Review of the recent literature, discussion with service leaders and other members of the community, and consultation are several strategies that can be useful.
2. Concurrently, review the 5- to 10-year trends in the internal and external environment that might affect the characteristics desired of the graduate. An example of such a trend is the changing characteristics of potential students.
3. Revise and refine desired characteristics of the graduate accordingly.
4. Identify philosophical beliefs and values of the faculty that are relevant to the curriculum, taking into consideration the mission and goals of the parent institution. Clearly identify characteristics and needs of potential students.

5. Clarify the main concepts identified in the philosophy. Clearly define each concept based on faculty beliefs. This statement will be the basis for all subsequent curriculum work.
6. Link the concepts into coherent propositions that form a conceptual **framework** for the curriculum. This might be eclectic or based on an extant framework for nursing (e.g., Orem, Roy, Neuman, Leddy).
7. Identify a structure for the curriculum that will accommodate general education, supporting (e.g., anatomy and physiology, general psychology), and nursing courses. Also reconsider the existing organization of the faculty, which should be consistent with the philosophy (e.g., a developmental organization, such as infants/children, adolescents, adults, elderly; or a health/illness continuum, such as health, chronic/long-term, acute).
8. Using the philosophy and program outcomes as guides, identify the vertical and horizontal strands of the evolving curriculum. Develop a **matrix** of these strands. For example, if leadership is one of the horizontal strands, an increasing complexity of leadership skills should be demonstrated as the student progresses vertically through the program.
9. Using the curriculum framework and the strand matrix as guides, determine names, placement, and objectives of courses.
10. Flesh out the course sequence with content, teaching/learning and evaluation activities. Ensure that all matrix strands are appropriately represented.
11. Identify an evaluation plan for the entire curriculum.

It is necessary for individual faculty members to be flexible. In addition, "curriculum must be flexible to accommodate work schedules; offer diversity in courses and programs; teach management of culturally diverse peoples, as well as delegation and negotiation skills; enhance verbal, written, and speaking communication skills; and enhance decision-making skills for the increasingly complex world" (Dillard & Laidig, 1998, p. 69).

Before detailing each of these steps, it is important to note that much of the success or failure of curriculum development is determined by the group communication processes of the faculty.

Faculty Communication Processes

"The greater the amount of participation of the faculty, the greater the degree of success" (Torres & Stanton, 1982, p. 7). Depending on the size and organization of the faculty, curriculum development may be accomplished by a committee of the whole, or by smaller committees that are assigned to various tasks. The total effort needs to "belong" to the total faculty, with each member accepting ownership. Otherwise, it is possible that disgruntled faculty will reject any curriculum change, and may even try to prevent successful implementation of the changes.

There are a number of strategies that can enhance the smooth and productive efforts of the faculty. Many of these strategies will enhance the communication among faculty members during various stages of the process:

1. There should be clear delegation of assignments to various committees. One person should make final decisions about the role and functions of committees.
2. There need to be realistic goals and adequate support and resources for the work of the committees.
3. A timetable for the total curriculum process should be developed at the start of the process. The amount of time needed will depend on the extent of the change anticipated, the curriculum experience of at least some of the faculty, and the other demands on faculty time. At least a year, and perhaps twice that much, will probably be needed to complete the process thoroughly and defensibly.

4. Faculty need to be proactive, active, involved, and enthusiastic. Creativity is essential, so faculty members need to brainstorm and promote a free flow of ideas and information.
5. To the extent possible, faculty should listen and not argue. Seek first to understand and then to be understood.
6. Think win-win. Curriculum revision should not be a power play but a mutual and noncompetitive process.
7. Avoid **negative synergy** because it is debilitating. It includes talking about other people dishonestly, politicking, rivalry, masterminding, and second-guessing outcomes for self-gain. Negative synergy can be contagious if not confronted, and can ultimately derail the process. Instead, celebrate accomplishments, no matter how small.
8. Take care of yourself. The curriculum process is time-consuming and may be associated with increased stress and uncertainty. Try to remain calm and peaceful, and stay up-to-date on information about the revision.
9. Try to provide a documented rationale to support the changes that you think should be made. This will help to avoid emotional defense of the status quo.
10. Group process among the faculty may need development through strategies such as small group work with a consultant, critical incidents/role play, or storyboarding.
11. Recognize and respect each person's unique contribution.

Bensusan (1997) developed an approach to learning that he labeled the escalator approach. This approach can be modified easily for faculty use in the curriculum development communication process. The steps of this approach include using imagination to brainstorm ideas and describe various perceptions about curriculum development; asking critical questions, giving constructive feedback, and verifying information; using creativity to ladder and frame ideas; and probing, refining, and recasting, considering various points of view and schools of thought.

Moreover, Goldenberg, Andrusyszyn, and Iwasiw (2004), suggest that curriculum development requires:

- Commitment of time, energy, and resources.
- Compatibility, which is the ability of the group to harmonize and function as a whole. This requires a focus on common ground and the curriculum as a whole rather than as individual courses.
- Communication. Consider having a facilitator to keep faculty on task and to referee conflicts. A gatekeeper can regulate communication and allow each person to be heard, set up the agenda, and summarize accomplishments. A harmonizer promotes group cohesion and diffuses tension (e.g., rejection, defensiveness), and a housekeeper can record minutes, secure and prepare meeting rooms, and serve as timekeeper. These roles should be rotated among the faculty members.
- Contribution. Curriculum development work requires consensus, which is derived from communication, compromise, and negotiation.

In turn, potential obstacles associated with group work include premature decision-making, individual dominance, conflicts, and unhealthy competition. (Tips to overcome these obstacles can be found in Box 5–1) Faculty members may resist curriculum revision because of:

- Fear of losing control of the curriculum.
- Misunderstanding due to lack of information or confusion about new vocabulary and jargon.
- Perception of lack of skill to progress with new demands on time and energies.
- Different views about what needs to be done.
- Lack of motivation to study the change.
- Lack of perception of a need to change ("if it isn't broken, don't fix it").

- Too many changes and too many demands related to the change process.
- Desire to be vindictive and make the leader look bad.
- Idea that "no one can tell me what to do."
- Threat to change current internal social support systems if faculty "teams" in some courses change.
- Lack of resources.
- View that formal methods used to facilitate change are barriers rather than helps.
- Lack of rewards (Dillard & Laidig, 1998, p. 79).

Curriculum Development Stages and Activities

Each of the steps of curriculum development will be discussed in this section.

Program Outcomes (Characteristics of Graduates)

"A focus on educational outcomes should be the pivotal point when redesigning a curriculum" (Daggett, Butts, & Smith, 2002, p. 36). The outcomes or goals of the program should be consistent with the philosophy of the faculty and should identify a level of behavior (Torres & Stanton, 1982). For example, it is not sufficient to say that the faculty members expect the graduate to be proficient in research. Do the faculty members expect the graduate to utilize evidence in practice? Will the graduate be expected to participate in practice-based research, or actually to conduct research? The development of educational outcomes of the program of study requires an understanding of the environmental forces internal and external to the program that will affect what outcomes will be desired in the next 5 to 10 years.

Environmental Forces and Issues

Environmental forces, such as changing student characteristics, financial influences, political effects, and trends in the delivery of health care, have a major influence on the curriculum development process. A number of sources, such as environmental scanning, forecasting, epidemiology, survey research, and consensus building can be used to identify trends that may influence desired educational outcomes.

Some of the types of issues that may need to be considered are sociological, political, and economic characteristics of the community, including setting and risk factors; demographic change; transformation of the American family; shift from resources to knowledge; rise of the global economy; multicultural diversity and ethnic understanding; and a shift from infectious to noncommunicable diseases.

Box 5–1 Tips to Overcome Obstacles to Curriculum Revision

1. Work actively with faculty colleagues so that you can retain a feeling of ownership of the curriculum.
2. Try to clarify the meaning of any new vocabulary or jargon.
3. Practice effective time management to deal with new demands on time and energy.
4. Strive toward consensus on different faculty views about what needs to be done.
5. Use self-talk to motivate yourself to study proposed curriculum changes.
6. Try to accept the necessity for change in order to progress.
7. Talk openly about your feelings.
8. Reframe negative thoughts as challenges and opportunities.
9. Negotiate for needed support and resources.

Another environmental consideration is context of the parent institution, including mission and traditions, the target client or constituencies, geographic area, goal of the institution (teaching, science, research), financing, and accountability and quality indicators. A state-supported college parent institution, for instance, may emphasize quality teaching at the baccalaureate level and open opportunity for diverse, commuter, and adult populations, whereas a private university may emphasize quantity of external funding for research, graduate study, and recruitment of a limited number of students with stellar academic qualifications. The mission and philosophy of the nursing program must be consistent with the mission and philosophy of the parent institution. The institutional mission is an internal environmental force that affects all elements of the nursing program.

In a study conducted in 1998 and 2003 (Bowen, Lyons, & Young, 2000), nursing program administrators were mailed questionnaires asking which courses, content, and/or electives were important in the curriculum now and which were projected to be more important in 2008. Administrators responded that they expect diversity of the student population, informatics, health-care costs/economics/finance/financial management, evidence-based practice, management/delegation, and health promotion/wellness care to be more important in 2008. Critical thinking and the changing health-care environment were deemed to be less important. Strategies such as simulation, case studies, **active learning** strategies, concept mapping, CD-ROM technology, distance learning, use of the Internet in courses, chat rooms, listservs, problem-based learning, cooperative/collaborative learning, mentoring, and videoconferencing were anticipated to be used more often in the future, whereas lectures were anticipated to be used less. Faculty members were perceived to be less interested in teaching critical thinking than in promoting it. Other future trends identified included computer adaptive testing, creative projects, critical analysis, and self-assessment, computer simulation, competency-based assessment, faculty/staff partnership models, use of computers, innovative teaching approaches, evidence-based teaching, use of adjunct faculty, use of clinical experts, and grant writing. Support services to retain students, recruitment at middle schools, and retention of diverse student populations were other perceived trends.

Environmental trends and issues influencing the practice environment also affect curriculum development. The rising number of unlicensed assistive personnel substituting for registered nurses (RNs) and the increase in part-time RNs, have created a necessity for understandable, reasonable, and accurate delegation of tasks, for example. Moreover, the increasing emphasis on evidence-based nursing practice requires an understanding of research methodology. Significant efforts at cost containment, restructuring, and downsizing of hospitals, influence of political and legislative activities, increasing dependence on technology, a shortage of registered nurses, shifting population demographics, and the movement of health-care delivery out of acute-care centers and into the community are significant trends that curriculum must reflect. Nurses in today's practice settings must learn how to manage their time, organize their jobs in light of shifting demands, and be able to prioritize assigned tasks (Bowen et al., 2000).

Reflecting many of the trends discussed above, The University of Louisville developed the following learning outcomes in its curriculum revision. The graduate will be able to:

• Communicate effectively orally with peers, clients, and other professionals.
• Communicate effectively in writing with peers, clients, and other professionals.
• Consistently demonstrate critical thinking, cognitive skills, and affective dispositions.
• Work effectively and cooperatively with groups.
• Select, use, and evaluate interventions for clients.
• Demonstrate personal and professional life skills and commitment to lifelong learning and service to the profession and the community.
• Use technology effectively in nursing practice (Freeman, Voignier, & Scott, 2002, p. 38).

In another example, faculty at Indiana University initially developed the following principles for characteristics of graduates. Graduates will be able to:

• Use resources in a more socially appropriate manner and design ways to offer services that will maintain or improve quality and lower costs.
• Improve access to care.
• Create less resource-intensive health care but more fulfilling lives for people as they age.
• Master information technologies.
• Develop **practice protocols** for new technologies that balance costs and benefits.
• Welcome the discipline of continuous improvement of quality.
• Understand the empowered role of the health-care consumer and develop skills to change individual attitudes.
• Move organizations, systems, and policies toward strategies that improve equity of resource distribution.
• Incorporate a more holistic perspective into care delivery (Daggett et al., 2002, p. 35).

The assessment of trends in potential student characteristics is also part of an environmental assessment.

Students

By "2020, the percentage of Americans of European descent is projected to decrease from the 75.1 percent reported in 2000 to 53 percent. The number of Asian Americans and Hispanic Americans is expected to triple, and the number of African Americans is expected to double" (U.S. Census Bureau, cited by Ruth-Sahd, 2003). Clearly, continuing population shifts will affect student diversity in schools of nursing.

In a 1992 survey of new RNs, 17% indicated a minority status (Richardson, 1998). All students in nursing schools need strong professional role models, but this need is especially important for minority students who may be the first in their families to attend college. Other considerations for a diverse nursing student body include:

• Increasingly older (adult) learners—These learners need to increase their self-confidence after years away from school in order to assume responsibility for learning and the use of resources.
• Married students with families—In the 1992 survey of new RNs, 57% were married and an additional 13% were divorced (Richardson, 1998). Married students often are part-time learners who need strong faculty-student support.
• Many students are now commuters who are geographically removed from the school campus. Identification with the school campus has been found to be strongly related to motivation and retention.
• Increasingly, students entering a nursing program have prior educational experiences, often a baccalaureate degree. These students need to have help to relate their prior education to nursing content.
• Students who have limited financial resources often attend school part-time, while working to earn tuition money and to help support their families. This is especially true of associate degree graduates.
• Men form a small but important cohort of students. Few studies have been done to identify similarities or differences in learning needs based on gender differences.
• Special-needs students form a significant proportion of the students in many nursing programs. These students may need tutoring, remediation for poor study skills, special advising, child-care on campus, and financial assistance.

Given the diverse backgrounds of today's students, it is necessary for faculty to know the characteristics (social, intellectual, and emotional) of students; their varied approaches to learning, skills, and knowledge; and their interests and cultural heritage. This aspect of environmental knowledge will help the faculty to adapt the curriculum to start where the student is. "Comparability among students is not a meaningful aspiration. . . . the good teacher, like the good school, increases rather than suppresses individual differences" (Eisner, 1990, p. 65).

Philosophy

"A curriculum **philosophy** is a speculative and analytical examination of beliefs which are logically conceptualized…[However,] beliefs are accepted opinions or convictions of the truth that are not necessarily supported by scientific knowledge…The purpose of the curriculum philosophy is to guide the educational process of the learner" (Torres & Stanton, 1982, p. 30). Given that **faculty philosophy** reflects the nature of the discipline of nursing and nursing education, it gives direction for the development of the curriculum. The beliefs affect the criteria from which to develop, teach, and evaluate learning (Dillard & Laidig, 1998). For example, a faculty that believes that its members are the content experts will emphasize lecture as a teaching method that efficiently imparts information to passive learners.

The nursing program's philosophy is based on the institution's stated mission, philosophy, and purposes or goals. The philosophy also includes beliefs of the nursing faculty about social and technology forces, concepts associated with learning, such as critical thinking and problem-solving, multiculturalism, and communication, and about four or five concepts a faculty has identified as the characteristics of the nursing metaparadigm (Torres & Stanton, 1982). "The philosophy provides a framework for discussion of answers to value-laden questions related to teaching and learning and a guide to all activities of the curriculum" (Csokasy, 2002, p. 32).

Torres and Stanton (1982, p. 33) identified some common beliefs about nursing that might appear in a program philosophy. These include:

- Nursing is a practice discipline.
- It involves a service to human beings.
- Human beings exist within a society.
- Nursing provides care and nurturance to human beings.
- Human beings are entitled to respect and dignity.
- A society has common interests.
- The discipline focuses on health.
- Nursing involves health promotion and maintenance.
- Health is the right of everyone in society.
- Nursing is humanitarian.
- Society should be responsive to the needs of human beings.

For example, the belief that human beings are entitled to respect and dignity would indicate a strong content strand of ethics in the curriculum. Basic faculty philosophic beliefs also affect the philosophy of the nursing program. Idealists emphasize the mind of the learner, whereas realists tend to structure the learner's environment through a behaviorist framework. Realists tend to emphasize content, and idealists tend to emphasize how students learn.

"Educators using an idealistic framework expect learners to be proficient in the mechanics of verbal and written communication and mathematics, and to demonstrate a strong foundation in the humanities, including history, art, music, and literature. Assessment strategies would provide opportunities for learners to demonstrate creative abilities within the humanities through application of the liberal arts. In the behaviorist-based curriculum and outcome assessment process, faculty [sic] help students strive toward mastery of information, with an emphasis on basic skills. The curriculum is usually designed to progress from the simple to the complex. Scientific objectivity and critical examination are important and when students exhibit these behaviors they are rewarded appropriately. Objective measures of knowledge are important in evaluation, and the teacher relies heavily on empirical data for decision-making"

(Csokasy, 2002, pp. 32–33).

Finally, with a humanist-based philosophy, there is heavy reliance on students' interpretation of their learning experiences. Humanist-based outcome assessment focuses on critical thinking and application of knowledge, with the role of teacher being to motivate and encourage experiential learning that will facilitate students' ability to seek their own goals (Csokasy, 2002).

It is usually very helpful for the faculty to develop a glossary for the philosophy that will define how the terms are being used. This leads to a common frame of reference, and more effective communication among faculty members as the curriculum process moves to identifying curriculum framework.

Curriculum Framework

A curriculum framework provides a way for faculty to conceptualize and organize knowledge, skills, values, and beliefs that are critical to the delivery of a coherent curriculum. An organizing framework also facilitates the sequencing and prioritizing of knowledge in a way that is logical and internally consistent (Finke & Boland, 1998). A framework organizes the curriculum, whereas a philosophy provides a belief and value base for the curricular structure and content.

Several models have been used by faculty for nursing curricula. For example, the medical model is still the dominant model used in schools of nursing, despite the fact that the model encompasses only those aspects of nursing that are shared with medicine. Content in such a model is usually organized by body systems (e.g., cardiovascular, orthopedic) or larger categories of medical specialties (e.g., medical, surgical, obstetrics). The model emphasizes medical diseases and pathophysiology, and relates nursing care to medical diagnoses.

The **behaviorist model** (based on the behaviorist philosophy mentioned earlier) is often applied within a medical model. There is a "focus on rule driven, predictable, outcomes for student learning...The teacher concentrates on teaching facts, directives, rules, theories, laws, and principles. . . At its core, it has information as its primary content and acquiring and using information in performance as its learning intent" (Bevis, 1989/1982, iii–iv). Lecture is a primary teaching strategy in this model. A behaviorist curriculum model is directive, under teacher control, and "tells" the student what and how to do tasks.

The **epistemological (concept) model** is organized by ideas and themes rather than subject matter or process skills (e.g., pain, delegation). The focus is on understanding and appreciation of systems of knowledge, key ideas, themes, and principles. For example, a pathophysiology course might focus on concepts such as edema, instead of the cardiovascular system, and on pattern recognition instead of each area of content being separated into body systems or medical diseases. The teacher's role is that of interactive questioner. Students focus on reading, reflecting, and writing. Teachers need to have in-depth knowledge about a field, and make connections to other fields. They need a consistent vision, perception, and insight (Van Tassel-Baska, 2004).

Faculty may also use an existing **nursing theorist model** to organize the nursing curriculum. The model may be derived from supporting sciences (e.g., stress/adaptation) or nursing (e.g., Orem, Roy, Leddy). An Orem-based curriculum, for example, would focus on providing care in a variety of situations where a patient might be unable to provide self-care. A Roy-based curriculum might emphasize stimuli and adaptive modes. And, a Leddy-based curriculum would focus on human being–environment mutual process and energetic patterning. A single theory may not reflect everyone's vision or language, however. Some faculties choose to develop an eclectic model, selecting concepts from several models or theories. For example, both the Roy and Neuman models emphasize the role of stimuli. It is necessary for the parent models or theories to share a common worldview, and attention needs to be paid to ensuring that the meaning of the concepts in the various model/theories is consistent with the original.

The use of theory encourages a structured line of reasoning. "A framework establishes boundaries and intent, which provides structure and direction for content" (Webber, 2002, p. 16). An organizing framework provides a meaningful picture of the knowledge that is important to nursing and how that knowledge is defined, categorized, sequenced, and linked with other knowledge. Acting as a blueprint, the framework structures knowledge in a meaningful way for faculty, students, administrators, evaluators, and others (Daggett, Butts, & Smith, 2002). It also reduces the influence of emotions, traditions, or rationalizations on faculty decision-making (Torres & Stanton, 1982).

Curriculum Matrix

A curriculum matrix is composed of vertical and horizontal content strands. Vertical strands represent content areas such as leadership that increase in complexity at each level of the curriculum. Horizontal strands are processes that apply the content throughout the curriculum, like clinical decision-making (Torres & Stanton, 1982). Vertical strands may be leveled by degree of difficulty, complexity, past experience, or frequency of utilization. Integrated content (e.g., teaching-learning) tends to be more easily included in vertical strands. Horizontal and vertical strands identify and structure the content of the educational process, and give a sequence to nursing learning experiences, prerequisite content, and supporting courses.

A matrix of curriculum content is a very useful strategy to permit visualization of curriculum content, and prevent overlaps or omissions of content. The matrix sequences content elements appropriately, and:

1. Identifies the specific content elements that should be taught within each course.
2. Allows the faculty to understand better what the students were previously taught, thus facilitating building the content in a progressive manner.
3. Gives the faculty and students a sense of direction because it shows which content elements will follow.
4. Gives structure to the differentiation of content elements from one course to another.
5. Assists in recognizing content areas not previously identified.

The matrix clearly identifies the general content that needs to be in the courses at each level of the curriculum.

Level and Course Objectives

Level and course **objectives** are derived from characteristics, or cumulative goals to be achieved by the graduate, and are informed by the curriculum matrix. They contain:

• The level of achievement expected at any given point within the program.
• The identification of content from the vertical strands.
• A process component from the horizontal strands, for example, the content might relate to the content of communication, while the process might be delegation of duties to auxiliary personnel. This might result in a course objective such as, "demonstrates effective communication skills when delegating duties to auxiliary personnel" within a level objective such as, "communicates effectively with other members of the health-care team."

After clarification and modification of previous steps in the curriculum development process, the curriculum matrix and curriculum framework are used to identify and sequence course requirements so that learning experiences are structured throughout the program. Many programs are congested with content that overwhelms students with too much content and detracts from learning. "Providing skills for learning and acquisition of information is better than mastery of content" (Speziale & Jacobson, 2005, p. 234). Some important considerations in the development of courses follow:

• About one-third of courses should be in general education, such as English and Humanities; one-third in supporting courses, and one-third in nursing courses.
• The flexibility of the curriculum should be enhanced by allowing free electives and limited prerequisites to courses.
• In a progressive design, more supporting courses, such as microbiology and nutrition, are offered early in the curriculum. Nursing starts early and increases as the student progresses through the program.
• In a parallel design, the same amount of nursing is offered in each year.
• In a collection-type curriculum, the kind most prevalent, each subject is treated as an independent entity having little or no connection to others.
• Areas about which faculty are most familiar usually require the greatest amount of content.

Criteria for course content include the following:

• The depth and breadth of the content must be appropriate for the learner.
• The validity of the content must be assessed (empirically tested).
• The content must reflect the emerging health-care system and the changing role of the nurse.
• Content that encourages generalizations, such as how to recognize patterns in health/illness manifestations, and how to link and synthesize content, should be emphasized.
• The content should be progressive, starting with areas that are more easily learned and foundational to areas of content that are highly dependent on previous learning and require synthesis. This should not be viewed as going from the simple to the complex, but rather as an approach in which emphasis is placed on the learner's ability to deal with specific pieces of information at any given period of time.
• The content should motivate the student to learn. It is not only how well the content is presented that is significant but also how such content relates to what the student perceives as essential in his or her learning.
• The content must reflect the level within the cognitive, affective, and psychomotor domains that is appropriate in relation to the stated objectives. Bloom's taxonomy (1956) of cognitive levels from simple to complex consists of knowledge (identifies steps); comprehension (differentiates among the steps); application (applies); analysis (relates to); synthesis (proposes interventions); and evaluation (determines priorities).

One framework that may assist faculty to identify course content is the knowledge/skills/ values/meanings/experience (KSVME) framework. In this framework, "nursing is defined as the desire, intent, and obligation to apply discipline-specific knowledge, skills, values, meanings, and experience (KSVME) for, with, or on behalf of those requiring and/or requesting assistance in achieving and maintaining their desired state of health and/or well-being" (Webber, 2002, p. 17). Nursing knowledge is defined as the cumulative, organized, and dynamic body of scientific and phenomenological information used to identify, relate, understand, explain, predict, influence, and/or control nursing phenomena" (p. 17). Nursing knowledge is discipline specific. Understanding and reasoning help to operationalize knowledge through some or all of the following content:

- Relevant scientific and phenomenological theory
- Discipline-specific theory
- Health
- Health promotion
- Health experiences
- Environment
- Diverse factors influencing care (age, gender, race, culture, family, religion, ethnicity, socioeconomic status, geographic region)
- Policies and procedures
- Factors influencing discipline/profession (research, health-care policy and economics, law and ethics, standards [national, specialty, institutional])
- Professional roles and responsibilities (manage and coordinate)
- Health-care delivery systems

Skills are deliberate acts or activities in the cognitive and psychomotor domain that operationalize nursing knowledge, values, meanings, and experience (p. 19). Some relevant skills include:

- Nursing praxis: Integration of KSVME in the delivery of therapeutic nursing interventions
- Safety
- Communication
- Critical thinking/reasoning (knowing, pattern identification, understanding)
- Collaboration
- Leadership/followership
- Delegation
- Creativity
- Learning/teaching
- Technology

"values are enduring beliefs, attributes, or ideals that establish moral boundaries of what is right and wrong in thought, judgment, character, attitude, and behavior and that form a foundation for decision making throughout life" (webber, 2002, p. 20). Relevant values include:

- Professional behavior (honesty, integrity, dignity, respect, ethics, morality, confidentiality, attitude)
- Role development
- Collegiality
- Holism
- KSVME of others

Meanings define the context, purpose, and intent of language, and may include:

- Nursing language
- Accountability/responsibility
- Accreditation/control forces (NLN, JCAHO, HCFA, AACN, specialty)
- Synergy
- Nursing history
- Registration/certification

Another framework that is increasingly being integrated into nursing curricula is care and caring. These concepts may include having concern for another, valuing, providing for, protecting, having responsibility for, helping, assigning importance to, serving, and being solicitous (p. 21).

Teaching/Learning Strategies

Teaching/learning strategies are the processes that are used for the actual delivery of the curriculum. The following list describes some principles that should be considered when choosing teaching/learning strategies. Teaching/learning strategies should:

- Clearly relate to the desired objectives and competencies, learning domain, and domain level.
- Be geared to and appropriate for the cognitive, affective, or psychomotor development of the students.
- Be challenging so that they move students to higher levels of cognitive and affective development.
- Be emotionally satisfying for students.
- Stimulate development of alternative perspectives of the problem or issue.
- Be sufficiently varied to prevent boredom, allow for and exploit the potential for individual student differences, and enable participation in transcultural experiences (Norton, 1998, p. 155).
- Articulate and allow application of some previous learning experiences within the same course as well as experiences from previous and concurrent courses.
- Provide a foundation for subsequent learning.

Creative curriculum development, the development of materials that faculty work with, should enable the faculty to provide students with activities that teach ideas, skills, or forms of perception that are educationally important, intellectually challenging, and stimulate higher-order thinking. Content is not restricted to text alone and the content students study should help them make connections with what they learn in other areas, including those outside of the school. For example, schools might consider requiring that students take a certified nursing assistant course before admission to the nursing program. That could effectively reduce the time and effort usually expended teaching and perfecting basic psychomotor skills.

Available materials should provide multiple teaching options, such as small-group discussion, role playing, independent study, out-of-class (e.g., Web-based) assignment, or laboratory practice for teachers to pursue (Eisner, 1990). See Chapter 10. Such options might include:

- Classroom activity (lecture, role playing, large-group activity), which provides the basic structure to guide learning, and is most economical in use of space and faculty time, but tends not to focus on individual learning styles, and supports greater student passivity.
- Small-group activity, which allows for greater interactions between faculty and students as well as between students, facilitates discussion of attitudes, and allows for a greater degree of activity on the part of the student, but is not as economical in use of time and space, and often does not play to faculty strengths.
- Independent activities (e.g., term papers, readings), which provide for reinforcement and greater clarity of previous learning on an individual basis, but often lack adequate faculty guidance to achieve optimum learning, and because this option is less directive in terms of learning, can cause duplications or vacuums in the content elements, and take up faculty time.
- Laboratory experiences (school, clinical), which reinforce knowledge and attitudes while allowing students to practice psychomotor skills, provide a "real" worldview of nursing, allow for the use of role models as a learning strategy, and are most supportive of the concept that faculty members are catalysts in the learning activity. They are difficult to control in terms of the vari-

ables that influence learning, require the greatest amount of time and energy on the part of faculty and students, and are the most costly.

"Active student participation in learning activities, accompanied by faculty feedback comprises one of the most powerful experiences in the learning process" (Norton, 1998, p. 153). Faculty members should be active participants and guides in learning, not mere lecturers (Dillard & Laidig, 1998). In active learning, there is less sustained lecture time, students are involved through stimulation to talk more, participate, and invest energy. Teaching methods, such as games, simulations, plays, newspapers, case studies, and reflective writing, foster active learning. Students need to be enabled to show more initiative by asking for student contributions, using more student ideas, giving students alternative courses from which to choose, providing more praise, accepting student feelings, being attentive to student comments, being accepting of different points of view, giving explanations of why praise or criticism is given, and providing structured (present a report, small group) and unstructured activities (Web-based or literature-based review).

In contrast, **passive learning** still has its role. These activities can present a great deal of information in a short time. Lecture notes, handouts, and audiovisual media can be prepared ahead of time and faculty members feel comfortable because they are in control. Students are socialized to these methods and little student cognitive effort is required.

Constraints in choosing and implementing learning activities include:

- Lack of faculty experience and knowledge
- Lack of understanding of students' knowledge and skills
- High faculty/student ratio
- Personal attributes (e.g., personality)
- Student stress and anxiety (resistance to active participation)
- Inability to use equipment/technology
- Inadequate time for activity and debriefing
- Inadequate funds for technology and equipment

Teaching methodologies are often based on the faculty member's perception of student abilities instead of on the objectives of the course. In addition, clinical hours may be set according to a predetermined schedule instead of the time needed to meet the course objectives. The emphasis should be on the ability of students to meet objectives, not on how the objective is to be met. Multiple learning activities with options should be offered, within the limits of available time and energy resources. Also, although it is rarely considered, both faculty and students need support systems to deal with the stress and anxiety of the educational program. The school administration and faculty colleagues are potentially most helpful here, but faculty should also use family and friend networks to diffuse some of the stress, and put it into perspective.

Once the curriculum has been developed, the last stage is to develop the plan by which the curriculum will be systematically evaluated.

Curriculum Evaluation

Curriculum evaluation is summative, or outcome-based, and judged by the characteristics of the graduate. Congruence with instructional goals, criteria, and standards, and use for planning is necessary. Evaluation of curriculum elements is necessary as the curriculum is being implemented; evaluation of the total curriculum is relevant after graduation of the first student cohort. The criteria for assessment of the curriculum process ensure consistency among the component parts, including:

- The flow of the content elements can be seen within all of the components, especially between the philosophy and learning experiences.

- The terms used may have a variety of meanings within the discipline but they must be consistent in their meaning within the specific program.
- The ideas expressed among and within each component are supportive rather than contradictory.

The evaluation process should consider the:

- *Context*, including mission and goals setting, internal and external forces, and beliefs of faculty.
- *Input*, including resources, students, program plan, curriculum organization, and support courses.
- *Process*, including courses, teaching/learning activities, and student learning.
- *Outcomes,* including general education outcomes, NCLEX-RN results, and communication and critical thinking abilities.

The evaluation process might include both (1) criterion-referenced evaluation that considers student achievement of content within objectives, and (2) norm-referenced evaluation that compares students to others at a similar level (e.g., NCLEX-RN results). Surveys can be mailed to representative groups of graduates, faculty, nursing and university administrators, and external constituents (e.g., nursing service staff and administration). Evaluation includes values and valuing about what is worth evaluating; is goal oriented; incorporates norms; is comprehensive and has continuity. Evaluation should be ongoing, frequent, recurrent, and continuous; have diagnostic worth, validity, and reliability; and the findings need to be integrated into ongoing curriculum revision and development.

Summary

Curriculum development is a linear process, a sequence of events that consists of a series of systematic, logical, dynamic, spiraled, and progressive stages (Torres & Stanton, 1982): program outcomes, a philosophy with an integrated framework, vertical and horizontal content strands for each course (curriculum matrix), level and course objectives, course content with teaching and learning strategies, and formative and summative outcome-based curriculum evaluation techniques. It addresses current situations that affect student make-up and selection, health-care changes, and is driven by professional organization requirements. Over the years, curriculum design has changed from a process-oriented approach to an outcome-oriented approach, which means that nursing faculty has to be "fine tuned" to the outcomes of not only their program but the community health-care need requirements as well. Development of the outcome-driven curriculum begins with desired endpoints or outcomes with content and teaching strategies changing to meet these endpoints. Faculty communication is essential throughout this process.

R e f e r e n c e s

Bensusan, G. (1997). The escalator. Retrieved November 3, 2005 from **http://ftp.newave.net.au/- michaelc/nw2001/esc,htm**

Bevis, E. O. (1989/1982). *Curriculum building in nursing: A process* (3rd ed). New York: National League for Nursing.

Bloom, B. S. (1956). *Taxonomy of educational objectives: The classification of educational goals. Handbook I: Cognitive domain.* New York: Longmans, Green.

Bowen, M., Lyons, K. J., & Young, B. E. (2000). Nursing and health care reform: Implications for curriculum development. *Journal of Nursing Education, 39*, 27–33.

Csokasy, J. (2002). A congruent curriculum: Philosophical integrity from philosophy to outcomes. *Journal of Nursing Education, 41*, 32–33.

Daggett, L. M., Butts, J. B., & Smith, K. K. (2002). The development of an organizing framework to implement AACN guidelines for nursing education. *Journal of Nursing Education, 41,* 34–36.

Dillard, N., & Laidig, J. (1998). Curriculum development: An overview. In D. M. Billings & J. A. Halstead (Eds.), *Teaching in nursing: A guide for faculty* (pp. 69–83). Philadelphia: Saunders.

Eisner, E. W. (1990). Creative curriculum development and practice. *Journal of Curriculum and Supervision, 6,* 62–73.

Finke, L. M., & Boland, D. L. (1998). Curriculum designs. In D. M. Billings & J. A. Halstead (Eds.), *Teaching in nursing: A guide for faculty* (pp. 117–133). Philadelphia: Saunders.

Freeman, L. H., Voignier, R. R., & Scott, D. L. (2002). New curriculum for a new century: Beyond repackaging. *Journal of Nursing Education, 41,* 38–40.

Goldenberg, D., Andrusyszyn, M. A., & Iwasiw, C. (2004). A facilitative approach to learning about curriculum development. *Journal of Nursing Education, 43,* 31–35.

Hull, E., St. Romain, J. A., Alexander, P., Schaff, S., & Jones, W. (2001). Moving cemeteries: A framework for facilitating curriculum revision. *Nurse Educator, 26,* 280–282.

Kelting-Gibson, L. M. (2005). Comparison of curriculum development practices. *Educational Research Quarterly, 29,* 26–36.

Norton, B. (1998). Selecting learning experiences to achieve curriculum outcomes. In D. M. Billings & J. A. Halstead (Eds.), *Teaching in nursing: A guide for faculty* (pp. 151–169). Philadelphia: Saunders.

Richardson, V. (1998). The diverse learning needs of students. In D. M. Billings & J. A. Halstead (Eds.), *Teaching in nursing: A guide for faculty* (pp. 17–33). Philadelphia: Saunders.

Ruth-Sahd, L. A. (2003). Intuition: A critical way of knowing in a multicultural curriculum. *Nursing Education Perspectives, 24,* 129–134.

Speziale, H. J. S., & Jacobson L. (2005). Trends in registered nurse education programs, 1998–2008. *Nursing Education Perspectives, 26,* 230–235.

Taba, H. (1962). *Curriculum development theory and practice.* New York: Harcourt, Brace & World.

Torres, G., & Stanton, M. (1982). *Curriculum process in nursing: A guide to curriculum development.* Englewood Cliffs NJ: Prentice-Hall.

Tyler, R. W. (1950). *Basic principles of curriculum and instruction.* Chicago: University of Chicago Press.

Van Tassel-Baska, J. (2004). *Curriculum for gifted and talented students.* Thousand Oaks CA: Corwin/Sage.

Webber, P. B. (2002). A curriculum framework for nursing. *Journal of Nursing Education, 41,* 15–23.

Wiggins, G., & McTighe, J. (1998). *Understanding by design.* Alexandria, VA: Association for Supervision & Curriculum Development.

REVIEW QUESTIONS

- What are the stages of the curriculum development process?
- What are faculty communication strategies that facilitate the curriculum development process?
- What are four "Cs" that the curriculum process requires?
- Why is it necessary to focus on education outcomes when redesigning the curriculum?
- What are some environmental forces or issues that play a major role in the curriculum development process?
- Why is it important to understand the characteristics of prospective students when redesigning the curriculum?
- How does the philosophy of the program influence curriculum design?
- Why is it important to use a curriculum framework when developing the curriculum?
- What is the importance of visualizing the curriculum matrix when reviewing curriculum content?
- How do level and course objectives factor into the curriculum development process?
- How are learning experiences identified for implementation of the curriculum?
- What are some principles to identify when developing teaching/learning strategies that are used for the delivery of the curriculum?
- What are strategic ways to evaluate the curriculum?

CRITICAL THINKING EXERCISES

You are asked to develop an accelerated nursing program. The students desired for this program already have a baccalaureate degree in biology, chemistry, or psychology. Select an existing traditional generic nursing program and identify those stages of curriculum development that will need curriculum redesign.

You are part of a team that will be evaluating a nursing program for accreditation. Select a nursing program and identify components of the evaluation process using context, input, process, and outcome criteria.

Review the syllabus and course objectives for a nursing course. Determine ways to enhance the skills, values, and meanings of the course objectives and content.

Think about the environmental forces or issues that currently exist that affect the education of future nursing students. Identify ways that these forces may be minimized in a nursing curriculum.

ANNOTATED RESEARCH SUMMARY

Slatter, J., & Carolson, J. (2005). Preparing an effective syllabus: Current best practices. *College Teaching, 53*(4), 159–165.

Syllabi can be useful in engaging students and creating an effective classroom atmosphere, yet discussions of their effective use rarely appear. In light of current research and theory on syllabi, we review their typical uses (structural, motivational, and evidentiary), commonly included components, and attributes that positively affect the teaching and learning process.

Statts, C. R. (2003). The development of a community-based baccalaureate curriculum model in a culturally diverse health care delivery area. *Nursing Education Perspectives, 24*(2), 94–97.

The nursing school at the University of Texas at San Antonio revised the curriculum using a community-based health-care model. More clinical experiences were offered in a variety of community settings and long-term relationships were developed with community health agencies.

Smith, A. J. (2006). Continued psychometric evaluation of an intuition instrument for nursing students. *Journal of Holistic Nursing, 24*(2), 82–89.

The purpose of this study was to evaluate the psychometric properties of a revised intuition instrument developed for nursing students. The method, principal component factor analysis, was used to establish construct validity and the Cronbach's alpha was used to examine reliability. The findings of the statistical analysis resulted in a 26-item intuition instrument with 6 factors accounting for 62% variance. The factors were labeled as Feelings That Reassure (27.7%), Spiritual Connections (10.9%), Feelings That Alert (8.4%), Feelings That Forewarn (5.8%), Physical Sensations That Alert (4.7%), and Reading Physical Cues (4.2%). Eigenvalues ranged from 1.100 to 7.225, and factor loadings ranged from 0.572 to 0.848. The overall Cronbach's alpha was 0.89 with a range of 0.73 to 0.85 for each factor. The conclusions revealed that the 26-item intuition instrument showed evidence of construct validity and reliability. The implications for the future suggest that the intuition instrument can serve as a stimulus to foster students' intuitive abilities.

Siu, H. M., Laschinger, H. K. S., & Vingilis, E. (2005). The effect of problem-based learning on nursing students' perceptions of empowerment. *Journal of Nursing Education, 44*(10), 459–469.

This study tested Kanter's structural empowerment theory within a university nursing student population. Differences in perceptions of empowerment among nursing students enrolled in either a problem-based learning (PBL) or a conventional lecture learning (CLL) program were examined, as well as the relationship between perceptions of structural empowerment in the learning environment and feelings of psychological empowerment. Participants completed measures of structural and psychological empowerment adapted to educational settings, as well as measures related to exposure to various learning strategies in their programs and clinical problem-solving abilities. Students in the PBL program (n = 41) had significantly higher perceptions of structural and psychological empowerment than students in the CLL program (n = 67). Regardless of academic program, structural empowerment was strongly positively related to psychological empowerment. The results of this are the first to support the applicability of Kanter's theory to nursing education settings.

Jones, E. A. (2002). Curriculum reform in the professions: Preparing students for a changing world. *ERIC Digest.*

This digest focuses on the major changes that college and university faculty have designed in their undergraduate professional education programs in three areas: accounting, nursing, and teacher education. Reforms in each of these programs are reviewed. The changes seen in these three professional education programs offer lessons for faculty in many different disciplines. Several thematic elements can be identified from this review of curriculum reform. Many reforms require students to be engaged actively in their studies, and students often work on real-world issues or problems. Problems are usually open-ended with no single correct answer, and all three field assessments of student learning are being used to gauge whether students are mastering the intended learning outcomes.

Chapter Outline

TAILORING TEACHING TO THE LEARNER

6

Vera Brancato

Learning Outcomes

On completion of this chapter, the reader will be able to:

• Describe factors that may affect readiness to learn.
• Identify the developmental characteristics of learners.
• Differentiate between the characteristics of millennial students and adult students.
• Describe factors that influence motivation and ways to enhance student motivation.
• Discuss the importance of emotional intelligence to nursing education.
• Describe strategies to help multicultural students learn.
• Differentiate among literacy, readability, and comprehension.
• Identify factors that can enhance or inhibit reading comprehension.
• Identify several strategies to help the learner learn.
• Explain resources that faculty can use to obtain feedback about learning.
• Discuss various learning style instruments.

Key Terms

Andragogy
Assessment
Classroom assessment techniques
Comprehension
Cultural competence
Emotional intelligence
Learning needs

Learning style
Learning style inventory
Literacy
Millennial students
Motivation
Readability
Readiness to learn

Traditionally, colleges and universities were viewed as institutions for the cultivation of new ideas and skills, occupational and professional training, and discovery about self and others. Teaching was conceptualized as the transmission of knowledge and facts about which learners previously knew little, for later application in the real world. Current research indicates a new perspective that embraces both faculty and student learning. A shift from a teacher-centered to a learner-centered paradigm focuses on creating a learning environment that enables students to realize their potential to learn through the discovery of knowledge for themselves. Research indicates that deeper learning occurs when students are engaged in, and aware of, their own learning experiences and have opportunities to reflect on and evaluate those experiences (Light, 2001). But even the best college teachers struggle with how to engage and make students aware that learning is occurring (Bain, 2004).

Parker Palmer (1998) suggests "that students who learn, not professors who perform, is what teaching is all about . . . . that students learn in diverse and wondrous ways, including ways that bypass the teacher in the classroom and ways that require neither a classroom nor a teacher!" (p. 6). Faculty must begin to act as facilitators of learning, guiding students on an inner journey to realize their own potential to learn. As a first step, faculty should strive to understand who their students are, their level of preparation, and their expectations. This chapter examines the characteristics of learners and how faculty can use this knowledge to assist students to learn. Faculty who develop a clear understanding of their students can facilitate the connections among their subjects, their students, and themselves.

Assessing the Learner

In a very broad sense, **assessment** of the learner begins with the faculty member attempting to get to know who the learner is while providing a safe, secure, and respectful environment. Assessment implies data gathering with interpretation so that learners' needs and characteristics can be identified and utilized to plan effective educational activities (Dean, 1994). Faculty members who develop an understanding of their students can use this information to maximize the learning opportunities for students. There is no guarantee that learners will learn by merely providing them with information. Finding out information about students (such as the learner's knowledge level, previous coursework, ability to read and comprehend the material, confusion about the reading assignment, etc.) provides the basis for building teaching strategies to meet their learning needs.

Learning needs can be described as internal forces that motivate the learner to pursue a goal that bridges the gap between one's present level of competence and the desired level of performance. When planning an assessment of learning needs, the faculty member must be able to identify the learner's current level of knowledge, attitudes, and skills as well as use her own professional judgment to decide upon the desired level of competency that is expected. Actively seeking input as to what learners' needs are encourages learners to feel that they have a personal investment in helping to guide decision-making about instruction (Bastable, 2003). Connecting new learning to students' previous learning also helps them to examine, challenge, and improve upon their understanding before they can begin internalizing or learning it. Various assessment strategies (Bastable, 2003; Haggard, 1989) can be used to identify the learner's needs, such as:

• Informal conversations or open-ended questions that encourage the students to reveal pertinent information about their learning needs

- Structured interviews that ask the learner specific questions about learning needs before instruction
- Focus groups that use group input about a certain topic to provide feedback about needs
- Self-administered questionnaires that permit the learner to write responses to questions about learning needs
- Pre-tests administered (can be online) before presenting the content, which can provide information about the learner's level of knowledge and **comprehension** of assigned readings

Readiness to Learn

Readiness to learn represents the degree to which the learner demonstrates an interest in and receptivity to learning (Bastable, 2003). Readiness to learn may be based on what learners want or need to know, their goals, and their expectations. Assessing the learner's readiness to learn should be accomplished before the actual teaching session because it represents a prime time for gathering information about the learner. Readiness to learn can be addressed using many of the same methods discussed under assessing learning needs, such as informal conversations, structured interviews, focus groups, self-administered questions, pre-tests, and observations. Readiness to learn can be influenced by a range of physical, emotional, and experiential factors and knowledge constraints that may or may not act as obstacles to learning. If faculty members assess readiness before instruction, these obstacles may be identified and potentially avoided or minimized.

Barriers to Student Readiness

One factor that affects readiness is the complexity of the task. Learning typically occurs from simple to more complex levels of difficulty. Therefore, faculty should be cognizant of presenting the material in an increasingly complex and logical sequence. Likewise, the physical and emotional environments also play an important part in contributing to the learner's readiness to learn. A secure, trusting, and stimulating environment tends to keep the learner interested and engaged in learning. Environmental effects (for example, excessive noise and uncomfortable room temperatures) can negatively affect concentration and the students' readiness to learn.

Learners also must be emotionally ready to learn. Anxiety can influence the learner either positively or negatively. Some degree of anxiety actually may motivate students to learn, but high anxiety or fear of reprisal may affect learning negatively. Being clear about expectations for assignments and course objectives can help to alleviate some of the anxiety that grades and unfamiliar requirements often have on learning. Peer support systems can also influence emotional readiness. Peer groups can provide emotional support or act as a study group to assist the student to learn, thereby helping to alleviate anxiety. Student motivation and a desire to perform successfully affect emotional readiness to learn and perform task mastery.

Experiential readiness (for example, whether previous learning has been positive or negative) may affect whether the student is motivated or willing to try to acquire new knowledge and skills. Learning disabilities and low-level reading skills may require special approaches to bolster readiness to learn. Students who are at risk for poor performance may become discouraged unless faculty recognize their special needs and help them to access resources to overcome their problems. Matching instructional tools and resources to the learner's special individual needs (such as various learning styles) helps to pique interest in learning and facilitate understanding and comprehension.

Cultural influences also may affect whether a student is ready to learn. Students who perceive that the material conflicts with their belief system may not be motivated to learn the material.

Language can also be a barrier if the learner is not fluent in the language used by the educator. Particularly problematic is the idiomatic dialogue that faculty or other students may use, making it difficult for some students to understand or comprehend. Striving to be clear, offering opportunities to clarify concepts and gain feedback about learning, and encouraging collaborative learning can all assist in minimizing barriers that affect comprehension.

Developmental Assessment

The American higher-education system enrolls a wide variety of students in many settings. Learners today are quite different from a few decades ago. Although the majority of students are the traditional 18- to 24-year-olds, larger numbers of older students add to the diversity of the student body. In order to facilitate learning, faculty is becoming interested in understanding where students "are coming from," literally and figuratively. What do faculty members need to know about these students so that they can develop an informed perspective and provide a more effective learning environment?

Millennium Characteristics

The **millennial student** (born after 1980) constitutes the largest cohort in our nation's history and the most diverse college-going generation (Coomes & DeBard, 2004). Several characteristics represent this generation of students. They are structured rule followers, protected and sheltered, confident and optimistic about their future, conventionally motivated and respected, cooperative and team-oriented, pressured by and accepting of authority, and talented achievers (Howe & Strauss, 2000). The millennial learner has been characterized as having a consumer mentality (he/she expects that if tuition is paid, a degree will be granted), has ubiquitous computer access, and is intolerant of nonengaging pedagogical techniques (McGuire & Williams, 2002). Thus, millennial students often do not seek knowledge that results from learning as the goal, but rather knowledge that is generated by the temporary rewards gained by demonstrating mastery of the knowledge (e.g., only interested in good grades on an exam rather than seeking knowledge retention). Faculty is challenged to emphasize the importance of learning as a process of self-discovery and growth in order to promote effective life-long learning (Wilson, 2004).

Faculty members need to be cognizant of millennial generational characteristics because the learners' expectations are often inconsistent with the institution's requirements. For example, even though millennial students have come to expect high grades, they characteristically only do what is expected of them (DeBard, 2004). In addition, although the percentage of students who spent six or more hours studying per week declined, students remained optimistic about success (DeBard, 2004). Such optimism without sufficient effort can become a source of conflict and failure. Students also lack study skills because they frequently learned the material in high school just for the examination rather than for comprehension, retention, and later application. In addition, as a result of the increasing number of students assuming jobs to help finance their education, less time is available to study. Overall, millennial students may have unrealistic expectations for what it takes to succeed academically and professionally.

The characteristics of the millennial learner not only provide challenges, but also provide opportunities for faculty to promote effective learning. Faculty should consider the following information and teaching tips (DeBard, 2004; Filene, 2005):

• Today's students grew up in child-centered families. Often, parents remain involved when these students leave to attend college. Carefully explain to students that they must give their consent so that faculty can discuss information about the student's classroom performance with parents.

- Students learn more readily when given structured assignments. They trust authority and count on authority. Because they lead very structured lives, they are often directionless without structure. To provide structure effectively, specifics about course responsibilities, assignments, and testing measures must be included in the syllabus, policy handbook, or as part of orientation to the course or program.
- Students respect cultural differences, accept high-stakes proficiency testing as a rite of passage, and are pressured from living in competitive environments. Students expect to be held accountable, and they have respect for objective evaluation. Providing feedback in a timely manner helps to allay anxiety for those who are pressured to succeed.
- Students are conventionally minded conformists who want to get along and are team-oriented. They are motivated by noble causes and readily volunteer to join groups of peers. Group activities that facilitate cooperative learning or service-learning activities work well to keep students motivated, interested, and engaged in learning.
- Students are focused on grades and expect high grades for compliance with academic standards. Alignment of assignments should be matched with a reward structure that is clearly explained, documented, and enforced.

Developmental Characteristics of the Millennial Student

In general, the developmental tasks of the young adult shift from the identity-seeking behaviors of the adolescent to finding one's place in broader society. Arthur Chickering (1969) describes seven "vectors" of development for the traditional-age college student: achieving competence, managing emotions, becoming autonomous, establishing identity, freeing interpersonal relations, clarifying purposes, and developing integrity. His framework of developmental tasks is flexible, indicating that individual students may move through the tasks at varying times. Faculty's awareness of these tasks can assist students who are struggling with them to become more autonomous, to develop an internal locus of control, and to determine how they will relate to self, others, and society. For example, students who are striving to become autonomous (not just learning how to live away from home and parents, but trying to make sound judgments) may benefit from role-play scenarios that require acting out problems and practicing how to devise potential resolutions.

As faculty, we need to be aware of developmental stages and acknowledge how these developmental needs affect instructional efforts. Therefore, faculty needs to assess tasks with which students are struggling at the time and how they can be helped to challenge their previous patterns of behavior and begin to formulate new ones that involve learning and higher level problem solving. In addition, developmental tasks affect how students perceive the learning situation and what they expect from it. Having an investment in understanding developmental tasks may give faculty added insight into more effective ways to connect with students to keep them engaged in the learning process (Davis, 1993). For example, students who work in groups on a project will need specific guidelines and expectations of participation so that all group members participate equally and the group knows what to do if a member is not participating. This aids in developing a sense of ethical identity in relation to completing a project, receiving equitable credit, and building team-work skills.

Understanding developmental stages could spur teaching that is targeted to challenge students to move into the next stage of development. For example, faculty should design critical-thinking assignments that challenge the student to move from seeing just one quick solution to a problem to being able to consider several alternative viewpoints and base a critical judgment on the evaluation of supporting data from several sources. Therefore, learning activities should inspire students to reflect and consider where they are and where they want to be.

Faculty members also need to provide a safe and supportive environment where students feel free to explore disequilibrium and challenges brought about by problem-solving activities without fear of sanctions.

Adult Learner Characteristics

Not all students are from the traditional 18-to-24-year-old group; some may be older and have other characteristics and developmental tasks to complete. In Fall 2003, college enrollment of students above the age of 25 was 36.8% (The Chronicle Almanac, 2005–6). Many are nontraditional students who are adults returning to school for one reason or another. Many return to college to obtain a degree or certificate in order to change careers or advance in their current profession (Hagedorn, 2005). This population provides many different challenges as well as opportunities for faculty. For instance, adult learners provide a rich source of experiences upon which to draw and share with other students; they seek to apply information that is learned; they often have time constraints; they often experience more anxiety about learning; and they have more diverse **learning styles.**

Knowles (1984) coined the term **andragogy,** the study of adult learners. He characterized adult learners as being self-directed, possessing years of experience and a wealth of information, being internally or intrinsically motivated, approaching learning with a desire to apply information to solve problems, and relating new knowledge to previously learned information and experiences (Baumlein, 2004). Several educational strategies can be used to maximize learning for students with these characteristics. For example, faculty can provide opportunities for group discussion that tap into the life experiences of the adult learner who can, in turn, become a rich resource for other younger students.

Faculty should provide material that is relevant and meaningful so that learners can connect new information to previously learned information and experiences with direct practical application (Caffarella, 1994). If direct application in clinical settings is not possible, then critical thinking exercises that provide opportunities to apply the material are essential. Adults generally want to apply information to current problems. For example, using case studies provides a good way to apply theory about a particular client scenario that the student is likely to encounter in the clinical setting. Likewise, having students conduct a health interview for an elderly person aids in transferring the concepts learned in class and provides the application that adults value rather than just reading about how to conduct the interview process.

Specific needs of adult learners also can be challenging to faculty. For instance, adult learners often have time constraints placed on them by family and work commitments. Strategies to assist with this might include helping to connect students with campus resources that might help with daycare needs, connecting them with other adult students who might be willing to share resources and provide peer group support, arranging for institutional services to be open in the evenings, using e-mail and other technology sources to provide alternative access to faculty to answer questions or provide course materials online.

Moreover, adult learners often experience more anxiety about learning because they perceive the educational environment to cater more to the younger student who often has fewer roles and responsibilities. Adults often have a greater fear of failing new educational endeavors especially if their previous educational experiences were not positive (Baumlein, 2004). Being cognizant of this fear, faculty can provide additional reassurance and support and can provide guidance to the student to seek campus resources and other support networks if needed. In addition, as adults they are often more complex and diverse in their learning styles and, therefore, necessitate that faculty use a variety of educational approaches to facilitate learning. Encouraging adult students to complete a **learning style inventory** and helping them to develop a variety of study skills will aid in alleviating some of their anxiety about how to study more effectively and about succeeding as they return to school.

A Developmental Perspective on Learning

Faculty should also consider the developmental views that students hold about learning. At the most elementary level is the learner who views faculty members as experts who impart knowledge that is to be memorized for future use. Faculty is seen as the keeper of the correct answers and depositors of knowledge into the learners' brains. Eventually, learners move into the next stage, recognizing that knowledge is often a matter of opinion and that experts can disagree. Some learners move to the next stage where they recognize that certain criteria are used as the basis for making sound judgments. Only at the highest level of learning is there consistent use of independent, critical, and creative thinking both in the classroom and in daily living. At this point, learners become aware of and have the ability to evaluate their own thinking. According to this developmental scheme, learners move forward and backward between levels rather than just upward to the highest level. Thus, faculty need to help learners alter their ability to view knowledge and learning as concrete and stagnant, and should adopt a variety of teaching strategies to assist in moving learners through this developmental scheme (Bain, 2004). Several teaching tips include:

- Challenging students with questions, such as "How do you know that?" "What questions are still left unanswered?"
- Case studies with complex problems
- Problem-based learning activities
- Critical thinking scenarios that encourage students to weigh evidence and make judgments

Motivation

Learning begins only when the learner is motivated to learn the material (Leamnson, 1999). Wlodkowski proposed that motivation refers to "those processes that can (a) arouse and instigate behavior, (b) give direction and purpose to behavior, (c) continue to allow behavior to persist, and (d) lead to choosing or professing a particular behavior" (1978, p. 12). **Motivation** is concerned with the will or desire of the student to put forth the effort to learn (Davis, 1993). To become motivated to learn, the learner must experience it as a need or feel a desire to know. Thus, learning can be effective if it satisfies a curiosity or natural interest. Faculty members need to capitalize on broad categories of motivators, such as individual improvement, needed employment competencies, or acquisition of a degree or certification requirements to influence or stimulate the student's motivation to learn (Greive, 2002).

Emotional Intelligence

Emotional intelligence is often recognized as a central characteristic of effective clinical nursing practice (McCormack, 1993; McQueen, 2004). Emotional intelligence (EI) has been defined by Freshman and Rubino (2002) as "proficiency in intrapersonal and interpersonal skills in the areas of self-awareness, self-regulation, self-motivation, social awareness, and social skills" (p. 1). Given that nurses encounter stressful events, such as caring for a dying patient, nurse educators should be mindful of teaching students to enhance their performance abilities related to EI. EI can be learned and developed and improved with age (Vitello-Cicciu, 2003). Debriefing and discussing emotionally charged clinical situations can help students to learn about the emotional sides of issues and to remain calm and think more clearly under pressure (Miller, 2005). First assessing and then enhancing EI can shield student psyches from emotional work that can be stressful and exhausting (McQueen, 2004). Unrelenting work of this nature otherwise can lead to burnout.

One part of EI consists of interpersonal intelligence, which encompasses such abilities as being able to organize groups, negotiate solutions, make personal connections, and engage in social analysis. The other aspect of EI is intrapersonal intelligence, which includes empathizing, trying to understand another's perspective, and engaging in counseling skills (McQueen, 2004). The ability to monitor one's emotions and the intelligent use of emotions to guide behavior and thinking enhances the effectiveness and outcomes in a given situation, which can ultimately lead to professional and personal success.

Evans and Allen (2002) suggest that nurses' abilities to establish a rapport with patients, manage their own emotions, and empathize with patients are essential to providing quality psychosocial care. EI, however, is often not emphasized in nursing curricula. Cadman and Brewer (2001) suggest that faculty should assess the EI of students before program admission and provide interpersonal skills training to build a sound emotional foundation to help students deal more effectively with the emotional labor involved in becoming a nurse and to function effectively as part of the interdisciplinary health-care team. The aim of incorporating EI training would not only be to improve the students' self awareness, self-regulation, self-motivation, social awareness, and social skills but also to augment their skills in the area of providing empathetic care to meet the psychosocial needs of patients. Learning to know oneself through self-reflection can lead to learning how to deal more effectively in challenging situations (Miller, 2005). Strategies should be used to enhance self-reflection and self-evaluation to enable students to explore their feelings and the emotional work involved in providing quality nursing care.

Developing EI does not occur simply by reading about it. First, self-awareness of ineffective behaviors must be identified and new behaviors must be rehearsed until mastered and used routinely. Faculty can act as mentors and role models giving accurate feedback about a student's behavior and performance during a stressful client situation. Some teaching tips include:

- In classroom and post-conference discussions, identify cause and effect behaviors that elicit ideas about alternative patterns of behavior to use when encountering difficult clients. This can lead to identification of one's emotional reaction and how it can affect another person, as well as identify other possible effective responses.
- Have students write a reflective journal to identify their own strengths and limitations regarding their empathy, respect for diversity, self-control, trustworthiness, adaptability to change, etc. Have students write their feelings and concerns about clinical assignments before and after taking care of their patient assignment so they can begin to evaluate their EI.
- Encourage students to pursue goals beyond what is expected of them. Mobilize them to seize opportunities and participate as leaders and initiators of projects within student groups or classroom activities.
- Role model empathy with patients and students to foster students' abilities to learn how to be attentive to emotional cues and listen empathetically.
- Offer frequent feedback, mentoring, and coaching to challenge students to objectively evaluate self and others.
- Employ cooperative learning strategies to emphasize the importance of team identity and modeling of behaviors associated with helpfulness and cooperation among students.

Multicultural Assessment of Students and Environments

College classrooms and clinical settings have become increasingly diverse and more reflective of globalization and immigration. Faculty needs to consider issues related to this increasing cultural diversity from two perspectives: being able to teach future nurses to care for the increasing numbers of clients from diverse cultural backgrounds and being able to meet the many challenges of preparing multicultural students to meet the health-care needs of a diverse society. It is imperative that faculty members begin to increase their own cultural awareness and **cultural competence** to help multicultural students to learn and all students to appreciate diversity. Cultural competence can be viewed as "a continuous process of cultural awareness, knowledge, skill, interaction, and sensitivity among caregivers and the services they provide" (Smith, 1998, p. 9).

The culture of nursing education and most of higher education continues to reflect a largely Eurocentric dominance, which adheres to the tradition of linear learning, deductive logic, hierarchical structure, and individualistic, competitive, time-oriented, and authoritarian dominance (Brennan, 1997). The cultural bias that may be caused by faculty teaching in this way may have deleterious effects on student learning. Frequently, faculty does not give enough consideration to the differences in ethnic cognitive and noncognitive variables that constitute the students' cultural differences. Therefore, given the increasing number of minorities being recruited into nursing, as well as represented in the population in general, faculty is challenged to relate to multicultural students who have varying learning styles and needs as well as various performance abilities. Factors that affect student learning relate to ethnic background, birthplace, immigration status, age, gender, lifestyle, educational and career background, and language proficiency (Williams & Calvillo, 2002). The obstacles faced by minority students include lack of ethnically diverse faculty who can serve as positive role models and mentors, lack of adequate financial assistance, and the need for increased educational support services (Billings & Halstead, 2005).

Non-native–English-speaking students offer challenges in the classroom. They may not participate in class discussions because they feel uncomfortable with the language, and may "lack linguistic proficiency, cultural conventions, or educational background" (Kim, 2005, p. 5). Several strategies can help such students to improve their listening and speaking skills. Faculty should speak clearly and at a reasonable pace, avoid the use of slang, encourage the use of audio taping, encourage peer discussion and sharing of notes, use visual aids for further enhancement of concepts, and use the Web or e-mail to post study guides and key points for further information and clarification (Kim, 2005). In addition, faculty should try to become familiar with students' backgrounds and invite guest lecturers from other cultures to attend class so that students can experience firsthand an appreciation of cultural competency in class discussions. Have students share their cultural beliefs, artifacts, and practices with their peers. Diverse backgrounds can provide enriching experiences and reduce cultural barriers. Be careful not to stereotype students or to overgeneralize (Billings & Halstead, 2005). Faculty must be careful not to overcompensate or appear to provide special attention and services to any specific group or individual, and must strive to treat everyone fairly and equally.

In order to achieve a proportionate representation of minorities in nursing, faculty should strive to make every effort to recruit students, retain them, and graduate them from nursing programs. Faculty plays a pivotal role in creating positive learning environments for all students. Strategies to enhance cultural competence follow:

• Get to know students early; find out any needs they may have. Be honest about lacking specific knowledge about all cultures. Encourage students to share their beliefs, values, and meaning of health-care concepts to facilitate learning about their culture.
• Incorporate known cultural information when discussing particular cultures. Ask students to relate to past knowledge of their own culture's beliefs and perspectives.
• Convey respect for all cultures. Avoid stereotyping and overgeneralizations.
• Discuss willingness to accept folk practices that are not harmful to adapt interventions to the needs of the client.

- Be a positive role model who views cultural differences as valuable rather than obstacles.
- Provide clinical assignments so that all students can have opportunities to care for culturally diverse patients.
- Use gaming, simulations, and role play to increase the comfort level and understanding about different cultures.
- Form study groups and connect with resources early. Provide specific and clearly written instructions for all assignments and encourage frequent contact with faculty to deal with misconceptions and misinterpretations early.
- Use guest lectures from a variety of cultures who can provide insight into specific health-care views and perspectives.

Literacy Assessment

The ability to read and write are unquestionably basic skills for academic learning and success. **Literacy** is a term that denotes the relative ability to use printed and written material or "the ability to read, understand, and interpret information written at the eighth-grade level or above" (Bastable, 2003, p. 192). Literacy includes both **readability** and comprehension. Readability of printed material refers to the ease with which the learner can read the written or printed material. Comprehension, on the other hand, refers to the degree to which the learners understand what they have read. Comprehension varies with the amount, clarity, and complexity of the material (Fisher, 1999). "The ability to read does not alone guarantee reading comprehension" (Bastable, 2003, p. 193).

Both readability and comprehension are affected by many factors. Faculty needs to be able to evaluate the learner's level of comprehension and the student's ability to read information from a variety of sources at an appropriate level for nursing. Factors limiting literacy skills can vary from limited educational opportunities, English as a second language, and learning disabilities. Developing a consensus as to what level of literacy is necessary for students to succeed in nursing is essential for the establishment of effective admission and promotion practices within the program (Hardy, Segatore, & Edge, 1993).

Strategies to Assist in Learning

Once the educator receives the assessment data about the students, several strategies developed by Knapper (1995) and Filene (2005) can facilitate a deeper appreciation of the material and connect the material that you want the learner to learn on the one hand to the learners' needs and what you intend the learning outcomes to be on the other.

- Decide upon the learning objective that you want to achieve in addition to the outcomes or what you want the learners to know.
  - Is the main goal of learning to emphasize knowledge mastery, skill acquisition, or attitudinal change?
- Identify the expectations you have for your students.
  - Communicate clear objectives that help the student examine what is done in the classroom.
  - Communicate what might contribute to learning outside of the classroom.
- Decide which activities will foster the learning that is desired.
  - How can students best achieve the objectives of the course?
  - Get frequent feedback to determine if learning is occurring.

- Match the aims of your teaching with learning activities to facilitate higher-level skills. For example, active learning strategies rather than passive learning approaches create an interactive process.
- Emphasize the process of learning that is involved in the activities and include instruction on skills necessary to carry out learning activities (for example, how to write essays effectively, perform research to complete assignments, work in groups, and read critically).
- Evaluate the amount of time necessary to fulfill learning activities required.
  - Applies to in-class and out-of-class activities so that students can prioritize and manage their time to study and complete assignments.
- Apply research findings about instructional strategies to teaching so that learning activities are sufficiently challenging to motivate achievement without overwhelming the students. The more you know about what the students bring to the classroom, the more attainable the outcomes.
- Apply learning theory in class by providing incentives, continuous feedback, and modeling one's own effective learning style. Treat and evaluate students fairly.

Understanding, Assessing, and Using Learning Styles

Research on learning styles has taken place over the past 40 years, beginning in the field of psychology and moving slowing into other disciplines, such as nursing (Cassidy, 2004). As educators, faculty members often teach students in much the same way they were taught, trying to provide the students with as much information and detail as possible to foster learning. The lack of student proficiency on examinations frequently suggests, however, that learning has not occurred equally for all students and that students may have different ways of processing and learning material. Learning style represents just one valuable insight into how students learn as individuals. Assessing learning styles can help educators design and develop effective instruction that meets the learners' needs best and facilitates more effective learning for individual students (Katz & Henry, 1993).

Billings and Halstead (2005) define learning style as "the unique way in which a person perceives, interacts with, and responds to a learning situation" (p. 27). Therefore, learning style refers to the preferred way by which an individual characteristically responds to or approaches different tasks or learning situations. Students should be encouraged to identify their preferences and use study and test-taking strategies based upon their preferences. At the same time, faculty should help students diversify their preferences so they are better able to enhance learning in a wide variety of settings. Faculty can help students expand their use of various styles by using a variety of teaching strategies. Adding alternative activities that supplement or replace traditional assignments or learning modalities affords students the chance to use different styles. Moreover, Leamnson (1999) emphasizes that content is often understood better by more students if it is repeated using different teaching strategies each time.

Research conducted on the more than 100 learning style inventories that have been developed has been inconclusive and inconsistent in identifying which single instructional method or learning style inventory works best for all students (Cassidy, 2004; DeYoung, 2003). With that said, Cassidy (2004) describes 23 different instruments that have been developed to assess various theories related to learning styles to provide faculty with the ability to make comparisons and better decisions about which instruments to use and when. A brief description of the most common instruments utilized in nursing education follows.

Specific Learning Style Instruments

Learning style instruments can be administered at any time during the student's matriculation in the program. Faculty can then use the information gleaned from the tool to assist individual students with remediation, tutoring, and counseling sessions. By taking a learning style instrument, students become aware of their own learning preferences, capitalize and incorporate this preference into their study strategies, and can work on developing additional strategies to facilitate their ability to learn in other ways. The following examples of instruments can be used to assess students' learning styles. Additional information can be obtained from The Policy Center on the First Year College Web site: http://www.brevard.edu/fyc/resources/Learningstyles.htm.

The Kolb Learning Style Inventory (1976) uses a 12-item sentence completion format that can be completed in approximately 15 to 20 minutes (Richardson, 2005). It is based on Kolb's (1976) view of learning as consisting of a four-stage cycle in which the learner moves from concrete experience (feeling), to reflective observation (watching), to abstract conceptualization (thinking), to active experimentation (doing). Concrete experiences (CE) versus abstract conceptualization (AC) and active experimentation (AE) versus reflective observation (RO) comprise the two pairs of polar opposites in this model. The combination formed from the learner's preference for one aspect in each of the two pairs constitutes the learning style (see Table 6–1). The four learning styles that exist in this model are:

1. Accommodative style: refers to the preference for CE and AE. Learners are characterized as being good at completing tasks; prefer doing things; seek opportunity and risks; solve problems using trial and error; and rely on others for information.
2. Assimilative style: refers to the preference for AC and RO. Learners prefer reasoning; creating theoretical models; and working with ideas and concepts rather than with people.
3. Divergent style: refers to the preference for CE and RO. Learners prefer organizing ideas into meaningful gestalt; are imaginative and sensitive; are good at generating ideas and implications; and are people-oriented and emotional.
4. Convergent style: refers to the preference for AC and AE. Learners prefer problem solving to interacting with others; prefer single solutions to problems; prefer to work on technical tasks; and prefer practical application of ideas (Davis, 1993; Forrest, 2004; Kolb, 1976; Richardson, 2005).

TABLE 6.1 Various Assessment Strategies

Informal conversations or open-ended questions that encourage the students to reveal pertinent information about their learning needs

Structured interviews that ask the learner specific questions about learning needs prior to instructions

Focus groups that use group input about a certain topic to provide feedback about needs

Self-administered questionnaires that permit the learner to write responses to questions about learning needs

Pre-tests administered (can be online) prior to presenting the content, which can provide information about the learner's level of knowledge and comprehension of assigned readings

Adapted from Haggard, 1989; Bastable, 2003.

The Dunn, Dunn, and Price Productivity Environmental Preference Survey (PEPS) (Dunn, Dunn, & Price, 1996) is a self-administered survey of 100 Likert-type statements that measure the following four categories:

1. Environmental: This category measures such factors as preference for environmental noise level, temperature, level of light, and formal verses informal setting.

2. Sociological: This category measures preference for studying alone or in a group, availability of a collegial or authoritative teacher, or a variety of either preference.

3. Physical: This category consists of a visual subscale (preference for reading to learn); an auditory subscale (preference for listening to learn); or a kinesthetic (tactile preference for practicing demonstrations or procedures). In addition, other preferences, such as time of day to study, frequency of breaks versus no breaks, or eating and drinking, and mobility are assessed.

4. Emotional: This category measures aspects such as responsibility, persistence, motivation, and need for structure/detail to complete assignments.

The PEPS instrument elicits self-diagnostic responses and takes 25 minutes to complete.

The VARK Questionnaire provides students with a quick online version to assess how they prefer to receive and process information: visual, auditory, reading/writing, and kinesthetic. There is no charge for this inventory. The strength of this questionnaire is that it provides a basis for students to reflect and discuss their preferences about learning practices including how to take notes and study for examinations (Fleming & Mills, 1992). To access the inventory, go to www.vark-learn.com/english/page.asp?p=questionnaire.

Learners vary in their preferences with regard to their use of different sensory learning modalities. Faculty members need to be sensitive to the variety of influences that affect learning and should strive to facilitate the students' awareness of their preferences. By identifying students' learning styles and suggesting study strategies based on their personal preferences, it may be possible to enhance student learning.

Teaching Tips to Help Students Use Their Learning Styles to Study More Effectively

- Use diagrams, PowerPoint presentations, videos, outlines, charts, concept maps, graphs, symbols, etc., to help students who are visual learners remember concepts. Encourage the use of index cards of different colors to help organize material to study and the use of different colored highlighters to underline important information in notes and handouts.

- Use cooperative learning groups to help auditory learners talk aloud and explain ideas to others. Encourage them to form study groups to ask each other questions, tape notes and read aloud to each other, and review course material with peers.

- Require writing assignments, such as listing concepts or rewriting ideas in own words, to help those students who prefer reading/writing. Give a variety of reading assignments and handouts, and encourage them to organize diagrams and charts into sentences. Have them summarize reading assignments in their own words.

- Have students actively work with content by using active learning strategies and give students an opportunity to practice what they learn in real-life settings (use scavenger hunts to find resources for the elderly community client or a windshield assessment to learn how to assess a community). Use field trips, role play, problem-solving activities, and flashcards to help them learn concepts. Allow them to move into different groups to work with a variety of students who learn differently.

Strategies to Enhance Motivation

Faculty can pre-assess students' motivation and attitudes about the course or topic through the use of questionnaires and small group discussion. In addition to interviewing students, the College Student Inventory (CSI), which is available in paper-and-pencil or online formats, provides an assessment in four areas: academic motivation, social motivation, general coping, and receptivity to support services (Hirsch, 2001; Stratil, 1988).

Motivation is internally derived, but can be enhanced or influenced by the faculty member's passion for the material. Making the material interesting to students who might not be excited about the topic is challenging, but faculty enthusiasm for the topic can motivate students to learn the material. Part of the faculty member's role is to model a positive sense of enthusiasm for the material and the students. Displaying emotion, energy, and animation in teaching sessions can help students catch the enthusiasm for learning. Humor is often effective to influence students who appear to be extremely unmotivated and difficult to reach. Using a cartoon or funny story related to nursing may be helpful to keep students engaged and receptive to learning the material.

Leamnson (2000) suggests "that the really difficult part of teaching is not organizing and presenting the content but rather in doing something that inspires students to focus on that content—to become engaged, to have some level of emotional involvement with it" (p. 39). Therefore, learning should become a more personal interaction between the faculty and the learner to facilitate or motivate the students' interest in the material. Teaching then becomes a process that encourages and reinforces curiosity and other modes of emotional involvement with the material.

Several other strategies can be used to help students become and stay motivated as well. Using authentic assignments, those that will actually lead to developing knowledge and skills that will eventually be used in later situations can be extremely motivating (Svinicki, 2004). For example, to teach students how to understand why it may be difficult for certain clients to make health-care appointments on time, consider assigning students to use public transportation, such as a city bus or subway.

Success itself can be a motivating factor. Faculty can structure assignments and tasks so that early success is likely and the learning is challenging and has interest value. Faculty who provide students with immediate feedback about their progress toward learning, help to reinforce the learner's efforts toward goal attainment. In addition, faculty can help students acknowledge their own efforts toward achieving success and to begin to perceive their errors or mistakes as learning opportunities. Giving encouragement and reflecting on the progress that students are making aid in enhancing motivation even in the face of obstacles and frustration (Svinicki, 2004).

Strategies to Enhance Literacy

While reading and comprehension difficulties are a part of academic risk, students often do not seek assistance specifically for these difficulties (Hirsch, 2001). Thus, illiteracy may often be a covert problem. Frequently students will complain of reading too slowly, but may also lack the comprehension skills that are actually more crucial to academic success. Various assessment tools can be used to assess reading difficulties. Reading rate can be calculated by having students read a passage from a textbook while being timed. The words per minute can be calculated from this sample reading. In addition, there are more than 40 formulas that can be used to measure the readability levels of written materials. Researchers suggest applying a number of readability formulas to any given piece of written material, and then using the results in conjunction with the reader's individual characteristics to determine the difficulty that students might have (Bastable, 2003).

Faculty can use two basic methods to evaluate reading materials. One method employs the use of one of a number of formulas to determine the average length of sentences and words (vocabulary difficulty). Examples of readability formulas include Spache, Flesch, Fog, Fry, and Smog, all of which have high reliability and predictive validity and are available on the Web (Bastable, 2003). In addition, newer computerized readability analyses are available to evaluate reading materials that can prove useful to faculty. These formulas function as a means to test written material, and the formula chosen should be geared to the specific learner population being tested. Many commercial software packages are capable of applying several formulas to calculate the reading level (Mailloux, Johnson, Fisher, & Petibone, 1995).

One strategy to help build reading and comprehension skills is to teach students to develop a system of active reading and note taking to reduce the text into what is most important to learn. This process involves surveying the material before reading, developing questions to answer before reading, reading small sections or paragraphs, summarizing the information in your own words within the margins of the text, and then reviewing to ascertain if the material has been retained (Hirsch, 2001; Stewart & Hartman, 2006). Helping students to find main ideas, highlighting the ideas, and developing one example to illustrate the idea are useful ways to help students focus on the material to be learned. Encouraging students to work collaboratively in groups to review and discuss reading assignments helps to broaden their comprehension of concepts and deepens their knowledge base. Helping students make the reading assignment personally relevant may increase comprehension, such as having them apply the material to a specific patient assignment or case study.

Literacy improvement takes time, effort, and practice. Reading a variety of materials, from textbooks to pleasure reading, can provide various opportunities to practice increasing reading speed and comprehension. By encouraging students to use a variety of techniques and to read frequently, students may benefit in their ability to transfer these practices to fit the demands of more difficult reading assignments and become more proficient in their literacy skills.

Assessing Learning

It is also important to assess learning so that instructors can better adjust and tailor strategies for future students.

Preadmission Assessment

Preadmission assessment information, such as grade point average, standardized test scores from such tests as the Scholastic Aptitude Test (SAT) and American College Test (ACT), and high school rank, often are used to admit students into nursing programs. These measures alone, however, are frequently not sufficient to determine the overall potential of students entering nursing programs today. Before entering into a program, pre-testing students in areas such as learning style preferences, mathematical abilities, reading and writing abilities, stress and coping strategy preferences, critical thinking abilities, and English as a second language (for example, the TOEFL exam) could help in planning for additional resources and to inform faculty about deficiencies that students may have before providing instruction (Billings & Halstead, 2005).

Feedback on Learning

Faculty can use a number of resources to determine what learning is actually taking place in the classroom so that course materials and methods can be adjusted accordingly. Traditionally, formal classroom assessment involved testing, which captures what students learned for the exam, but does not identify how they learned throughout the course. Low scores would indicate too late that students did not learn as much or as well as faculty intended or expected. Angelo and Cross (1993) identify 50 different methods that faculty can use to "obtain useful feedback on what, how much, and how well their students are learning. Faculty can then use this information to refocus their teaching to help students make their learning more efficient and more effective" (p. 3). Such methods give faculty ways to monitor learning throughout the course to help students before they begin to flounder.

Classroom assessment techniques (CAT) are tools that have the following characteristics: learner-centered, teacher-directed, mutually beneficial, formative, and context-specific (Angelo & Cross, 1993). Classroom assessment is learner-centered, which shifts the emphasis from teaching to learning. CAT can be used to provide students with feedback to inform them whether they have grasped the material or if they need to adjust their study habits to enhance their learning. Teacher-directed refers to the faculty member's responsibility for describing when, how, and what to assess. It is the individual faculty member's own judgment that is used to determine which CAT is used and when.

Classroom assessment is mutually beneficial. By participating in the assessment, students learn if they have accurately grasped the material or if they need to improve or alter their study strategies. Likewise, faculty members can gain insight into their students' learning and alter or improve their teaching based upon this input.

Classroom assessment techniques are context-specific, meaning that what works well with one class or group may not work well with another class or group. Thus, faculty members need to consider using a variety of techniques. Faculty can use a CAT before beginning class, during class, and/or at the end of class to determine how well students comprehend the information and to discover gaps in understanding before moving to the next topic.

Specific Instruments

Seven of the most widely used, quickest, and simplest techniques to assess content knowledge in almost any discipline follow:

- Background knowledge probes: These can be a pre-test or short answer questionnaire to use before presenting or introducing a topic. They are designed to elicit specific background knowledge from the student on the topic so that the faculty member can determine how and where to begin the formal instruction of the material. This technique also serves as a preview to focus the students' attention on the topic.
- Focused listing: This is used to determine what students recall about important terms or concepts by having them list several ideas that they remember about the term or concept.
- Misconception/preconception checks: These use specifically designed tools to uncover common incorrect or incomplete assumptions that students have about a topic and that may act as barriers to new learning. A questionnaire or pre-test designed to uncover commonly held incorrect knowledge is an example.
- Empty outlines: These work well when large amounts of facts and principles are regularly presented. The empty or partially completed outline is given to the students who must complete it within a designated amount of class time.
- Memory matrix: This provides feedback in the form of a blank rectangle divided into columns and rows that the students fill out with recalled information and use to illustrate relationships in the material. Faculty can quickly scan and analyze the matrix to assess the student's understanding of concepts.
- Minute papers: These enable students to write on a note card their responses to what was the most important point learned in class or what question still remains unclear or unanswered. This useful feedback provides manageable amounts of information about student learning that can help faculty adjust their teaching for the next class. The minute paper requires students to do more than just merely recall what they heard or did; it asks them to evaluate what they understood or did not understand.

- Muddiest point: This involves having the faculty pose a question such as "What is still unclear or muddy?" Students write the answer to the question anonymously so that students will be honest and not fear reprisal. This input can help faculty to clarify misconceptions and provide remedial recommendations.

The minute paper and the muddiest point have been identified as resources that assess higher level thinking.

Summary

This chapter cues faculty into the importance of assessing and promoting learning. Learning is an extremely complex concept that varies for each individual student. Students learn in diverse ways and need to be assisted to develop additional learning skills in order to be more successful in a variety of learning environments. Faculty should strive to facilitate and guide students to realize their highest potential to learn by encouraging connections between themselves, their students, and the material that students are expected to learn.

R e f e r e n c e s

Angelo, T., & Cross, K. P. (1993). *Classroom assessment techniques: A handbook for college teachers* (2nd ed.). San Francisco: Jossey-Bass.

Bain, K. (2004). *What the best college teachers do.* Cambridge, MA: Harvard University Press.

Bastable, S. (2003). *Nurse as educator: Principles of teaching and learning for nursing practice* (2nd ed.). Boston: Jones and Bartlett.

Baumlein, G. (2004). The cyberstudent. In L. Caputi & L. Engelmann (Eds.), *Teaching nursing: The art and science* (pp. 434–446). Glen Ellyn, IL: College of DuPage Press.

Billings, D., & Halstead, J. (Eds.). (2005). *Teaching in nursing: A guide for faculty* (2nd ed.). St. Louis: Elsevier Saunders.

Brennan, J. (1997). Nursing education for the 21st century—Preparing culturally diverse minority nurses. In V. Ferguson (Ed.), *Educating the 21st century nurse: Challenges & opportunities* (pp. 153–169). New York: National League for Nursing.

Cadman, C., & Brewer, J. (2001). Emotional intelligence: A vital prerequisite for recruitment in nursing. *Journal of Nursing Management, 9*(6), 321–324.

Caffarella, R. (1994). *Program planning for adult learners: A practical guide for educators, trainers, and staff developers.* San Francisco: Jossey-Bass.

Cassidy, S. (2004). Learning styles: An overview of theories, models, and measures. *Educational Psychology, 24*(4), 419–444.

Chickering, A. (1969). *Education and identity.* San Francisco: Jossey-Bass.

Coomes, M., & DeBard, R. (2004). A generational approach to understanding students. In M. Coomes & R. DeBard (Eds.), *Serving the Millennial generation* (pp. 5–16). San Francisco: Jossey-Bass.

Davis, J. (1993). *Better teaching, more learning: Strategies for success in postsecondary settings.* Phoenix: The Oryx Press.

Dean, G. (1994). *Designing instruction for adult learners.* Malabar, FL: Kreiger Publishing Company.

DeBard, R. (2004). Millennials coming to college. In M. Coomes & R. DeBard (Eds.), *Serving the millennial generation* (pp. 33–45). San Francisco: Jossey-Bass.

DeYoung, S. (2003). *Teaching strategies for nurse educators.* Upper Saddle River, NJ: Prentice Hall.

Dunn, R., Dunn, K., & Price, G. (1996). *Learning style inventory.* Lawrence, KS: Price Systems.

Evans, D., & Allen, H. (2002). Emotional intelligence: Its role in training. *Nursing Times, 98*(27), 41–42.

Filene, P. (2005). *The joy of teaching: A practical guide for new college instructors.* Chapel Hill, NC: The University of North Carolina Press.

Fisher, E. (1999). Low literacy levels in adults: Implications for patient education. *Journal of Continuing Education in Nursing, 30*(2), 56–61.

Fleming, N., & Mills, C. (1992). Not another inventory, rather a catalyst for change. In D. Wulff & J. Nyquist (Eds.), *To improve the academy: Resources for faculty, instructional, and organizational development* (Vol. 11, pp. 137–155). Stillwater, OK: New Forums, Inc.

Forrest, S. (2004). Learning styles. In L. Caputi & L. Engelmann (Eds.), *Teaching nursing: The art and science* (pp. 388–405). Glen Ellyn, IL: College of DuPage Press.

Freshman, B., & Rubino, L. (2002). Emotional intelligence: A care competency for health care administrators. *Health Care Management, 21*(4), 1–9.

Grieve, D. (2002). *A handbook for adjunct/part-time faculty and teachers of adults* (4th ed.). Elyria, OH: Info-Tec.

Hagedorn, L. S. (2005). Square pegs: Adult students and their "fit" in postsecondary institutions. *Change, 37*(1), 22–29.

Haggard, A. (1989). *Handbook of patient education.* Rockland, MD: Aspen.

Hardy, L., Segatore, M., & Edge, D. (1993). Illiteracy: Implications for nursing education. *Nurse Education Today, 13*(1), 24–29.

Hirsch, G. (2001). *Helping college students succeed: A model for effective intervention.* Philadelphia: Taylor & Francis Group.

Howe, N., & Strauss, W. (2000). *Millennials rising: The next generation.* New York: Vintage Books.

Katz, J., & Henry, M. (1993). *Turning professors into teachers: A new approach to faculty development and student learning.* Phoenix: American Council on Education and The Onyx Press.

Kim, S. (2005). Teaching international students. *The Teaching Professor, 19*(4), 5.

Knapper, C. (1995). Understanding student learning: Implications for instructional practice. In W. A. Wright and Associates (Eds.), *Teaching improvement practices: Successful strategies for higher education* (pp. 58–75). Bolton, MA: Anker.

Knowles, M. (1984). *Andragogy in action.* San Francisco: Jossey-Bass.

Kolb, D. (1976). *Learning style inventory: Technical manual.* Boston: McBer.

Leamnson, R. (1999). *Thinking about teaching and learning: Developing habits of learning with first year college and university students.* Sterling, VA: Stylus Publishing.

Leamnson, R. (2000). Learning as biological brain change. *Change, 32*(6), 34–40.

Light, R. (2001). *Making the most of college: Students speak their minds.* Cambridge, MA: Harvard University Press.

Mailloux, S., Johnson, M., Fisher, D., & Petibone, T. (1995). How reliable is computerized assessment of readability? *Computers in Nursing, 13*(5), 221–225.

McCormack, B. (1993). Intuition: Concept analysis and application of curriculum development. *Journal of Clinical Nursing, 2*(1), 11–17.

McGuire, S. & Williams, D. (2002). The millennial learner: Challenges and opportunities. In D. Lieberman & C. Wehlburg (Eds.), *To improve the academy: Resources for faculty, instructional, and organizational development* (Vol. 20, pp. 185–196). Bolton, MA: Anker.

McQueen, A. (2004). Emotional intelligence in nursing work. *Journal of Advanced Nursing, 47*(1), 101–108.

Miller, R. (2005). Emotional intelligence. *Advances for Nurses, 7*(19), 35–37.

Palmer, P. (1998). *The courage to teach: Exploring the inner landscape of a teacher's life.* Philadelphia: Jossey-Bass.

Richardson, V. (2005). The diverse learning needs of students. In D. Billings & J. Halstead (Eds.), *Teaching in nursing: A guide for faculty* (pp. 21–39). St. Louis: Elsevier Saunders.

Smith, L. (1998). Concept analysis: Cultural competence. *Journal of Cultural Diversity, 5*(1), 4–10.

Stewart, T., & Hartman, K. (2006). *Investing in your college education.* Boston: Houghton Mifflin.

Stratil, M. (1988). *College student inventory.* Iowa City, IA: Noel-Levitz.

Svinicki, M. (2004). *Learning as motivation in the postsecondary classroom.* Bolton, MA: Anker.

The Chronicle Almanac, 2005–6: College Enrollment by Age of Student, Fall 2003. Retrieved October 3, 2005, from **http://chronicle.com/weekly/almanac/2005/nation/0101501.htm.**

Vitello-Cicciu, J. M. (2003). Innovative leadership through emotional intelligence. *Nursing Management, 34*(10), 28–33.

Williams, R., & Calvillo, E. (2002). Maximizing learning among students from culturally diverse backgrounds. *Nurse Educator, 27*(5), 222–226.

Wilson, M. E. (2004). Teaching, learning, and millennial students. In M. Coomes & DeBard (Eds.), *Serving the millennial generation* (pp. 59–71). San Francisco: Jossey-Bass.

Wlodkowski, R. (1978). *Motivation and teaching: A practical guide.* Washington, DC: National Education Association.

REVIEW QUESTIONS

- What factors should the faculty consider when assessing the learner?
- What factors affect readiness to learn?
- What are several barriers to learning?
- What are several characteristics of millennial students and how do they affect the educational environment?
- What are several characteristics of adult students and how do they affect the educational environment?
- What are several strategies that affect student motivation and what strategies can be used to overcome the barriers to motivation?
- What is the importance of emotional intelligence to nursing education?
- How can an instructor evaluate the readability of materials?
- What strategies can faculty use to help learners learn?
- What is meant by the term learning styles?
- What is meant by the term classroom assessment techniques (CAT)?

CRITICAL THINKING EXERCISES

Interview a millennial nursing student about her learning needs and goals, readiness to learn, learning style preference and study habits, motivation to learn, and literacy issues. Compare and contrast this information with that of an adult learner or yourself.

Find an educational pamphlet that is used in the hospital setting for adults and children and apply a readability formula to determine the reading level. Then, in several textbooks such as biology, chemistry, medical-surgical nursing, psychiatric nursing, etc., determine the readability level for a few paragraphs in each book. Compare and contrast the level in the pamphlet with the textbook. Analyze how different concepts are explained with regard to the discipline.

Decide on a relevant content area that you could teach. Develop a creative way to teach a new concept that would include how you would assess the learner's previous knowledge of the subject and the learner's readiness to learn the subject. Develop a teaching plan that would incorporate a variety of learning styles and provide your rationale for the use of various modalities. Identify how you might use a CAT to assess if the students are learning the material.

ANNOTATED RESEARCH SUMMARY

August-Brady, M. M. (2005). The effect of a metacognitive intervention on approach to and self-regulation of learning in baccalaureate nursing students. *Journal of Nursing Education, 44*(7), 297–304.

This quasi-experimental study found a significant difference in the deep approach to learning and self-regulation of learning for nursing students who used concept mapping, compared with the control group who did not use concept mapping. These findings suggest that metacognitive strategies, such as the use of concept mapping, promote deeper learning and greater control over that learning.

DiBartolo, M. C., & Seldomridge, L. A. (2005). A review of intervention studies to promote NCLEX-RN success of baccalaureate students. *Nurse Educator, 30*(4), 166–171.

A review of studies that focus on interventions to promote success on the NCLEX-RN demonstrated that researchers were often limited in their ability to connect specific interventions to passing scores. Future research is indicated that uses more rigorous designs and includes larger and more diverse student groups for testing specific interventions that help them prepare to pass the NCLEX-RN exams.

Johnson, S. A., & Romanello, M. L. (2005). Generational diversity: Teaching and learning approaches. *Nurse Educator, 30*(5), 212–216.

This article promotes the understanding of generational diversity so that all learning is valued by both faculty and students. The context, characteristics, and learning styles of each generation are included, along with suggestions to enhance teaching and learning. Faculty can use these ideas to promote student learning in multiple ways.

Peter, C. (2005). Learning—Whose responsibility is it? (2005). *Nurse Educator, 30*(4), 159–165.

This study describes the Learn for Success (LFS) program's outcome for at-risk students who demonstrated better-than-expected academic achievement and decreased attrition rates at a baccalaureate nursing program. This program included a comprehensive range of retention strategies based on Pintrich and Schrauben's learning model. Included were learning strategies, motivational strategies, and self-management strategies.

Chapter Outline

MANAGEMENT STRATEGIES IN THE EDUCATIONAL SETTING

7

Robert G. Mulligan

Learning Outcomes

On the completion of this chapter, the reader will be able to:

- Explain the four "pillars" of classroom management.
- Discuss strategies to increase student motivation.
- Design a classroom environment that facilitates learning.
- Develop strategies that foster student accountability.
- Integrate strategies that keep students engaged in the learning process.
- Redirect students engaged in distractive behaviors.
- Display behaviors that develop professional "mentoring" relationship with students.

Key Terms

Accountability
Cognitive perspective
Emotional intelligence
Extrinsic motivation
Group alerting
Humanistic perspective
Inner discipline

Intrinsic motivation
Motivation
Overlapping
Ripple effect
Smooth transitions
Social perspective
Withitness

Instructors play various roles in the typical classroom setting, but none is more important than that of classroom manager. Effective instruction cannot take place in a poorly managed classroom. If students are disorderly, disrespectful, unprepared, and no rules or procedures guide behavior, little real learning takes place and students cannot learn the inner sense of discipline needed to be true professionals. In these situations, both students and teachers suffer. The instructor struggles to teach, and students learn much less than they should. Well-managed classroom environments, on the other hand, provide an environment in which teaching and learning can flourish. A well-managed classroom environment does not happen by accident. It takes a great deal of planning and effort. The instructor is charged with creating an environment that is conducive to learning.

Classroom Management in the Nursing Education Setting

Creating such an environment is a dynamic process. The effective nursing instructor performs many functions. These functions can be described as the four "pillars" of classroom management: (1) choosing effective instructional strategies to meet the needs of the student, (2) designing a classroom environment that facilitates student learning and uses time and resources wisely, (3) choosing strategies that respond to students who are uncooperative or who are not performing at a level necessary to meet their professional standards, and (4) making effective use of classroom management strategies to support the previous three pillars and keep the momentum going throughout the semester. Communication and positive relationships between instructors and students also are critical components of effective classroom management.

The First Pillar: Instructional Strategies

The first pillar deals with instructional strategies. Effective instructors are able to use a variety of instructional strategies, including both deductive and inductive approaches. They are skilled at the use of cooperative learning and group work. They are skilled in the use of effective questioning techniques, graphic organizers, note taking, and effective planning. They assign meaningful homework, laboratory exercises, and practicum observations. In addition to these skills, they know which strategy is appropriate for a particular student or a particular content area. Although a lecture may be appropriate for one subject, group learning, or an inductive "discovery" approach may be a better approach for another lesson. Good instruction includes "content knowledge" but also includes "pedagogical knowledge" or the "how to" of teaching. Pedagogical knowledge includes knowledge of creative ways of teaching, knowledge of how to give assessments that accurately evaluate students' progress, and being aware of which aspects of the discipline are difficult or easy for students to learn.

Included in the concept of instructional strategies is also curriculum design. This means that the effective nursing instructor can identify and articulate the proper scope and sequence as well as pacing of content. Rather than relying totally on the scope and sequence identified in the course syllabus or the course textbook, they must consider the needs of their students both as a class and as individuals. Instructors must determine the content that requires emphasis and the most appropriate presentation of that content. They must also be skilled at constructing and arranging learning activities that present new knowledge in new and exciting formats, such as stories, explanations, demonstrations; and different media like oral, written, video, the Web, simulations, and hands-on practical experiences. See Box 7–1.

Box 7-1 Authentic Assessment

111

Traditionally, the university instructor has relied on lecture and laboratory experiences to teach concepts. Nursing students were expected to memorize concepts, participate in laboratory exercises, and "parrot" back information to the instructor on tests, lab reports, or "rounds." Today's instructor is skilled at assessing student knowledge and *understanding*, by alternative or "authentic" ways, which include presentations, models, PowerPoint presentations, portfolios, models, case studies, or demonstrations. Authentic assessment ensures that students know concepts but more importantly, have the ability to apply concepts and take concepts to the next level—the level of independent thinking and problem solving.

Motivation

Knowledge of student **motivation** is key to choosing effective instructional strategies. Motivation has been defined as those processes that energize, direct, and sustain behavior. Students who are motivated are energized, directed, and sustained. But what motivates students?

Different perspectives on motivation include: behavioral, humanistic, social, and cognitive. According to the behavioral perspective, student motivation is based on external rewards and punishments. Incentives are positive or negative stimuli or events that can motivate a student's behavior. Incentives can add interest to the class, direct attention toward appropriate behavior, and discourage inappropriate behavior (Emmer, Evertson, Clements, & Worsham, 2000). Incentives include grades and feedback about the quality of student work, recognition or awards, and allowing students to complete a preferred activity.

The **humanistic perspective** is founded in the student's need for personal growth, freedom to choose, and positive growth. This perspective is most familiar in the work of Abraham Maslow (1954, 1971). According to Maslow's hierarchy of needs, students' needs must be satisfied in order for students to reach their full potential:

• Physiological: hunger, thirst, sleep
• Safety: survival, protection from harm
• Love and belongingness: security, affection, attention from others
• Esteem: feeling good about ourselves
• Self-actualization: realization of our full potential

The humanistic perspective is also seen in the work of William Glasser (1986). In his book *Control Theory in the Classroom*, he states, "our behavior is always our best attempt at the time to satisfy at least five powerful forces which, because they are built into our genetic structure, are best called basic needs" (p. 14). Glasser described these needs as:

• To survive and reproduce
• To belong and to love
• To gain power
• To be free
• To have fun

Glasser indicates that students will behave properly only in classroom environments that allow them to experience a sense of control or power over their learning. In *The Quality School: Managing Students without Coercion*, Glasser asserts, "For workers, including students, to do quality work, they must be managed in a way that convinces them that the work they are asked to do satisfies their needs. The more it does, the harder they will work." (Glasser, 1990, p. 22). In order to satisfy these needs, instructors must, among other things, choose tailored and appropriate instructional strategies.

The **social perspective** on motivation is seen in the need for affiliation. This is the motive to be connected with other people. Students who are high in the need for affiliation or related-ness have a strong desire to spend time with their peers, develop strong friendships, are closely connected with their parents, and have a strong desire to have a positive relationship with their teachers. Students in schools with caring and supportive interpersonal relationships have more positive academic attitudes, and are more satisfied with school (Baker, 1999; Stipek, 2002). Other research has shown that an important factor in student motivation and achievement was students' perception of a positive relationship with their teacher (McCoombs, 2001; McCoombs & Quiat, 2001).

The **cognitive perspective** on motivation emphasizes that students' thoughts guide their motivation. This perspective focuses on students' internal motivation to achieve, their attributions about success or failure and effort required for a task, and their beliefs that they can control their environment effectively (Werner, 1986, 2000). The cognitive perspective on motivation also stresses the importance of goal setting, planning, and monitoring progress toward a goal (Zimmerman, Bonner, & Kovach, 1996).

The current interest in the cognitive perspective on motivation also looks at students as extrinsically or intrinsically motivated. **Extrinsic motivation** is motivation to obtain something, such as rewards or punishments. **Intrinsic motivation** involves the internal motivation to do something for its own sake or because the student enjoys it. For this type of student, working long hours in a course is enjoyable because he or she enjoys the content of the course. Psychologist Mihaly Csikszentmihalyi (1990, 2000; Csikszentmihalyi, Rathunde, & Whalen, 1993; Nakamura & Csikszentmihalyi, 2002) has described this type of learner in _Flow: The Psychology of Optimal Experience (1990)_. He states that students experience _flow_ when they experience feelings of deep happiness and enjoyment in their work. This happens when a student experiences a sense of mastery and when the student is deeply absorbed in her work. Flow is most likely to occur when students are challenged and perceive themselves as having a high degree of skill. Choice of instructional strategy plays a crucial role in flow.

The Second Pillar: Proactive Planning to Facilitate Learning

The second pillar is designing a classroom environment that facilitates student learning and uses time and resources wisely. The effective classroom manager is proactive. This type of instructor plans, organizes, and designs the class before the first student ever sets foot in the classroom or laboratory. The proactive teacher will reap the benefits of extensive planning. Classes will run smoothly, students will be prepared and cooperative, time will be used efficiently, and authentic instruction will take place. The reactive teacher will waste time responding to interruptions and will spend an inordinate amount of time "disciplining" students rather than instructing them.

COMP

A widely used classroom management system is the Classroom Organization and Management Program (COMP) developed by Carolyn Evertson at Vanderbilt University (Evertson, 1995; Evertson & Harris, 1999). The program emphasizes rules and procedures, but also addresses techniques for organizing the classroom, developing student **accountability,** planning and organizing instruction, conducting instruction, maintaining momentum, and getting off to a good start.

Some strategies for getting off to a good start according to Evertson, Emmer, and Worsham (2003) in COMP are:

- Establish expectations for behavior and clear up student uncertainties.
- Make sure that students experience success. Difficult tasks can be assigned later.
- Be available and visible. Let students know that they can approach you.
- Be in charge. Establish the boundaries between what is acceptable and not acceptable in your classroom.

The main points of COMP are that a carefully planned system of rules and procedures is the best way to communicate teacher expectations. Rules focus on general expectations or standards of behavior. They are usually few in number and deal with general welfare, courtesy, and safety. Procedures apply to specific activities aimed at accomplishing something. Procedures are not aimed at stopping something but rather should be stated in the positive. Procedures are generally greater in number and may vary with the activity described. Procedures include collecting assignments, due dates, use of equipment, laboratory or classroom safety, procedures for entering and leaving the classroom, emergency procedures, and materials safety. Procedures should be written as "do" statements and not as "do not" or "never" statements. For example, "Always wear protective eye wear and intact latex gloves when exposed to blood or body fluids," is better than "Do not handle blood or body fluids with your bare hands."

The COMP program also requires that the teacher develop systems of accountability that focus on managing student work, communicating assignments, monitoring student progress, and providing student feedback. Students should be taught to take responsibility for their own behavior and use techniques of self-monitoring and self-evaluation. COMP checklists for student accountability might include:

- What standards will you set to guide students in succeeding?
- How will you post assignments?
- How will you collect and hand back student work?
- How will you keep track of completed assignments?
- How will you and the students keep track of work in progress?
- How will students make up missing work?
- How will absent students know about assignments?
- How will you give feedback to students?
- How will you grade assignments?
- How will students manage their own assignments and progress?

At the beginning of the semester these rules and procedures should be taught to the students and should be reinforced and even re-taught throughout the semester. On the first days of the semester the critical features of the management system should be introduced to the students in a way that involves the students. One module focuses on specific suggestions regarding room arrangement, storage, or equipment and materials, and procedures for individual and group participation in the course. Student involvement in the creation of rules or in these orientation activities encourages students to take responsibility for their behavior.

While Evertson and her colleagues emphasize prevention in the COMP program, Jacob Kounin (1977) has also described a system of proactive classroom management that is more useful on a day-to-day basis. Kounin's approach to classroom management is often described by a term that he coined in his research *"withitness."*

113

The Second Pillar: Proactive Planning to Facilitate Learning

The main points of Kounin's theory are that prevention of misbehavior is more important than handling misbehavior. He also believes that instruction and discipline are closely connected. Lesson management and variety are integral to a well-managed classroom. Effective teaching influences classroom management more than classroom management strategies. When instructors and students create environments where students feel safe and comfortable and where academic and personal skills are maximized, learning is enhanced and effective skills are developed. The most important classroom management strategy, according to Kounin, is to keep students actively engaged and accountable for their own behavior and academic performance.

Kounin's main points are as follows:

- **Withitness:** being aware of what is going on in the classroom and on top of the situation
- **Overlapping:** dealing with more than one thing at a time—multitasking, working with a small group, but still knowing what is happening in the rest of the classroom
- **Smooth Transitions:** keeping things running smoothly in the classroom to minimize down time and keeping the momentum going—things moving along
- **Ripple Effect:** behavior ripples or spreads; a teacher needs to be timely at dealing with negative behavior and encourage positive behavior
- **Accountability:** keeping students involved and attentive by calling on them regularly
- Variety and Interest: implementing lessons that are enjoyable and varied, and actively involving the students; keeping up teacher enthusiasm
- **Group Alerting:** gaining and focusing students' attention and communicating expectations

Physical Environment

The last proactive strategy is often overlooked even by experienced instructors. The physical environment of the instructional setting is extremely important. Four basic principles identified by Evertson, Emmer, and Worsham (2003) include:

- Reduce congestion in high-traffic areas. Separate work areas and make them as accessible as possible.
- Make sure that you can see all students easily. All instructors, and nursing instructors in particular, must be able to monitor all students. You must have clear sight lines to see all students and all work areas.
- Make often-used teaching materials and student supplies accessible. This will make preparation time and cleanup time easier as well as save precious instructional time.
- Make sure that students can see and observe classroom presentations. Establish a particular place where you and all students will make presentations.

Equally important is one's classroom management style, which affects both teacher performance and ultimately the strength and personality of the students with whom they interact.

Classroom Management Style

Classroom management style is also a critical part of creating a positive classroom environment. Classroom management style may be defined as how the instructor keeps order and brings about the appropriate student learning outcome. Is the instructor warm and friendly? Is the instructor personal or aloof? Is the instructor supportive or punitive? Although not a strategy per se, classroom management style affects classroom climate and also has demonstrable results in student learning. After analyzing hundreds of parenting studies, Diana Baumrind (1971) has identified four parenting styles: authoritarian, authoritative, neglectful, and indulgent. These styles may be analogous to classroom management styles. These same styles have been applied to teachers (Santrock, 2001):

- Authoritarian classroom managers are restrictive and punitive and focus mainly on keeping order in the classroom rather than on instruction or learning. Students in authoritarian classrooms tend to be passive learners, fail to initiate activities, have anxiety about living up to teacher expectations, and have poor communication skills.
- Authoritative classroom managers encourage students to be independent thinkers and doers but still provide effective monitoring. Authoritative teachers engage students in verbal give-and-take and show a caring attitude toward them. They do know how to set limits when needed. Their students tend to be self-reliant, get along well with their peers, and show high self-esteem.
- Permissive classroom managers allow students a great deal of autonomy but provide them with little support for developing learning skills or managing their behavior. Students in permissive classrooms tend to have inadequate academic skills and low self-control.
- Indulgent classroom managers, similar to permissive classroom managers, are highly involved with their students but place few restrictions on their behavior. They believe that placing few restrictions on students will produce creativity. Students in indulgent classrooms also tend to have inadequate academic skills and lack organizational skills and self-control.

The Third Pillar: Dealing With Misbehavior

Despite our best planning and proactive strategies, some student will misbehave. Choosing strategies that respond to students who are uncooperative or who are not performing at a level necessary to meet their professional standards is the third "pillar" of classroom management. Having a variety of practical strategies to deal with misbehavior will help the nursing instructor to feel that he is prepared to deal with almost any situation. The instructor who intervenes early and intervenes effectively with student misbehaviors will have fewer incidents later in the semester. These "corrective" strategies will solve problems at the moment of misbehavior. But long-term solutions also need to be considered. These will be discussed in the fourth "pillar" of classroom management.

Sociology and psychology have contributed a great deal of theory to the question of why students misbehave. Freudian psychologists emphasize the role of parents as role models. Behavioral psychologists emphasize the role of reward and reinforcement of inappropriate behaviors or the role of modeled behavior.

One of the earliest theorists to conclude that students choose their own behavior was Rudolf Dreikurs (Driekurs & Cassell, 1972; Dreikurs, Grunwald, & Pepper, 1982). Driekurs emphasized that students choose their own behaviors. If this is the case, the goal of the instructor is to develop the attitude that every student can change her behavior and that with help from the instructor every student can learn responsible behavior. One of the most important roles of the instructor is to help the student to develop social interest and social competence so that they are motivated to choose socially useful behaviors. Students must receive a great deal of encouragement. Teachers should use a democratic or collaborative discipline style to allow the student to flourish. Effective classroom management and responsible student behaviors will not flourish in an autocratic or permissive classroom.

Dreikurs has identified four "mistaken goals" that he believes are behind most misbehavior:

1. *Attention.* If students are not getting the attention they need for good behavior, they will seek attention through inappropriate behavior. These students would benefit from more attention

paid to their responsible behavior choices. Students who seek attention will talk out, show off, interrupt others, and demand teacher attention. The instructor may choose to acknowledge only appropriate behaviors and to ignore inappropriate behaviors.

2. *Power and control.* The student repeatedly misbehaves to become the center of attention. These students would benefit from some legitimate avenues for control in the classroom. When seeking power, students may drag their heels, make comments under their breath, or tell the instructor that they are unwilling to perform a task. Students who delay or refuse to complete a task may be given a choice to do it now or later or be shown the consequences for their choices in a logical manner.

3. *Revenge.* The student feels the only way to get attention is to retaliate against adults. The student feels he has been treated unfairly. These students would benefit from learning to deal with hurt feelings in more socially constructive ways. When seeking revenge, students may try to get back at the instructor and other students by lying, subverting class activities, or maliciously disrupting the class. Again, giving students a choice or pointing out the inadequacies of their passive aggressive behaviors may be of help to the instructor and the class.

4. *Helplessness and inadequacy.* Students who feel they are not a member and do not have a sense of belonging would benefit from a great deal of encouragement and positive reinforcement. When displaying inadequacy, students withdraw from class activities and make no effort to learn. Instructors who use positive reinforcement, shaping and gradual reinforcement of appropriate skills, and mentoring can help these students.

The instructor should attempt to discern the reasons behind student misbehavior. What needs of the student are not being met? Meeting student needs both in the proactive classroom management plan and in the corrective plan will prevent much misbehavior and enable the instructor to deal with misbehavior quickly. For some strategies to handle misbehavior in the classroom, see Box 7–2.

A similar perspective on meeting the needs of students within your classroom management strategy is seen in the work of C. M. Charles (2002). He sees students as having seven basic needs that must be met in the classroom in order to create a classroom learning community. These needs are dignity, enjoyment, power, security, hope, competence, and acceptance.

The main points of Charles' *Synergetic* approach are:

• Teaching that actively involves students in the learning process results in little misbehavior. Invite your students to work with you in creating and maintaining an interesting, inviting program for learning, one that is free from fear and based on personal dignity and consideration for others.

Box 7–2

Dreikurs also recommends that instructors react with logical consequences rather than punishment:
• Students have a sense of belonging because they help the instructor set limits on their own (the student's) behavior.
• They help set the limits until they can completely set their own limits.
• Natural consequences are ones that occur naturally. Logical consequences are desirable and the results of the student's own actions.
• Logical consequences usually require the student to make right what has gone wrong.

- Methods for helping students to behave responsibly can be implemented in a gentle, but still very effective manner. Cooperatively establish a set of agreements about how the class is to function and class members are to conduct themselves.
- Classroom conditions need to be established that increase motivation and energy. Discuss and demonstrate conditions that elevate class spirit and energy. Ask the class to identify topics in which they have great interest and would like to study in more detail.
- Teaching and discipline need to be approached from a unified perspective to be effective. Discuss the factors that are known to lead to misbehavior in the classroom. Ask the students to work with you to eliminate or reduce these factors.
- Preventing and redirecting misbehavior is essential. An instructor who knows and understands the causes of misbehavior and who recognizes that these causes begin with unmet needs is practicing "preventive" classroom management.
- Looking at the cause of misbehavior is important. Teachers need to prevent misbehavior by limiting its cause and correct misbehavior by attending to its causes.
- The usual causes of misbehavior are probing boundaries, mimicking others, boredom or frustration, strong distraction, desire for attention, desire for power, no sense of belonging, residual emotion from an outside event, threats to personal dignity, disagreements that escalate and/or egocentric personality.
- The main purpose of discipline is to help students. In Charles' *Synergistic Discipline,* student responsibility is increased. Students and teachers are on the same side working to prevent misbehavior and addressing misbehavior when it does occur. His system does this without offending the student and producing the negative feelings often felt by students in systems of discipline based on punishment.

Keeping students' seven needs in mind, the teacher needs to entice cooperation, rather than force it. Students do cooperate for teachers they trust. The teacher needs to create a classroom with heightened enthusiasm and a sense of purpose. The tools to accomplish this include: teacher ethics, trust, charisma, communication and interest; class agreements; and procedures for problem resolution. When problems occur, the teacher should say something, such as, "Is there a problem I can help you with?" or "Can you help me to understand why this is happening?" The focus is on helping the student to choose responsible behavior rather than punishing. Keeping reactions under control when conflicts arise is an integral part of Charles' *Synergetic* approach.

High-Need Students

Be aware of the needs of different types of students (Marzano, 2003). Although the nursing education instructor is not in a position to directly address severe problems, instructors with effective classroom management skills are aware of these high-need students and are able to come up with a variety of responses to such problem students.

Categories of high-need students include:

- Passive
- Aggressive
- Attention problems
- Perfectionist
- Socially inept

Passive students are characterized as follows:

- Fear of relationships
  - May be victims of abuse (physical/verbal)

- May suffer from medical problems
  - For example, depression, social phobias, etc.
- Fear of failure
  - Students may suffer from a deeply engrained belief that they do not have the requisite skills to succeed in school

Possible ways to deal with the passive student include providing safe peer relations and protection from aggressive people, assertiveness and positive self-talk training, rewarding small success quickly and withholding criticism.

Aggressive students may present themselves as:

- Hostile
  - Poor anger and impulse control, low empathy, sense of entitlement, inability to see the consequences of their actions, low self-esteem, thrill seeking, aligning themselves with deviant peer groups, and committing criminal behavior
- Oppositional
  - Consistently misbehaves, argues with adults, inappropriate language, apt to criticize, blame, and annoy others
- Covert
  - Often around when trouble starts, never quite do what is asked of them

Possible solutions to deal with an aggressive student include helping the student to recognize his/her behavior, contracting with the student to reward correct behaviors and giving consequences for incorrect behavior, giving the student responsibilities to help the instructor and other students in order to foster successful experiences, and keeping in mind that aggressive students are often masking hidden fears and inadequacies.

Attention problems appear in the following ways:

- Hyperactive (attention-deficit hyperactivity disorder [ADHD])
  - Poor impulse control
  - Inability to stay seated or work quietly
  - Tendency to blurt out questions/answers
  - Trouble taking turns
  - Tendency to interrupt others
- Inattentive (attention-deficit disorder [ADD])
  - Fails to pay close attention
  - Rarely appears to listen
  - Forgetful
  - Easily distracted

Possible solutions include contracting with the student to manage behaviors; teaching skills of concentration; study and thinking skills; helping the student with planning, outlining, and time management skills; and rewarding successes.

Perfectionist students may have the following characteristics:

- Closely resembles the diagnosis of obsessive compulsive disorder (OCD)
  - Drive to succeed that is close to unattainable
  - Self-critical
  - Low self-esteem
  - Deep-seated feelings of inferiority and vulnerability

• Only way they feel loved, respected, or get attention is to be perfect
• Believe they are liked for what they can produce, not who they are
• Can be self-destructive

Possible solutions include showing the student that mistakes happen and that they may be acceptable, teaching the students that mistakes can be a learning experience, and having this type of student tutor other students.

Socially inept students:

• Have difficulty making and keeping friends
• Stand too close
• Talk too much
• Make "stupid" or embarrassing remarks
• Are well-meaning students but try too hard to relate to others
• Often feel sad, confused, and different from others
• Are often labeled immature, tactlessness, and insensitive

Possible solutions include teaching the student social skills, such as appropriate physical distance or politeness; teaching the student to recognize the meaning of facial expressions, such as anger or hurt feelings; and making suggestions regarding hygiene, dress, mannerisms, and posture.

Responding Appropriately to Levels of Misbehavior

Barbara Coloroso is another theorist whose views are consistent with recent thought that students must take a more active role in taking responsibility for their own behavior. She believes that students should work with instructors to develop **"inner discipline."** She defines inner discipline as the ability to behave creatively, constructively, cooperatively, and responsibly without being directed by someone else. She bases her teachings on the "golden rule" saying, "I will not treat a student in a way that I myself would not want to be treated" (Coloroso, 1994).

Coloroso states that teachers should try to use "proper discipline," which includes:

• Showing students what they have done wrong
• Giving them ownership over the problems they have created
• Providing them ways to solve the problems
• Leaving their dignity intact

She states that the consequences of behavior need to be "reasonable, simple, valuable, and practical (RSVP)" (Charles, 2002, p. 149). She divides misbehavior into three levels: "mistakes, mischief and mayhem." Mistakes are described as errors in judgment or trust. Instructors should deal with these students after the class. A simple question posed to the student may be, "I want to be able to trust you again. How can we do that?" The mischief level of misbehavior involves showing students what they did wrong, giving them ways to make restitution, making them responsible for their actions, and helping them to save face and leave the related problem with their dignity intact. The mayhem type of misbehavior may result in serious harm to other students. Coloroso suggests that to fix their behavior, students could take the following routes: restitution, or making good; resolution, preventing it from happening again; or reconciliation, healing the students who were harmed. Coloroso would emphasize that any solution to a discipline problem must leave the dignity of both the instructor and the student intact. She would strive for a "win-win" solution to problems and disputes.

The Fourth Pillar: Supporting Learning and Student Success

The fourth and last "pillar" of effective classroom management is making effective use of classroom management strategies that *support* the previous three pillars and keep the momentum going throughout the semester. Some instructor goals supported by this pillar include:

- Getting students back on track through signals, expressions, and gestures
- Showing interest in student work by observing, commenting, and discussing
- Restructuring work that is too difficult
- Assisting students in learning appropriate social skills
- Facilitating students' self-control
- Redirecting students' focus to academic tasks
- Encouraging peer support and appropriate classroom behaviors
- Relieving tension by injecting humor (not sarcasm)

These goals might be simplified into three main areas: teaching responsibility, teaching students that they are capable, and developing a professional "mentoring" relationship with students.

Teaching Responsibility

Teaching responsibility can be described as teachers modeling and actively lending assistance to help the students achieve valuable prosocial behaviors. Teaching content is always the primary focus of an instructor but for a nursing student to go out into the world and work with others, he also needs to know how to live and work with others and to apply what he has learned in the university in his interactions with others. Patricia Kyle and Lawrence Rogien (2004) in *Opportunities and Options in Classroom Management* list the following behaviors that instructors should actively teach and model to their students. These prosocial behaviors may be seen in Table 7–1.

Dr. Goleman's 1995 book, *Emotional Intelligence,* argues that human competencies like self-awareness, self-discipline, persistence, and empathy are of greater consequence than intelligence quotient (IQ) in much of life, that we ignore the decline in these competencies at our peril, and that teachers can and should teach these abilities.

According to Goleman, the five main components of **emotional intelligence** are:

1. **Self-awareness:** knowing what you are feeling, and using your awareness to make good decisions
2. **Handling your emotions:** keeping yourself in good spirits, coping with anxiety, handling anger
3. **Self-motivation:** persistence and zeal; getting yourself started and keeping yourself going, even in the face of setbacks and discouragement
4. **Empathy:** reading people's feelings without them telling you
5. **Social skills:** handling your emotions in relationships

Hundreds of articles and books have been written demonstrating the importance of Goleman's concept of emotional intelligence in the nursing profession (Goleman 1995; Habel 2005).

Teaching Students That They Are Capable

Students who dwell on the "I can't" messages in their heads will not succeed in the nursing classroom. Lew and Bettner (1995) emphasize the importance of making students feel capable by:

TABLE 7–1 121

Prosocial Behaviors	Description
Character development	Instilling character virtues basic to the development of good character: accountability, caring, charity, citizenship, compassion, consideration, courtesy, diligence, fairness, good judgment, impulse control, honesty, loyalty, responsibility, understanding
Communication skills	Listening skills, paraphrasing another's ideas, clarifying information, and summarizing
Social skills	Skills needed to interact effectively with people: greetings, taking turns, disagreeing graciously, sharing materials and equipment
Anger management	Recognizing anger and its sources: identifying triggers, developing strategies to deal with anger constructively
Conflict resolution	Knowing steps to avoid conflicts, and using them when conflicts arise
Responsibility for one's actions	Developing the ability to take responsibility for one's own actions even if it means accepting the logical consequences of one's choices; learning from mistakes
Self-control	Learning to recognize that one is losing control of one's emotions, having coping strategies to gain control of emotions and choosing appropriate behavior
Decision-making skills	Making decisions within structured choices in order to practice effective decision-making and learning from poor decisions as well
Emotional intelligence	Emphasizes the emotional development of students; their awareness and control of their own emotions, their empathy, and relationships with others

- Making mistakes a learning opportunity
- Focusing on improvement, not perfection
- Building on student strengths
- Allowing students to struggle within their ability level
- Acknowledging the difficulty of the task
- Analyzing past successes, and then focusing on the present
- Breaking the task into smaller instructional parts
- Working on positive self-talk
- Celebrating accomplishments

To change "I can't" messages to "I can" messages is a gradual process of change in attitude that must be accomplished over time. This includes creating an environment in which students know that they can make mistakes. It also means pointing out areas of improvement to the student and showing the student how to make step-by-step improvements. These students also must learn positive self-talk and positive self-image. If a task is difficult, students should be taught to accept the difficulty of the task and to use problem-solving and planning skills to accomplish the task. Both realism and optimism can be combined in order to focus on student growth.

Developing a Professional Mentoring Relationship With Students

A positive instructor/student relationship should be built from the first day of class. Positive relationships with students have an effect on the entire class and also influence the choices that students make in their behavior. Positive relationships are a motivator to students that influences responsible behavior choices and academic achievement. Instructors must believe that all students are good and that all students can succeed. Instructors must believe that all students can *learn* responsible behavior if they are not already practicing responsible behavior.

Relating to your students on a personal level is important. Not only caring about them, but also showing caring by demonstrating interest in their hobbies, families, areas of research and study builds a health "rapport" with students. A caring instructor not only demonstrates "report" talk but also "rapport" talk.

Creating a classroom where you want to be and where your students want to be is much easier than teaching a classroom where students are often off task and being corrected frequently. "Supportive" rather than "corrective" strategies build a classroom conducive to learning and a classroom that is enjoyable both to the instructor and to the student. Another aspect of supportive classroom management is effective communication skills.

Communication Skills

Communication with students means speaking fluently, pointing out key points, giving clear explanations, using examples, checking for comprehension, and highlighting lessons with clear closure. Table 7–2 provides examples for each of these categories.

To support classroom management and ensure that all aspects of effective teaching, preventative classroom management, and corrective classroom management continue throughout the

TABLE 7–2   Communication Skills

Speak clearly	No vagueness—precision Language that learners understand Clarify technical terms
Point out key points	Give cues such as "this is important" Write points on board or project points onto screen Give students an outline
Give clear explanations	Cover information step by step Show logical connections Consider the learner's perspective
Use examples	Concepts are best taught by examples and "non" examples
Check for under-standing	Formative checks for understanding should be made frequently
Highlights of the lesson should be used as lesson closure	Highlights of the lesson are a way to bring closure but are also an excellent strategy from the standpoint of cognitive psychology • Repeat • Review • Summarize

entire semester or course, an effective teacher-student relationship must be established. Just as teaching involves the interplay of both "science" and "art," effective classroom management involves the interaction between dominance and cooperation.

The Dynamics of an Effective Teacher-Student Relationship

Robert J. Marzano in his book *Classroom Management That Works* (2003), cites the research of Theo Wubbels and his colleagues (Brekelmans, Wubbles, & Creton, 1990; Wubbles, Brekelmans, van Tartvijk, & Admiral, 1999; Wubbles & Levy, 1993), on the dynamics of an effective teacher-student relationship. They identify two dimensions whose interactions define the relationship between teacher and students. One dimension is dominance versus submission; the other is cooperation versus opposition. According to Marzano, the optimal teacher-student relationship is one of high dominance and high cooperation. Quoting Wubbels and his colleagues (1999), Marzano writes:

> Teachers should be effective instructors and lecturers, as well as friendly, helpful, and congenial. They should be able to empathize with students, understand their world, and listen to them. Good teachers are not uncertain, undecided, or confusing in the way they communicate with students. They are not grouchy, gloomy, dissatisfied, aggressive, sarcastic, or quick-tempered. They should be able to set standards and maintain control while still allowing students responsibility and freedom to learn (Wubbles, p. 167).

These teacher characteristics may be seen in Table 7–3.

Emotional Objectivity

A final aspect of teacher disposition that should not be overlooked in creating a supportive classroom management plan is "emotional objectivity." Marzano (2003) states than an effective classroom manager implements and enforces rules and procedures, executes disciplinary actions, and cultivates effective relationships with the students without *interpreting* violations of classroom rules and procedures, negative reactions to disciplinary actions, or lack of response to forge relationships as a personal attack. These instructors act as professionals and look upon learners as

TABLE 7–3

Teacher Characteristic	Ideal Interaction	Extremes (No Interaction)
High Dominance	Clarity of purpose	Lack of attentiveness or concern for students
High Submission	Guidance	Lack of clarity of purpose
High Cooperation	Concern for the needs and opinions of others	Inability or lack of resolve without the approval of others
High Opposition		Active antagonism toward others and a desire to thwart their goals

people with whom they interact on a daily basis. They do not overreact. They do not see the students as "the enemy." In addition, they do not take misbehavior personally.

This means maintaining a balance between psychological distance and aloofness. It means carrying out classroom duties without becoming emotionally involved regarding the outcomes. This means taking the "middle ground" and not "personalizing" the actions of students. A healthy emotional tone is a characteristic of many theories of classroom management including COMP (Evertson, 1995) and others.

Summary

Understanding and practicing the four pillars of classroom management are key components of managing teaching and learning. Strategies for increasing learning, motivation, responsibility, and achievement are addressed throughout this chapter. As teachers it is important to connect with the students, plan an effective environment for learning, and to model and encourage professional mentoring relationships. The unique interactions between teacher and students form the basis of effective teaching.

References

Baker, J. (1999). Teacher-student interaction in urban at-risk classrooms: Differential behavior, relationship quality, and student satisfaction with school. *The Elementary School Journal, 100,* 57–70.

Baumrind, D. (1971). Current patterns of parental authority. *Developmental Psychology Monographs, 4*(1, Part 2).

Brekelmans, M., Wubbels, T., & Creton, H. A. (1990). A study of student perceptions of physics teacher behavior. *Journal of Research in Science Teaching 27,* 335, 350.

Charles, C. M. (2002). *Building classroom discipline.* Boston: Allyn and Bacon.

Coloroso, B. (1994). *Kids are worth it! Giving your child the gift of inner discipline.* New York: Avon Books. Revised edition, (2002) New York: Harper Collins.

Csikszentmihalyi, M. (1990). *Flow.* New York: Harper and Row.

Csikszentmihalyi, M. (2000). Creativity: An overview. In A. Kazdin (Ed.), *Encyclopedia of psychology.* Washington, DC and New York: American Psychological Association and Oxford University Press.

Csikszentmihalyi, M., Rathunde, K., & Whalen, S. (1993). *Talented teenagers: The roots of success and failure.* Cambridge, UK: Cambridge University Press.

Dreikurs, R., & Cassel, P. (1995). *Discipline without tears.* New York: Penguin NAL. Originally published in 1972.

Dreikurs, R., Grunewald, B. B., & Pepper, F. C. (1982). *Maintaining sanity in the classroom: Classroom management techniques.* New York: Harper and Row.

Emmer, E. T., Evertson, C. M., Clements, B. S., & Worsham, M. E. (2000). *Classroom management for successful teachers* (4th ed.). Boston: Allyn and Bacon.

Evertson, C. M. (1995). *Classroom organization and management program: Revalidation submission to the Program Effectiveness Panel, U.S. Department of Education.* (Tech. Report). Nashville, TN: Peabody College, Vanderbilt University. (ERIC Document Reproduction Service No. ED403247).

Evertson, C. M., Emmer, E. T., & Worsham, M. E. (2003). *Classroom management for elementary teachers* (6th ed.). Boston: Allyn and Bacon.

Evertson, C. M., & Harris, A. (1999). Support for managing learner-centered classrooms: The classroom organization and management program. In H. J. Freiburg (Ed.), *Beyond behaviorism: Changing the classroom management paradigm* (pp. 59–74). Boston: Allyn and Bacon.

Glasser, W. (1986). *Control theory in the classroom.* New York: Harper and Row.

Glasser, W. (1990). *The quality school: Managing students without coercion.* New York: Harper and Row.

Goleman, D. (1995). *Emotional intelligence.* New York: Bantam.

Habel, M. (2005). CE 373: Emotional intelligence helps RNs work smart. *Nursing Spectrum* (*Greater Philadelphia / Tri-State edition*). *14*(16), 17–19.

Kounin, J. (1977). *Discipline and group management in classrooms.* Revised edition. New York: Holt, Rinehart, & Winston.

Kyle, P. B., & Rogien, L. R. (2004). *Opportunities and options in classroom management.* Boston: Pearson-Allyn and Bacon.

Lew, A., & Bettner, B. L. (1995). *Responsibility in the classroom: A teacher's guide to understanding and motivating students.* Boston: Connexions Press.

Marzano, R. J. (2003). *Classroom management that works: Research-based strategies for every teacher.* Alexandria, VA: Association for Supervision and Curriculum Development.

Maslow, A. H. (1954). *Motivation and personality.* New York: Harper and Row.

Maslow, A. H. (1971). *The farther reaches of human nature.* New York: Viking Press.

McCoombs, B. L. (2001, April). *What do we know about learners and learning? The learner-centered framework.* Paper presented at the meeting of the American Research Association, Seattle.

McCoombs, B. L., & Quiat, M. A. (2001). *Development and validation of norms and rubrics for the Grade 5 assessment of learner-centered principles. (ALCP) surveys.* University of Denver Research Institute, Denver.

Nakamura, J., & Csikszentmihalyi, M. (2002). The concept of flow. In C.R. Snyder & S. J. Lopez (Eds.), *Handbook of positive psychology* (pp. 80–105). New York: Oxford University Press.

Santrock, J. W. (2001). *Educational psychology* (2nd ed.). Boston: McGraw Hill.

Stipek, D. J. (2002). *Motivation to learn* (4th ed.). Boston: Allyn and Bacon.

Werner, B. (1986). *An attribution theory of motivation and emotion.* New York: Springer.

Werner, B. (2000). Motivation: An overview. In A. Kazdin (Ed.), *Encyclopedia of Psychology.* Washington, DC & New York: American Psychological Association and Oxford University Press.

Wolfgang, C. H., & Glickman, C. D. (1980). *Solving discipline problems: Strategies for classroom teachers.* Boston: Allyn & Bacon.

Wolfgang, C. H., & Glickman, C. D. (1986). *Solving discipline problems: Strategies for classroom teachers* (2nd ed., p. 330). Upper Saddle River, NJ: Prentice Hall.

Wubbels, T., Brekelmans, M., van Tartvijk, J., & Admiral, W. (1999). Interpersonal relationships between teachers and students in the classroom. In H. C. Waxman & H. J. Walberg (Eds.), *New directions for teaching practice and research* (pp. 151–170). Berkeley, CA: McCutchan.

Wubbles, T., & Levy, J. (1993). *Do you know what you look like? Interpersonal relationships in education.* London: Falmer Press.

Zimmerman, B. J., Bonner, S., & Kovach, R. (1996). *Developing self-regulated learners.* Washington, DC: American Psychological Association.

Review Questions

- Provide examples of how each of the motivation strategies can be used in a classroom setting in a (1) behavioral perspective, (2) humanistic perspective, (3) social perspective, and (4) cognitive perspective.
- Discuss how Dreikurs' mistaken goals may be minimized in a classroom setting.
- Explain how to create a classroom with heightened enthusiasm and a sense of purpose.
- Develop strategies to help the perfectionist student succeed in the classroom setting.
- Select three prosocial behaviors identified by Kyle and Rogien and discuss how you use them in developing a professional mentoring relationship with students.

Critical Thinking Exercises

▶ You are a newly hired instructor for an Accelerated BSN Program. The chairperson assigns you to teach a new course in Pharmacology. Using COMP as a foundation:
  a. Give examples of rules and procedures for your classroom.
  b. Discuss ways to foster student accountability. How can you make students keep track of their own progress or lack thereof?
  c. Integrate actively Kounin's theory and concepts into your curriculum plan.
▶ Role play how emotional intelligence can be used in the classroom.

Annotated Research Summary

Maxwell, B., & Reichenbach, R. (2005). Imitation, imagination and re-appraisal: Educating the moral emotions. *Journal of Moral Education, 34*(3), 291–307.

No observer of research currents in the human sciences can fail to detect a new appreciation for the contribution of emotions to descriptions of such wide-ranging psychological phenomena as moral judgment, personal and social development, and learning. Despite this, we claim that educating the emotions as a dimension of moral education remains something of a taboo subject. As evidence for this, we present three categories of interventions that fit unmistakably into the category of the education of the emotions, but which go generally unrecognized. In the light of the fact that emotional education is held not just to be possible, but is in fact commonplace, we present an error theory to explain its general occlusion. Next, we argue that the taboo surrounding the education of the emotions helps to explain the lack of recognition that relevant kinds of emotional reactions, especially guilt and shame, seem indeed to be a better measure of successful moral education than moral acts. This, we take it, is one of the suppositions of the old classroom management device called the "shame corner." In the last section we propose a comparative analysis of the shame corner and its pedagogical descendant, the "time-out corner," in terms of their assumptions about the structure of moral judgment and the significance of moral emotions. Without recommending the reinstitution of the shame corner, we conclude that, far from constituting progress in moral education, the time-out corner is, from this perspective, apparently wrong-headed and confusing.

Chambers, S. M., & Hardy, J. C. (2005). Length of time in student teaching: Effects on classroom control orientation and self-efficacy beliefs. *Educational Research Quarterly, 29*(3), 3–9.

This study used the classroom management framework conceptualized by Wofgang and Glickman (1980, 1986) to explain the various dimensions of classroom management. This framework defines three broad areas—instructional management, people management, and behavior management. It appears that the lengthened student teaching experience does not have an impact on classroom management styles and/or self-efficacy. Results support the continued use of the one-semester student teaching option. The authors recommend further study, particularly pre/post-test studies examining the impact of student teaching experiences on classroom management skill acquisition. Initiating data collection efforts during program induction is suggested. Additional research regarding instructional management and self-efficacy is also encouraged.

Weinstein, C. S., Tomlinson-Clarke, S., & Curran, M. (2004). Toward a conception of culturally responsive classroom management. *Journal of Teacher Education, 55*(1), 25–38.

Given the increasing diversity of our classrooms, a lack of multicultural competence can exacerbate the difficulties that novice teachers have with classroom management. Definitions and expectations of appropriate behavior are culturally influenced, and conflicts are likely to occur when teachers and students come from different cultural backgrounds. The purpose of this article is to stimulate discussion of culturally responsive classroom management (CRCM). We propose a conception of CRCM that includes five essential components: (1) recognition of one's own ethnocentrism; (2) knowledge of students' cultural backgrounds; (3) understanding of the broader social, economic, and political context; (4) ability and willingness to use culturally appropriate management strategies; and (5) commitment to building caring classrooms. In the final section of the article, we suggest questions and issues for future research.

Vitello-Cicciu, J. M. (2002). Exploring emotional intelligence: Implications for nursing leaders. *Journal of Nursing Administration, 32*(4), 203–210.

Emotional intelligence is being touted in the popular literature as an important characteristic for successful leaders. However, caution needs to be exercised regarding the connection between emotional intelligence and workplace success. The author contrasts two current models of emotional intelligence, the measurements being used, and the ability of emotional intelligence to predict success. Implications for the workplace are discussed.

Cummings, G. (2004). Research leadership. Investing relational energy: The hallmark of resonant leadership. *Canadian Journal of Nursing Leadership, 17*(4), 76–87.

Recent research has shown that hospital restructuring that included staff layoff has adversely affected the role, health, and well-being of nurses who remained employed. Further research found that nurses working in environments that reflected resonant (emotionally intelligent) leadership reported the least negative effects to their health and well-being following hospital restructuring. What remained unclear was the mechanism by which this mitigation occurred. The purpose of this paper is to explore additional findings from this leadership research and discuss one explanation unique to the academic literature for the mitigation variable—the investment of relational energy by resonant nursing leadership to build relationships with nurses and manage emotion in the workplace.

Chapter Outline

USING TECHNOLOGY IN NURSING EDUCATION

Marilyn Stoner

8

Learning Outcomes

On completion of this chapter, the reader will be able to:

- Understand the use of technology in the educational field.
- Appraise different types of technology for its contribution to the curriculum outcomes.
- Develop confidence in online terminology.
- Evaluate online methodologies for effectiveness in facilitating learners' goals.
- Synthesize new technologies as an enhancement to current teaching strategies.

Key Terms

Emoticons
Ergonomics
Information competence
Information literacy
Intellectual property
Security
Social engineering
Syllabi
Technological hardiness
Technostress

Technology permeates all forms of education. Whether you are using the computer on your desktop, sending e-mail via a network, searching the Internet, or finding directions to your university, technology is involved. Technology greatly enhances student learning. It increases the interactivity and access to other students and faculty; it allows nursing faculty to produce custom learning objects; and it has led to the clinical lab, which presents new methods of simulating patient care. This chapter will provide educators with a brief snapshot of many of the uses for technology. Although there are continuous advances in technology, this chapter presents helpful suggestions and resources guiding safe and effective use of today's technology. Most of the computer technology discussed in this chapter is for Windows users, but many applications are also available for Macintosh users.

The focus of this chapter is on the application of technology, understanding how different types of programs work, and how they might be used in a variety of courses. It is not possible to master everything in this chapter at once. As you read through the chapter, make notes about what sounds interesting and doable given your current resources. The two primary resources you will need are time and money. Often, mastering new technology requires more time than money. The good news is that many computer applications are available for free for limited periods of time.

Overview of Types of Technology

All forms of educational technology are used in one or more of four basic ways as listed in Table 8–1.

This chapter will explore the first three uses of technology. Simulations of live patient care will be covered in Chapter 9.

Technology Used to Connect People and Services

Colleges and universities use technology extensively and many people first get to know a university through a Web site. Many colleges use Internet-based services for the entire admission, registration, and student management processes. Perhaps the most commonly used networked service on a campus is the library. Newer online services include learning labs and tutoring services. The most common overall use of computers is electronic mail (e-mail). In addition to e-mail, university networks include Web-based directories of users, departments, and services.

Technology Used to Create Learning Objects

Faculty use technology to create a wide variety of learning objects. Most commonly these objects include documents such as **syllabi** and visual presentations using PowerPoint. A large repository

 TABLE 8–1 Forms of Educational Technology

1. Technology is used to connect users to other users, products or services.
2. Technology is used to create learning objects, such as multimedia presentations, documents, and Web sites.
3. Technology is used to support or house the learning environment, in learning management platforms. (The most common platforms or systems are Blackboard, Web CT, and e-college.)
4. Technology is used to simulate live patient care. (Examples of patient simulators are available in many forms including infants, adults, and surgical simulators to name a few.)

of learning objects can be found at the Multimedia Educational Resource for Learning and Online Teaching (http://www.merlot.org). This chapter will provide examples of basic and advanced techniques for creating learning objects of all types. Faculty members who teach online know that it is an effective and challenging method of instruction. The most common concern expressed by faculty is the increased amount of time it takes to facilitate high-quality learning experiences online. As with e-mail and other technology issues discussed in this chapter, it is best to be proactive when creating or conducting an online class. Table 8–2 outlines tips for developing a system of managing time and effort in an all-online class and provides an example of a 5-day class schedule.

 TABLE 8–2 Time Management Tips for Online Classes

- Students will feel more at ease if you keep a schedule and they know what to expect.
- Find your own style and use **emoticons.**
- Save announcements from one semester to the next; you can set them up to display for a week.

Week or Day No.	Activity
1	Announcement: Welcome Announcement. Send this announcement to everyone who is enrolled in the course via the e-mail function. Forums: Post your introduction. Respond to the introductions of students. Read all forums and respond. Offline Preparation: Keep paper and pencil notes about student information—where they work, etc. Whatever you might like to include in postings when responding to them. Send a private e-mail to each student as they post their introductions.
2	Forums: Respond to introductions in public forum. Check forums of Technical Angst (TA), questions about the course. Offline Preparation: Maintain class log of information.
3	Announcement: Announce next week's activities, also send this announcement in an e-mail to student's private e-mail and include: • List where next week's activities will be conducted • What is due now • Bridging comments about what was done this week and what needs to be done next week • Review what papers and activities should have been done Forums: Read and respond to all forums. Other Online Preparation: Check the course statistics stats—find out who's on and who is not. Use this to find out who has not been in class and then call or e-mail them. Look to see who are the high and low "accessers" to the class. Intervene if you think there is something that needs to be addressed. For example, someone who has accessed the course many times and not posted much may not understand where to post work.
4	Announcement: Remind everyone where the course activities are this week. Forums: Post introduction for week 2 in the forums for that week. Post the learning activities in the forums.

(table continued on page 132)

TABLE 8–2 Time Management Tips for Online Classes (continued)

Week or Day No.	Activity
	Use the "collect" feature and respond to students by collecting responses, pointing out the similarities and differences, or whatever you usually point out. <u>Other Online Preparation</u>: Post grades for previous week. Archive the discussions for week one, check course statistics for the last classes. Create next forum.
5	<u>Forums</u>: Check forums of Technical Angst (TA), questions about the course. Respond to previous postings in forum.

The research shows that students learn best when the class, any type of class, is highly interactive. Online courses are perhaps the most interactive courses as students must participate to be counted as present. Students can be silent in a traditional class, however, they cannot be silent in a well-designed online class.

Technology: What Students and Faculty Need to Know

Although technology is integral to the learning and teaching experiences, it is also a source of great frustration, especially for novice computer users (Lindsay & McCluren, 2000). Nursing faculty must include instructional content that supports the use of technology in the educational experience. The term **technological hardiness** is a concept to use in teaching faculty how to promote the skills and insights necessary for the effective use of technology. Technological hardiness (TH) is defined as the affective, cognitive, and psychomotor skills necessary to utilize technology in all of its forms effectively, without undue physical, mental, or cognitive stress.

Students and faculty now routinely begin their day with reading and composing electronic communication, searching online databases, and accessing the Internet. The most complicated equipment in education used to be the car driven to campus. Now there are virtual campuses, libraries, and meeting rooms. "Attending" class is no longer straight forward. Students must learn to use a personal computer, navigate the Internet, compose postings for e-mail and class discussions, create files for a variety of purposes, and stay electronically safe while doing it all. This requires a high level of TH skill and insight.

Psychomotor Considerations

Computer users must consider the lifetime effects of viewing monitors and sitting at desks and other locations with computers. Muscles, joints, bones, and eyes are all affected by computer use (Clark, Frith, & Demi, 2004). As a result, students must learn to use appropriate posture and adequate lighting, and to take frequent rest periods while using a computer. It is even more important that students with disabilities understand **ergonomics** and methods of adapting home computer work stations to meet their unique needs. Faculty can promote student awareness of ergonomics by suggesting a simple intervention such as placing a small mirror on a computer desk area so the user can occasionally glance over at the mirror to check posture. Users also can set timers to ensure that rest periods are taken.

Frustration arises when students are unable to complete online tasks as assigned (O'Regan, 2003). There are innumerable reasons why any given technologically mediated assignment cannot be completed. Problems with clearing the computer cache, server malfunctions, unstable connections to the Internet, and Web page and database design flaws are a few of the many reasons. The result of the inability to get technology to do what we want is referred to as ***technostress,*** a term coined by Bron in 1984. He defined technostress as a "modern disease of adaptation caused by inability to cope with the new computer technologies" (Weil & Rosen, 1997). Technostress is a major health factor for faculty and students.

Many computer users assume that user error causes computer problems, and they experience negative changes to self-esteem when they cannot complete projects as directed (Klein, Moon, & Picard, 2002). Users erroneously think that all technology problems are related to their own inabilities and knowledge deficits. In reality, problems are often related to programming and design issues. Remembering that technology itself may be faulty when problems arise can be very helpful for students and faculty as they strive to maintain confidence related to computer skills.

In order to avoid as much frustration as possible, faculty can design assignments using proven technology that itself utilizes a low threshold of technical sophistication. When using technology, it is important to use the lowest threshold activity, which is generally the most stable. This ensures that students with even dial-up or telephone connections will be able to access the learning objects.

Beyond helping students reach instructional goals, there are other practical considerations. Technological frustration can relate directly to an important concern of faculty: the evaluation of teacher effectiveness. Technical problems can have a dramatic negative effect on how students evaluate instructors. Integrating additional technical assistance into a course will be appreciated by students. As a result, a student may be more willing to separate the inability to complete a class assignment due to technology problems from the evaluation of the faculty member's teaching skill.

Realizing that there are many complexities in the design, development, and production of hardware and software is a crucial component of developing TH. A sense of humor is also invaluable in coping with computer frustrations. Faculty can model a sense of humor by including humor in text and graphics. Large supplies of computer-related comics are available for use (with permission) on national cartoonist Randy Glasbergen's website http://www.glasbergen.com.

Simple metaphors and visuals can also reach students on affective as well as cognitive levels. Include music and relaxation techniques, such as deep breathing, in your instructions for assignments. Encourage students to manage their time effectively using a timer and breaks and to relax while completing work. These interventions also help to promote time management skills and physical health.

Faculty can also invite students to share their technical stresses and triumphs with them and the class. Spending a few minutes discussing frustrations is helpful to understand student errors in thinking and identify ways to modify assignments. Social support is critical in developing a sense of connectedness. In an online course, this is easily done by creating a discussion thread that invites postings from students. Sharing stories is a powerful way to learn about and affirm oneself (Wurman, 2001). Invariably, students respond with, "I thought it was just me who had that problem!"

Cognitive Considerations

Trial and error is not an effective method of learning technical skill, because computers require new vocabulary, models of thinking, and problem solving. Although students do not need to become computer experts, it is time well spent to master some basic information about computers. It is important to include only proven technology in course design and program functions. Utility rather than novelty should be the guiding principle when using technology (Roueche, Milliron, & Roueche, 2003).

Cognitive aspects of TH are fostered by providing a technology orientation to the course and to the technology and support services on campus. When giving instructions about an assignment, be sure to include instructions on how to develop the technical skills required for assignments.

Understanding the limits of computers and how to problem solve is critical to success in using technology. Perhaps the area in which students need the most additional information is how to get help when they run into problems. A support program to help students, especially those who are anxious about computers, has been found to be helpful (Marcoulides, Stocker, & Marcoulides, 2004). Giving students explicit information on the technology specifics needed for each class has been effective in teaching students how to navigate not just online classes but other technologically mediated functions (Ko & Rossen, 2001). This includes library searching, use of online plagiarism detection services, registering for classes, and the like.

Developing technological hardiness in ourselves and our students has many rewards. Students who feel capable of using a computer have been more successful in both distance and campus programs. Technically capable students express more satisfaction on mid- and end-program evaluations, and have been less likely to drop out of programs (Britt, 2006). Competence in this area makes teaching and learning more satisfying.

Teaching With Technology

Using technology to facilitate learning is the ultimate goal. The time spent learning new programs and applications becomes worthwhile when students learn new concepts as a result. Incorporating new forms of technology into instructional practices expands what we can teach. Technology also helps us reach learners with a variety of learning styles (Fuszard, 1995). Uploading learning objects within learning management platforms and to Web pages gives students greater access to the objects we've created. See Table 8–3 for a list of myths about technology.

 TABLE 8–3 Myths of Technology

1. Technology will always work.
2. You have to understand how it works to use it.
3. Technology (e-mail, ichat, etc.) is a replacement for traditional communication (telephone, face to face).
4. The newest technology is the best.
5. Technology always saves time.
6. You can "master" all the technology you will use.
7. Computers are smart—they "know" what you want them to do.
8. Every new piece of software will work with every existing piece of software (and hardware) you own.

Using Technology to Produce Your Own Learning Assets

Learning just a few simple programs can greatly expand your repertoire of learning objects. There are many programs, PowerPoint for example, that give faculty members more options in teaching.

Box 8–1 Technical Failures   135

The best way to plan for technical failure is to take steps to prevent it. There are several important strategies you can incorporate into your instructional strategies to help you prepare for many technical problems. First and foremost, back up all of your files. This is the most important action you can take and it is often overlooked. Every university routinely backs up files, but many faculty members do not. It may be necessary for you to set up a system for backing up files on your office computer. You will also need to develop a system to back up the files on your home computer. You can create backups by copying files to a CD or to external hard drives. Insist that students do the same.

You can create a narrated streaming media presentation simply by using a PowerPoint presentation you've already created by using Camtasia. You can upload the video presentation to a Web page by learning management system such as Blackboard.

Other multimedia authoring tools include Microsoft's Producer and Movie Maker, which are available at no additional charge from Microsoft. Macromedia also makes a number of entry level and advanced authoring tools. Many nursing educators are taking the time to learn to use the higher level tools produced by Macromedia because they are becoming the production standard. Campus support services are often invaluable in assisting students and faculty. Box 8–1 discusses how to prepare for technical failures.

Games: Crosswords and Other Word Puzzles, Question and Answer

Students love online games of all types. Question and answer, all types of word puzzles, and jig-saws can be created for use in the classroom or online. In fact, many of the applications to create these puzzles are free. The use of games is supported by both adult (Knowles, Holton, & Swanson, 1998) learning principles and best practices. Web-based games can increase an instructor's repertoire of skills and provide more creative ways of disseminating and reinforcing content. Word games are especially helpful in building vocabulary for English as a second language students.

Examples of these free games and their intended support of learning comprehension level can be found in Table 8–4 . Examples of game programs for purchase are listed along with their complexity for use in Table 8–5. Online games can support learning in relation to Bloom's taxonomy and many of the word games cited can easily be created and implemented within an hour.

TABLE 8–4 Free Game Programs to Enhance Online Teaching Effectiveness

Game	Implementation	Learning Comprehension Level
Word Search	Easy to develop and use. Created with Mike Hall's Word Search. http://www.1archive.com/game/wordsearch/	Knowledge and comprehension
Crossword puzzle	Easy to develop and use. Created with Crossword Compiler. This example is used in nursing theory. http://www.crossword-compiler.com/	Knowledge and comprehension

(table continued on page 136)

TABLE 8–4 Free Game Programs to Enhance Online Teaching Effectiveness (continued)

Game	Implementation	Learning Comprehension Level
Jigsaw puzzle	Easy to develop and use. Created with JigZone. This example is used in a computer science class. http://www.awrjl.com/AWC/sdlc_jigsaw_puzzle.htm	Knowledge and comprehension
Drag-and-drop	Medium complexity for development. Easy to use. Created with in-house programming. This example was created for a child's botany class. http://arboretum.fullerton.edu/grow/drag-drop/plant_parts.asp	Application and analysis
Library puzzler	Difficult to develop, easy to use. Created with in-house programming. http://guides.library.fullerton.edu/introduction/puzzler/puzzler.htm	Application and analysis
Moral dilemma	Difficult to develop, easy to use. Created with in-house program. http://www.dushkin.com/connectext/psy/ch03/kohlberg.mhtml amming.	Synthesis and evaluation
Simulation and critical thinking	Difficult to develop, medium difficulty to use. These examples are the manufacturer's and change frequently. http://www.halfbakedsoftware.com/quandary_tutorials_examples.php	Synthesis and evaluation

 TABLE 8–5 Examples of Game Programs for Purchase

Tool	Description	Complexity of Use
Crossword Compiler	Creates free-form and structured crosswords and vocabulary puzzles. http://www.x-word.com	Easy
Hot Potatoes	Creates quizzes, crossword puzzles, and other word games. Free to educators and nonprofit organizations. http://halfbakedsoftware.com/hot_pot.php	Easy
Macromedia Flash	Creates Web movies and games with animation and sound. http://www.macromedia.com/software/flash/	Easy to difficult, depending upon complexity
Mike Hall's Word Search	Creates word searches. Free with acknowledgement. http://javaboutique.Internet.com/WordSearch/	Easy
Quandary	Creates decision-making and critical thinking games. http://www.halfbakedsoftware.com/quandary.php	Easy to difficult, depending upon complexity

Jeopardy

Box 8–2 Low Threshold Activities Are Best **137**

When designing and creating learning objects, it is best to start with "low threshold" activities (LTA). An LTA is one that requires the lowest level of effective technology. An excellent resource on LTAs is found at the Learning, Teaching and Technology Group (TLTG) Web site: http://www.tltgroup.org/.

Knowledge and comprehension can be supported by using crossword puzzles, word search, and other word-based games as well as jigsaw puzzles. Application and analysis skills are enhanced by games using question and answer, and simulations (Blenner, 1991). Synthesis and evaluation can be enhanced by more complex decision-making and critical thinking games implementing any of these word games requires design and planning. Box 8–2 discusses some of the best types of activities to start with.

Best Practices and Tips of Computer Users

The following offers tips for more effective and productive use of technology.

Managing Files and Folders

The first thing people who use computers notice is that a large number of files and folders are created in a short time. As files are used and edited, the challenge to find the folders and files for any project becomes difficult. Developing a strategy for naming folders and files is crucial to being an effective computer user. In order to manage folders and files, be sure to use a disciplined approach to creating and saving documents.

Always spell names of files and folders correctly, so that you can effectively use search tools to find them. Moreover, think about all the types of files you will be collecting before you have a large number. You may want to put all similar documents in the same folder. It does not matter what you call the folders as long as you can remember the names.

Naming Files

It takes a disciplined approach to naming files to be able to find them. It is best to use a descriptive term when you name a file. This will make it much easier to find later. It is also important to avoid special characters such as \ / : * ?" < > | in file names as the file may not open properly in learning management systems. The letters before the "." Are the filename and the letters after the "." are the extension (i.e., doc or PowerPoint). Do not change the extension unless you must for some compelling reason.

File names can be a couple of hundred characters long but it is rarely necessary to have the names longer than a few letters. Remember that the longer the file name, the more you have to type. The longer the file name, the greater the chance for a typo.

Word Processing, Editing

Word processing is the most common function related to education performed on a computer. It is surprising how much a word processing program can do. As mentioned earlier, it is best to get acquainted with the help index in all programs so that you can become familiar with the thousands of functions built into a program.

Nursing instructors use some specific features of word processing programs more than others. In addition to creation of documents, you can insert comments or corrections into a student's papers by using "track changes" or "insert comments" in Microsoft Word.

Keyboard Shortcuts

People learn to use computers and software on a "need to know" basis. As a result, many helpful features of a computer or software are never "discovered" and go unused. There are several things you can do to make sure you are always exploiting the useful features of your computer. Take time to look at the online help for the computer or software. The technical assistance index is usually accessed through the "help" link on the application toolbar or desktop of your computer. Make it a habit to search for additional information on common functions used. For example, everyone likes to save time—put the term "shortcuts" in the search box under Help. You will find several selections related to shortcuts. Select the link for "keyboard shortcuts." You find a lengthy list of keyboard shortcuts to save you time.

Another important feature of Windows and Macintosh operating systems is the ability to search for files and folders from the start menu. Assuming all files were named with a correctly spelled title, and you can remember it, you can search for files from the start menu or desktop. This saves you large amounts of time when you have hundreds of files stored on your computer.

Screenshots

Screenshots are an excellent learning tool for presentations, technical assistance, and demonstrating competence in computer skills. To take a picture of the computer screen at any given time press the "PrtScn" usually found on the top right of your keyboard. Place your cursor where you want to insert the screen shot. Think of it as a graphic. You can use screen shots to teach students how to use software; you can ask them to take screen shots of their completed online projects and place the images in PowerPoint presentations for many purposes. You can edit the size and crop sections of the image for use by right clicking the image to bring up the picture tool bar.

Templates and Macros

There are many timesaving features in most word processing and database applications. Taking the time to learn about these features is worthwhile. Templates are preformatted designs used in presentations, Web pages, documents, and spreadsheets. You can usually download additional templates from the developer and third-party providers. Some will be free, others will be available for a fee.

Macros, like templates, save users a great deal of time. Macros are small automated programs that help you execute common tasks with a few keystrokes. Use the help menu in the program to learn more about these features. Practice with simple functions to get accustomed to how they work then graduate to larger tasks.

Security and Privacy

There is no way to overemphasize the need for ensuring that your computer is secure and that all of your data files are backed up. There are many ways that you can easily back up files. The simplest and least expensive is to back up files on CD or other magnetic media. Newer forms of back up include external hard drives of all kinds. You can choose the size of the external hard drive to buy by assessing your budget and whether you want to back up the entire contents of your computer or only the data files. Programs are available to create a mirror image of your hard drive when there is a complete crash of the system or simply files you have created. You can copy and paste the files from your desktop computer to your portable hard drive or buy any one of a variety of software programs to do it automatically.

Security

Threats to your computer's safety and to your identity are part of the downside of the Internet. If you never use the Internet you have no problem, but once you open up e-mail, buy something online, or visit Web pages, your computer is vulnerable, as are you by unintentionally revealing private information about yourself. Although the threats are big, there are some low-cost ways to prevent the majority of potential attacks to you and your computer.

The most important **security** updates you will get are to the Microsoft Windows operating system. Be sure to set your Windows preferences to ask you automatically about installing updates. Routinely check Microsoft for security patches if you do not set the software to check for you automatically. Every piece of software you are using gets updated by the manufacturer on a regular basis. You will find it necessary to keep software updated to ensure that it works properly and you are able to get the most out of it. It is likely that you will need to download plug-ins to view multimedia or other Web content. Table 8–6 lists the most commonly used software plug-ins.

Antivirus software is an essential tool for anyone who opens e-mail attachments and visits Web sites. There are many commercial and free software programs available. Many campuses provide these programs free or at discounted rates. Viruses and other manmade creations that could destroy your files can also be stopped by firewall hardware, such as a router, which is relatively inexpensive and available at a local computer store. When you have a router installed, it creates a "wall" to the Internet. You can access the Internet, but Internet users cannot access your computer without your permission. Nevertheless, you can still have creators of Web sites place "spyware" on your computer. Spyware includes small files that track varying degrees of your Web surfing habits. There is "anti-spyware" software that is free or low-cost.

The bottom line of security and privacy is that a few ounces of prevention will save you many hours of headaches and frustration. Be sure to maintain up-to-date antivirus software, a firewall router, and anti-spyware software on your computer at all times.

Passwords and Hackers

It won't be long before you have a collection of user names and passwords for all types of Internet resources. It is critical that you manage these passwords in a way that protects your privacy. Most of us have far more than we can remember without writing them down. Do not keep them in your Outlook or other Internet accessible database.

Hackers often do not need to have expert programming skills to gain access to computers. They use **social engineering** principles to get access to confidential information in order to commit fraud, to destroy networks, or participate in other criminal activities. Social engineering is defined as the art and science of getting people to comply with your wishes. Social engineering

 TABLE 8–6 Common Software Plug-Ins

Multimedia plug-ins: Real Player, Windows Media Player, MPeg
Java for running online games
Shockwave
Macromedia Flash
Winzip or other unzipping utility

uses two primary areas of attack. First, someone posing as a student, staff, or faculty member may ask questions about passwords and access codes. Social engineers may ask one faculty member how many digits are in a password and call someone else and ask about the syntax or structure of a password. The second type of activity is someone simply watching how you use your computer. Perhaps someone comes to your office to pose as a student and get information about the program. The would-be hacker may be watching how and what you do to gain access to your university account. Position your computer away from doors so that people cannot watch your keystrokes or other computer activity.

Searching the Internet

The Internet is the most extensive collection of information ever created. Search engines such as Google, Yahoo, and Microsoft use very sophisticated and innovative programming intended to help us find what we are looking for in as short a time as possible. Search engines make their money from advertising sponsors. Although they are technically free to use, you will be exposed to many organizations trying to sell you products and services. The places you visit on the Internet, the length of time you stay at a site, and what you do there are all sources of valuable information to advertisers.

At the time of this publication, Google is considered the premiere search engine. Google uses your "search terms" much like a library database to locate what you want. There is a very extensive collection of instructions and tips for using Google at the site http://google.com. Spending an afternoon reading through some of the basic information on searching strategies will save you hours of time.

Accessing and Securing Help

No matter how many classes you take or books you read, you will still need to get additional help from time to time. The best place to get answers to your computer-related question is your university's help desk. Do not be discouraged if an answer is not immediately forthcoming when you ask a question. It may be that your question is the tip of a technological iceberg that is just attacking the university network. You may also be using a unique piece of software that does not communicate well with the established software on campus. Some questions will take time to answer properly. By posing questions, help desk staff can be alerted to potential widespread problems.

Always consult the online help in any software programs you have as well. Granted, it is often a challenge to find the right search terms, but you will never get an answer if you don't at least search the files. The next best source is posing questions in online groups. Start with users groups sponsored by the manufacturer of the product or the software developer.

Typically, the technical skills required include accessing the Internet, composing postings, managing attachments, organizing files and folders, and record keeping. Additional skills, outside of the nursing class, include searching library databases, using online plagiarism detection services, and completing other interactive online activities.

Technology Support of Higher Education

Universities use an impressive array of technology to manage student services, produce grades, secure networks, analyze data, support databases such as the library and student records, not to mention regulate sprinklers and lighting. This chapter focuses primarily on the uses of technology that provide learning management systems, produce content, or connect students and faculty. But it is worth a few paragraphs to discuss other campus uses of technology to introduce faculty who might be new to teaching. Three primary uses will be discussed: enrollment management systems, library services, and learning centers.

Enrollment Management

Students can apply, be admitted, take courses, and apply for graduation using the Web. In between, faculty members can look up student records of courses for advising, search for class lists, and get phones numbers of students, just to name a few of the hundreds of pieces of information available in university student record databases. You will find that there are many more security measures when using these systems than with e-mail or learning management systems.

Library

Libraries provide support to students and faculty in innumerable ways. Library databases—often password protected to download articles and other copyrighted information—are vast resources of information. Library technology changes as quickly as clinical and educational technology does. Be sure to plan time to visit your library and attend workshops. Start with a long look through the library Web site.

Learning Centers

University learning centers provide students with all types of support. Many traditional face-to-face services are now offered online. Be sure to check out the learning center at your college. Key tutoring services, such as writing assistance, are now readily available online. Students can upload their papers to the learning center Web site, have them reviewed and returned via e-mail.

If your university does not have online assistance with studies skills, such as writing or nursing content, consider using a text from a publisher that provides online help. Many textbook publishers are now bundling online tutoring services with text books.

Common Software Used in Teaching

Faculty typically uses a handful of computer programs routinely. In nursing, the most common software programs are Word and PowerPoint and calendar organizers, such as Outlook that also manage e-mail and contacts.

Electronic Mail

The good news is that e-mail provides us with instant access to people all over the world. The bad news is that e-mail provides us with instant access to people all over the world. As with most technology, it makes sense to take a proactive approach to e-mail. See Table 8–7 for an example of e-mail guidelines to give students. Be proactive yourself and use common methods of communication, such as blogs, threaded discussions, and Web pages to answer common questions.

Students will e-mail instructors to get answers to questions without thinking that time management is an issue for faculty, too. Because students have direct access to instructors by using e-mail 24/7, it is important to educate students regarding the proper behavior for seeking help and contacting faculty. Without knowing faculty expectations, students may overwhelm instructors' ability to answer individual e-mails.

TABLE 8–7 E-Mail Guidelines for Students

I. Use these guidelines to help you determine how to communicate best with your instructor. Each instructor will have her own standards for e-mail communication; be sure to ask each instructor.

II. Students need information on how to communicate best via e-mail with faculty. E-mail communication should only be used to gather information; it cannot be used to reach decisions. Examples of appropriate e-mail communication include setting a time for a phone appointment, obtaining clarification, or providing additional information as requested. Use all information sources at your disposal, BEFORE using e-mail. These include course syllabus, other students, texts and course readers, and "Questions about the Course" online discussion forum.

III. E-mail "do's"

- Create a signature in your e-mail program that will automatically include your name and phone number at the bottom of each e-mail; regularly update your antivirus program (Zone Alarm, Norton, McAfee), so that you can be sure your e-mail is secure and that you are protected from most viruses and worms.
- When you compose an e-mail, it must include the following:
  - Your full name and course number in the subject line
  - Text with complete sentences that thoroughly present your question or comment
  - All the previous communication on the subject (AOL users and others will have to set this option in their preferences)
  - Correct spelling and grammar
  - Professional tone
- Whenever you are responding or composing an e-mail, be sure to change the subject line as necessary.
- Wait 48 hours (Monday to Friday) before asking your instructor a second time if she got your e-mail.
- Always read your e-mail one more time before pressing the "Send" button.
- In all of your electronic conversations with instructors, remember that all of your instructors receive about 50–100 e-mails a day. When teaching online classes, the number can go up dramatically.
- If you receive an e-mail that causes a strong negative reaction, assume it is honest miscommunication, ask clarifying questions to check if your understanding of the e-mail content is correct.

IV. E-mail "don'ts"

- Don't send an e-mail without all the required information.
- Never send instructors a chain e-mail.
- E-mail is not for discussions about grades or course content. Office hours are for those discussions. You can come to the instructor's office during office hours or request a phone appointment at a mutually convenient time.
- Don't send an e-mail inquiring about your grade on a given assignment until 1 to 2 weeks after the assignment is due.
- Never open an attachment from someone you do not know.
- Don't use html coding in e-mails. Turn off the cute pictures, music, and graphics. These take a long time to download and are the biggest source of viruses.
- Don't expect an answer to e-mail over a weekend.

V. E-mail security

- You must actively maintain the security of your computer.
- You can download ZoneAlarm for free or your can buy Norton or Macafee antivirus programs.
- You also need to update your Microsoft products regularly. You can set your computer to do automatic updates; you do not have to do all of them, but always do the critical updates.

PowerPoint is the most commonly used presentation software. Some would say the most *overused* software. Even National Public Radio aired a show critiquing the overuse of PowerPoint in education (http://www.npr.org/templates/story/story.php?storyId=1467589). There is an emerging body of research about what makes a PowerPoint presentation that students remember. The most important point to remember is PowerPoint is an adjunct to the learning process and should be a support to the presentation of material. Suggested guidelines for PowerPoint are available on many Web sites. Ask a staff member in the faculty development department or multimedia services to help you design effective PowerPoint presentations. The rule of the day is *less is more*, when it comes to PowerPoint content. One Web site with clear directions is: http://info.wlu.edu/presentation/powerpoint.html.

One often underutilized tool in PowerPoint is the use of the pen while presenting the show. Find the pen by right clicking on the slide when you are in the slide show view. A menu will come up with several options. Select the "pointer options," then select "pen." Use the pen to mark slides. These marks are temporary; they will disappear once the slide is advanced. This can be a very helpful option to help call attention to specific parts of a slide.

Referencing and Formatting Software

There are a variety of software programs, both stand alone and add-ins to Word, that help organize references and format papers in APA and other styles. Some templates can be found free at the online Microsoft template gallery, but most are available for purchase. Check out the university bookstore on your campus for information and cost for programs such as Format Ease, Citation, Reference Manager, and EndNotes.

Statistical Software

Many faculty members use statistical software in research and evaluation of their teaching effectiveness. SPSS is the most common statistical software program used on campuses. Version 16.0 is currently available and can analyze just about any type of data used in the social sciences (Boslaugh, 2005).

Faculty and Student Web Pages

Web pages are the most convenient and effective way to deliver online content to campus and distance students. Students do not have to search around in online classes to find material such as grading tools, technical assistance, and course links. Consider starting your use of technology with a simple Web page. Templates are readily available. In a couple of hours you could have a basic Web page with your contact information and study guides for a class. One tip—always put your e-mail address in a text box so "bots" or automated tools that collect e-mail addresses off the Web cannot find it easily. This will save you from some spam or unwanted e-mail. Table 8–8 and Box 8–3 discusses the computer and the environment.

Technological Quicksand–Intellectual Property

Technology has made a lot of tasks much easier. Most of these tasks, like searching library databases, used to be time-consuming. Now students can search library databases easily from home any time they like. Finding information on the Internet is easy. There are unlimited sources of

Nursing is a profession based on caring, not only for patients but for the environment. Using computers actually threatens the environment in many ways. First, toxic materials are used in the creation of a computer. Materials such as lead, mercury, and arsenic are examples of a few of the *many* hazardous materials inside a personal desktop computer (www.handyharman.com).

Computers and related products become obsolete very quickly and become "e-waste." Often e-waste is produced in higher volumes than other consumer types of trash. More and more computers and other electronic material are considered disposable and individuals replace the equipment rather than repair it as in years past. "The average lifespan of a computer has shrunk from 4 or 5 years to 2 years (Hara & Kling, 1999; National Safety Council, Electronic Product Recovery and Recycling Baseline Report).

Another important consideration in using computers is the rate of paper use. Students can be taught simple techniques for cutting down on the use of paper. Techniques such as always using "print preview" before printing will alert them to issues with formatting or other problems that would require multiple attempts at printing a document. See Table 8–8 for some environmentally friendly suggestions.

information at the tips of a computer user's fingers. But with all of this information, students need to understand how to evaluate information of all kinds for accuracy and relevance. Such an evaluation is called **"information competence"** or **"information literacy."**

The American Library Association. *Presidential Committee on Information Literacy. Final Report* (Chicago: American Library Association, 1989) defines "information literacy" as a set of

TABLE 8–8 Environmentally Friendly Suggestions for Using Your Computer

- Use print preview instead of printing drafts—read from the screen.
- Use both sides of paper for drafts.
- Use recycled paper products only.
- Use recycled ink cartridges and soy-based inks when possible.
- Recycle your own ink cartridges.
- Set the printing on your computer to "draft" or the setting that uses the least amount of ink.
- Statistics vary on the amount of electricity used by computers; they range from 2% to 8% of the world's energy. Turn off your computer when not in use.
- Sign up for distributed computing, which means that your computer's unused space can be used for advancing science. Consider being a part of research through http:ud.com—this organization unites computer users all over the world in cancer research.
- When you buy new equipment be sure to dispose of your computer appropriately; there is hazardous material in computers.
- Insist that the manufacturer of your computer products dispose of old equipment in this country rather than shipping to third world countries. (Exporting the Harm: The High Tech Trashing of Asia http://www.svtc.org/cleancc/pubs/technotrash.htm)
- Join the Clean Computer Campaign: http://www.svtc.org/cleancc/pubs/technotrash.htm
- Even computer disks can be recycled. Contact Green Disk at http://www.greendisk.com/ to get information on how to recycle computer disks.
- Share Technology helps find sources to donate or recycle old computers. http://sharetechnology.org/

abilities requiring individuals to "recognize when information is needed and have the ability to locate, evaluate, and use effectively the needed information." Unfiltered information includes the Internet, political action groups, and all types of print and broadcast media. Teaching students to evaluate the accuracy, validity, and reliability of information is crucial to developing effective habits for lifelong learning. Without understanding some basic concepts of information literacy, the shear amount of information available to students will easily confuse and overwhelm them.

Academic Dishonesty

A second and equally worrisome aspect of using technology in education is the ease of copying information and using it improperly. All forms of academic dishonesty are on the rise, but plagiarism is becoming increasingly commonplace. Two types of plagiarism include paper recycling and the "copy and paste" method of using information on the Internet without including an attribution to the original author or source. Although technology makes this easier, technology also provides some possible solutions to enhancing academic integrity and identifying plagiarism. Students react positively to using it when the entire purpose is described to them in advance of using the service. They upload and download their own papers and results and receive additional information on the incidence of plagiarism and how to avoid it. Talking about plagiarism is an excellent introduction to the need for learning formatting techniques, such as those presented by the American Psychological Association (APA).

Teaching Using Distance Technology and Distance Learning

Students in general have high expectations of instructors. In online classes, students often expect 24/7 access to instructors. Be clear with students about when and how often you will be online. Let students know how to contact you if they are having difficulty. Student ratings of instructional effectiveness are often the key to continuing employment, not to mention tenure. Students are more likely to rate an online instructor positively when the expectations are clearly spelled out in class. Using the seven Principles of Undergraduate Education will help guide you in developing your own teaching style. The seven principles can be found at http://www.tltgroup.org/programs/seven.html. Students often have misconceptions about online education. The most common misconception is that an online class is easier and less time-consuming than a traditional class. ←yes!₀

Distance Learning

Distance learning is a broad category of instructional methods that involves a multitude of technology. Programs often include more than one distance learning technique. The first distance learning programs were correspondence courses. Since those first programs were started, distance nursing programs now involve interactive video, online, and combinations of the methods.

Technology is best used when it enhances interactivity between faculty and students and students and students. Technology must be used effectively so that learning occurs with a reasonable expenditure of time and effort on the part of the students and faculty. Distance learning programs must maintain the same high academic standards as traditional courses. New instructors may mistakenly think that distance courses have different outcomes based on the technology used. But the nursing program curriculum should not be influenced by the technology used. Of course, adaptations of learning methods must occur when technology is used. Best practices also incorporate strategies to support diverse methods of learning. As with traditional courses, distance learning is most effective when multiple methods of instruction are used. Importantly, students should receive prompt feedback on their work. The following discussion describes practical methods for applying the best practices in nursing education programs that use technology.

Interactivity

Interactivity is accomplished relatively easily using distance technology. Many instructors incorporate online communication strategies into traditional courses to augment the communication. There are many types of technologically mediated online discussions. The lowest threshold communications strategies are discussion boards on a faculty Web page, e-mail listservs, or Web logs also called blogs. These methods of increasing interactivity are all very effective. Discussion forums in learning management systems, online group chats, and Web casts are examples of other technologies that can be used to bring students and faculty closer together virtually.

Blogs

Web logs, also known as blogs, are emerging as a writing tool that is easy to use. They are Internet-based, and can enhance health professionals' writing, communication, collaboration, reading, and information-gathering skills. Students from different disciplines, such as medicine, public health, business, library science, and journalism, garner knowledge from blogs as innovative educational tools. The use of blogs as an interactive and effective educational method, has not been well documented by nurse educators. See Table 8–9 on giving writing instructions to students.

Student to Student

Several techniques can be used to increase student-to-student interaction in distance programs. Threaded discussions around course content provide the backbone of interactivity between students and faculty in a distance learning program. Threaded discussions can be designed to include the entire class or groups. Creating group assignments, with clearly described individual responsibilities, is an effective way to increase student-to-student interaction online. Students can be held accountable for threaded discussions by providing them with clear expectations and grading criteria (see Tables 8–10 and 8–11).

Other types of discussion forums can be used to increase informal interactivity. Using the learning management system, Web page or blog, a threaded discussion can be created that focuses on "Questions About the Course." This threaded discussion saves the faculty time spent answering e-mail questions about general course-related topics. It also helps students answer questions about the course for other students. It is necessary to monitor this discussion thread to ensure that

TABLE 8–9 SOAP for Online Discussions

When you are composing instructions for writing anything, it is important to include all the necessary information in the instructions. The SOAP acronym is well known in the documentation of patient care. However, the SOAP acronym is also used to ensure your writing prompts give students all the information they need. Consider using the SOAP acronym to design the prompt for online discussions.

S	Subject: information regarding who or what the piece is about
O	Occasion: the writing situation
A	Audience: the intended audience
P	Purpose: to express, to inform, to persuade

TABLE 8–10 Discussion Participation Guidelines

In order to receive full credit for posting:

Include references to the text and other required reading material.

Do not respond to every posting individually. Use the collect feature and consolidate postings.

Change the subject line to reflect your posting.

You can ask questions, suggest alternative explanations for another student's interpretation of material.

Let your thinking show. Show off how much you know about a course. Give examples from your clinical experience.

Do not simply post, "I agree."

For longer postings, use your word processor so you can use spell checker.

Use emoticons and other changes in words and space to emphasize your meaning.

Remember, ALL CAPS is reserved for strong emphasis, usually when you are angry.

Post page numbers and references when answering questions.

Show how you apply the concepts from readings (the text and articles) in your answers.

Spelling and grammar are correct.

The postings are timely.

You can compare and contrast various student points of view.

Maintain consistency with the thread discussion.

The posting should follow the main thread, rather than creating a new posting.

---

the responses are accurate. Not only does this save instructor time, but it also is a great source of information to an instructor when updating a course syllabus; the instructor can include answers to common questions in future syllabi.

A second threaded discussion called "Student Lounge" or something similar helps students get to know each other and eliminates social discussion from course-related discussions. Students, especially students new to online communication methods, may not stick to a specified topic. Threaded discussions for the purpose of socializing give students an outlet to communicate about issues not specified in the curriculum. Instructors should make sure students know if instructors will be participating in these discussions.

 TABLE 8–11 Grading Online Discussions

Open up the "item" you are grading so only one shows at a time.

Be sure to sort the discussion forum by author so you can see quickly if the student met the guidelines for participation. To do this, scroll to the bottom of the page and click on "sort by" author.

Moving between the discussion board and the grade book, you can respond to groups of answers and grade the postings at the same time.

To begin the grading, use the collect feature and select one thread of five to six postings.

Several postings will then show up (remember you will not be able to view attachments using this method).

You can respond to only one posting when using collect.

You will be able to acknowledge these postings easily and then move on to the next small group of postings.

Move between your open windows by clicking on the names of the programs you want (review grading rubric for discussions in Chapter 12).

"Technical Angst"

Another type of online discussion forum can be called something to the effect of, "Technical Angst." This forum presents an opportunity for students to express their technical frustrations. Often, new computer users experience a steep learning curve when using new forms of learning technology. The technical angst threaded discussion is an informal method for venting frustration. Instructors should read this discussion and offer advice and tips.

When you are using online communication it is important to make a few decisions about the course structure related to breaches of netiquette and flame wars. Students should know in advance if you will be deleting any inappropriate messages or if you will request that they delete a message, Web page, or posting. If you are using a learning management system such as Blackboard or Web Ct, you can set a preference for the threaded discussion to be locked or to be edited by the user. Some instructors reserve this right for themselves. The point is to think about it and let students know what your standards are and how inappropriate postings will be addressed.

Make students feel welcome in distance classrooms. Students form quick first impressions in distance classrooms just like in traditional classrooms. It is important to have your online course and your interactive video classroom ready to receive students from the first class. Just a few teaching methodologies that work well in a distance class are listed in Table 8–12.

Interactive Video Instruction

Interactive video is a widely used form of technology that uses audio and video feeds to sites distant from the campus. Interactive video connects the video presence of the instructor with one or more (sometimes eight to 10) sites at campuses anywhere in the world. Often, the courses are supported by an online course site in Blackboard, which eases the challenge of getting documents to distance sites. This section will review some of the key issues for nursing faculty using this method of instruction alone or as a hybrid with other instructional methods.

Advance Preparation

As with all courses, teaching using interactive video instruction (IVI) requires thoughtful preparation in advance of the course. Often this preparation includes providing directions for the facilitator at the distant site or for students if there is no facilitator.

The guidelines discussed earlier are as relevant in the IVI course as any other. Effective teaching strategies allow students from all sites to interact with each other, with the faculty, and make use of multiple instructional techniques. Making students feel welcome and individually noticed can be the most challenging in an IVI classroom as you are often only able to see one or a few sites at a time. There are some techniques, however, that you can use to get to know students at other sites.

TABLE 8–12 Examples of Lessons Used in Distance Classes

Debates
Dialogues
Role play
Death awareness

Full instructions on these various teaching-learning strategies are listed in Appendix A.

1. Who drives the farthest to get to their site?
2. How many students have a nurse as a mother or other relative?
3. Who has the most children?
4. When was the last time someone in the class was publicly acknowledged for a job well done?
5. Who has the oldest living parent?
6. Who has the most pets?
7. Who was born the farthest from the campus?

Use some type of informal interaction during the planning stage of the class. Use the list of general questions in Table 8–13 to help students get to know each other and learn more about the instructor.

To make the IVI classroom more personal, consider starting classes with humorous actives, like singing, juggling, or playing humorous short clips from movies. There is no end to the creativity that can be used to get students excited about learning.

The biggest challenge in the IVI classroom is handling student questions. It is necessary to plan, in advance, how you will handle student questions. You may have students hold questions until certain points in the presentation or you may also have students submit questions via e-mail if there is computer access. The point is to assess the resources you have and use them to both encourage and manage interaction with students. Use a method that first increases student-to-student interaction. This can be done by leaving periods of time that let students ask and answer questions at each site. The students can then ask you questions that cannot be answered by others in the class.

Plan time to practice with the technology you will be using. Have the technicians who will be helping you record a presentation arrange it so that you can see yourself giving a class. Watch IVI courses delivered on public television, cable, or satellite services.

Preparation for Each Class Session

The preparation for IVI classes is similar to that of traditional classes. Preparation starts by arriving on time to ensure that the room is set up for the class and video is connected to all sites. The most common challenge is the dilemma of whether to start if all sites are not hooked up at the beginning of class. All of the classes are videotaped by the staff in the control room. It is possible to send copies of the entire lecture to sites that were not hooked up. Those tapes can also be posted on a secure Web site for repeated viewing by students.

During the Class

Start the class with an ice breaker described previously or design your own. This will give students time to settle into class and get to know each other. Help the facilitator ensure that students respect each other and maintain the same behavior standards as a traditional classroom. You may even want students to design their own behavior guidelines to reinforce their ownership of the classroom and commitment to each other.

When students speak, ask them to refocus the camera on the person speaking. Have students give their names when they speak. Encourage them to wait just a moment before speaking as it takes a couple of seconds for the camera to train on the person speaking and activate the sound transmission. Other important guidelines for IVI classes are listed in Table 8–14.

TABLE 8–14 Important Guidelines for IVI Classes

Keep the microphone muted when not speaking.

Microphones only send the sound over the transmission line; they do not amplify your voice like traditional microphones, be sure to speak up.

Use a Web site, e-mail, or online course system to ensure that students have the necessary support material for each class.

Intervene early when students are disrupting the class, discuss appropriate classroom behavior with the entire group. Call student after class when behavior is not acceptable.

Follow the same reporting guidelines for disruptive student behavior that are used on the campus.

Ensure that everyone has the technical assistance phone numbers and contact information.

Send an e-mail to all students welcoming them to the class and giving your contact information.

Keep copies of the tape recordings of classes; you can use these recordings to demonstrate your teaching skill and evaluate your presentation skills.

Know the facilitators at the distant sites, keep in regular contact with them, remind them about the objectives for class each week and their role in ensuring success for the students.

Carefully prepare PowerPoint material. Your image is often projected on top of the slides, in one of the corners. Leave room on your slides to ensure your video image does not obscure the material on the slide.

When students are going to make presentations in the video classroom, be sure to help them know what type of media is available and how to prepare the technical aspects of their presentation.

Provide students with a set of guidelines such as those in Table 8–15. Other guidelines also are important to consider. Fair use and copyright guidelines must be followed in the IVI classroom. Showing commercial videos and other media must meet the fair use standards. Check with your campus **intellectual property** officer if you are not sure what can be shown in an IVI classroom. Do not be afraid to ask publishers for permission to show their instructional material.

Assessment Strategies

Every class should involve some type of informal or formal assessment strategies. One important consideration in getting ready to use technology is to become knowledgeable about your department's assessment plan. Ask to see assessment reports and other evaluations of course design. You might also ask for a colleague to come to your class, whether online or other format, to give you feedback on your techniques.

Other Supportive Methods of Instruction Using Technology

Although this chapter presents many uses for different types of technology, there are still many more. The following is a list of potential uses of technology that are suitable for any type of course format.

Virtual Office Hours

Students may not be able to talk to you during your regular office hours. Using online chats, instant messaging, or other online tools can be an excellent way to talk to students about course content, advise them about their course of study, or give other forms of support.

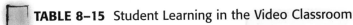

TABLE 8–15 Student Learning in the Video Classroom

Learning in the video classroom is similar to learning in traditional classrooms in many ways. There are, however, some important differences that you need to understand.

Similarities to a Traditional Classroom
There are other students in the classroom with you.
There is an instructor leading the class.
You can ask questions of the instructor.
You will be asked to respond to questions by the instructor.

Differences from Traditional Classrooms
Your classroom is not the only one connected to the instructor; there can be as many as eight other sites connected at the same time.
You will see the instructor, but not other students who are also connected.
The instructor only sees the last group of students who spoke.
In order to be heard, you need to use a microphone.
When you are submitting assignments, you may be submitting them online, via the facilitator in the room, or other means.

Your Role in the Video Classroom
Your role as an actively involved student in the video classroom is similar to other classrooms.
Come to class prepared to participate.
Do not speak while the instructor is speaking.
If you will be making presentations, be sure to come early and practice with the technology in the room.
Keep a copy of everything you turn in.
Pick up after yourself.
Don't move microphones, tables with microphones attached, or cameras unless directed by facilitator.
Treat all equipment with care.
When speaking to the instructor, either asking a question or responding, realize there is a slight delay in the sound and video transmission; make a couple of introductory sentences and wait for the instructor to acknowledge you.
If you experience difficulty hearing or seeing the broadcast, notify the facilitator immediately.
If you have individualized questions or issues with the broadcast faculty member, contact her individually.

Chats, Test Preparation, Test Review

More and more faculty members are encouraging students to study using the online chat feature in learning management systems. Faculty may or may not participate in these sessions. Chats work well for preparation and review for quizzes and tests. An added feature of most chat tools allows for you to save a transcript of the discussion; this transcript can help you prepare students more effectively for tests in the future.

Summary

Technology has developed to the point of being a wonderfully innovative and unavoidable addition to the educational process of nursing students. Using technology has vast possibilities for nursing faculty. Technology in the right doses, format, and with the appropriate resources can effectively address the cognitive, affective, and psychomotor learning domains of the student. Technology can be integrated into every aspect of the teaching process for nurses. It can be used to assess learning needs of the student, plan innovative ways to facilitate learning, use a variety of methodologies to accomplish teaching-learning objectives, and be an evaluation mechanism alone or with traditional strategies. Many of the "how to" and "where to go to find" aspects have been included in this chapter to assist the novice and advance the expert nurse educators in their quest for teaching excellence but the possibilities for the use of technology in nursing education are endless. Technology is and will remain an intricate and innovative part of nursing education. By following some of the links and ideas provided in this chapter you have taken steps to enhance the education process for future nurses. Table 8–16 gives many ideas for creative teaching exercises.

TABLE 8–16 Debates, Dialogues, Role Play, and Death Awareness Exercises

Before the debate, your group must thoroughly research the area of debate. Although you will be presenting content you have prepared ahead of time, you will also be responding to the argument presented by the other team. It is necessary for you to have as comprehensive an understanding of your topic as possible. It is also important to know something in advance about the "other side" of the issue so you can anticipate what facts, analogies, and arguments will be presented by your opponents.

All of your preparatory material should be posted online and shared with your instructor, via the drop box. You also will need to post a sheet with all references, APA style 5th edition. Each issue will be debated by a panel of students. Size of teams will vary according to the number of students at a site. Each team thus has the following primary responsibilities.

The Pro Side

The pro side will be primarily responsible for stating the position taken by its group. Members will bring up, point by point, the issues inherent in each part of the argument. A prepared written statement is required. The pro side should post a formal document that outlines the key issues of the debate. The initial statement should be two to three screen lengths.

Think of this as a comprehensive introduction to the topic. Introductions outline what will be presented and define the scope of the argument. An analogy of this portion of a debate is the opening argument of a trial.

The Con Side

This is the substantive part of the argument and ALL members of the team must participate equally in its development. The con side will be responsible for citing relevant research to back any of the statements given by the stater. Members must have intimate knowledge of the empirical (objective) content of the positions taken and should understand the research supporting the side chosen.

The way you present an argument in a paper, is much the same as the way you present your argument on the topic in the format. You propose a thesis statement and then systematically develop or substantiate the thesis statement. The initial statement should be three to four screen lengths.

The Critiquers

Critiquers will be responsible for probing the opposite team for weaknesses in its arguments. They may question data, disprove, counter, and use any rational method to discredit the opposition's position or data. An appreciation for research design and data analysis may help the critiquer. It is also strongly suggested that the critiquer be very familiar with the articles and materials being used by the opposing team.

TABLE 8–16 (continued)   **153**

The Audience

The students not involved in a debate are still a part of the situation. Two kinds of audience participation will be expected: clarification and question. The rest of the students in the class are expected to evaluate the debates and question participants at the end of the presentation to ask questions and clarify issues.

The Procedure

Day One: Pro and Con sides upload their position statements.
Day Two: Students read postings, make notes, and find errors and omissions from the arguments.
Day Three: Pro and con sides upload their responses to the appropriate forums.
Day Four: Students read postings, making notes, and find errors and omissions from the arguments.
Day Five: Critiquers upload their responses to the arguments of the pro and con sides.
Day Six: All students complete evaluation forms and submit to the instructor. Online discussion is held and the rest of the students ask questions and make comments. Be sure to include issues you found in the arguments in your critique.

Where to get information on your topic:

Texts—current and prior

Online library—journal articles

Internet, only if the site meets intellectual standards

Interviews with experts in the field

Professional standards

Position statements

Government documents

Guide to fallacies in arguments: http://www.intrepidsoftware.com/fallacy/toc.htm

Site to evaluate Web data: http://www.indiana.edu/~librcsd/eval/review.html

Active Learning Through Dialogue

The famous physicist David Bohm described a form of communication that is aimed, not at solving problems, but at creating understanding. Bohm said: "… it is proposed that a form of free dialogue may well be one of the most effective ways of investigating the crisis which faces society, and indeed the whole of human nature and consciousness today." (See http://www.muc.de/~heuvel/dialogue/index.html.)

I have found this to be a powerful tool in helping students and others become aware of factors affecting their own lives and the lives around them. It is also a very effective method for obtaining input from the voiceless members of a group who rarely speak or have cultural backgrounds that inhibit sharing their own ideas, contradicting figures of authority, and other patterns of demonstrating autonomy.

Procedure

Have students sit in a circle. After you explain the rules, there is no discussion until the first participant speaks, it can be anyone. Once someone has spoken, participation moves to the left of the first person to speak. Each member of the group has a turn to share. If someone does not want to speak when her or his turn comes, the person says "pass."

Rules

See http://www.muc.de/~heuvel/dialogue/dialogue_proposal.html#

All conversation stays in the room (can be hard if supervisors and staff nurses are present together).

No interrupting, wait your turn.

(table continued on page 154)

TABLE 8–16 Debates, Dialogues, Role Play, and Death Awareness Exercises (continued)

You may talk about whatever is on your mind.

No judging of comments.

No speaking directly to someone else—no conversations, say what is on your mind, do not answer questions posed by someone else.

Use "I" statements.

The facilitator may want to pose a question if there are time limits, for example: What are the stresses and tensions of returning to school?

The dialogue proceeds around the room until everyone has spoken once or however many turns you have time for. In my experience, students often cry. There is so much tension in their lives that even a few seconds of silence and reflection provokes a strong emotional reaction. You may want to have facial tissue available if you think your group is very stressed.

Role-Play Example
Objectives

To give students, especially those from backgrounds of white privilege, insight into the experience of other cultures.

To appreciate some of the issues in cross-cultural communication.

Develop an understanding of at least one other culture norms, values, language, customs

Preparation: Students:

Students self-select or are assigned a cultural group to research and present.

Students are instructed to research their cultural group, in preparation for an online course assignment. The assignment can be directed or nondirected. For example, you may want the students to "simply" introduce themselves in a group discussion and learn as much as they can about others in the group. You may want them to discuss a specific topic pertinent to the course using the frame of reference of the culture as they understand it.

Assignment: Online

Students reenroll in the course, using a name they have selected based on their research. During the duration of this assignment, this is the login name they use.

A forum is set up where the discussion takes place. All discussion is restricted to this area of the online course.

On the first day of the assignment, students introduce themselves with their new name, giving information about:

• Where they are from in their country of origin.

• Their family or origin, who their mother and father are, and siblings.

• Are other family members residents of the household?

• You could suggest they give career goals, life goals, anything that brings out where the student is in relation to their culture of origin. The student is encouraged to reflect on whether their own goals reflect the larger culture or have they chosen their own way?

• The students should also be engaging other students in a discussion of their culture and what they are presenting to the group.

Ideas for discussion questions:

Newspaper headings

Birth control, child birth practices

Access to health care

Access to higher education

Professional roles

Gender issues

Issues related to aging

Death bed practices

Once the activity is over (I would suggest a week-long discussion), then you can have a period of reflection on what it was like to be "from another culture."

TABLE 8–16 (continued)   155

Death Awareness Activity

All students make a random list of the following information:

Two people you love the most

Two roles you want to continue the most

Two most cherished dreams

Two most important possessions

Two activities most desired

Once everyone has written down the list, and numbered them from 1 to 10, the instructor randomly directs students to cross off half of the list, or more

Online

The instructor will leave a message in the forum and announce "Cross off #3."

Or the instructor can say in a chat—cross off #3.

Continue with this until the activity is done.

Throughout the activity encourage students to reflect on what losing these items means to them.

Once the activity is done, talk about how this experience parallels the experience of dying for some people, especially those who gradually lose their abilities. Ask students to describe what is left of their life. They can talk about if the remaining items on the list would make a meaningful life or not.

Students can reflect on their experiences caring for people who are close to death and the amount of suffering they expressed.

R e f e r e n c e s

Blenner, J. (1991). Researcher for a day: A simulation game. *Nurse Educator, 16*(3), 32–35.

Bloom, B., Englehart, M., Furst, E., Hill, W., & Krathwohl, D. (1956). *Taxonomy of educational objectives: The classification of educational goals. Handbook I: Cognitive domain.* New York, Toronto: Longmans, Green. Available at: **http://chiron.valdosta.edu/whuitt/col/cogsys/bloom.html.** Retrieved December 18, 2005.

Boslaugh, S. (2005). *An intermediate guide to SPSS programming: Using syntax for data management* (p.231). Sage Publications.

Britt, R. (2006). Online education: A survey of faculty and students. *Radiologic Technology, 77*(3), 183–190.

Clark, D., Frith, K., & Demi, A. (2004). The physical, behavioral, and psychosocial consequences of Internet use in college students. *Computers, Informatics, Nursing, 22*(3), 153–161.

Chikering, A., & Gamson, A. (1987). *Seven principles for good practice in undergraduate education.* AAHE Bulletin. Available at: **http://www.aahe.org/bulletin/sevenprinciples1987.htm.** Retrieved July 25, 2004.

Flashlight Online available at **http://www.tltgroup.org/** Retrieved December 18, 2005.

Fuszard, B. (Ed.). (1995). *Innovative teaching strategies in nursing.* Gaithersburg, MD: Aspen Publishers.

Hara, N., & Kling, R. (1999). A case study of students' frustrations with a Web-based distance education course. *First Monday, 4*(12). from: **http://www.firstmonday.org/issues/issue4_12/hara/index.html.** Retrieved on July 25, 2004.

Klein, J., Moon, Y., & Picard, R. (2002). The computer responds to user frustrations. *Theory, Design and Results, 14,* 119–140.

Knowles, M., Holton, W., & Swanson, R. (1998). *The adult learner.* Woburn: MA: Butterworth-Heinemann Publications.

Ko, S., & Rossen, S. (2001). *Teaching online: A practical guide.* New York: Houghton Mifflin Company.

Lindsay, W., & McClaren, S. (2000). The Internet: An aid to student research or frustration? *Journal of Educational Media, (25)* 2; 115–128.

Marcoulides, G., Stocker, O., & Marcoulides, L. (2004). Examining the psychological impact of computer technology. *Educational and Psychological Measurement, (64)* 2; 311–318.

O'Regan, K. (2003). Emotion and E-Learning. *Journal of Asynchronous Learning Networks, 7*(3). Retrieved July 26, 2004 from **http://aln.org/publications/jaln/v7n3/index.asp.**

Ridley, R. T. (2004). Classroom games are COOL: Collaborative opportunities of learning. *Nurse Educator, 29*(2), 47–48.

Roueche, J. E., Milliron, M. D., & Roueche, S. D. (2003). *Practical magic: On the front lines of teaching excellence.* Washington, DC: American Association of Community Colleges. Retrieved July 26, 2004 from **http://www.eduweb.com/likelearn.html.**

Wargo, C. (2000). Gaming to reinforce learning about disseminated intravascular coagulation. *Journal of Continuing Education in Nursing, 31,* 149–151.

Weil, M., & Rosen, L. (1997). *Coping with technology: @home @work @play.* New York: Wiley.

Wurman, R. S. (2001). *Information anxiety 2.* Indianapolis, IN: Que Publications.

W e b   R e s o u r c e s

The BEST comics around—ask for permission to use! **http://www.glasbergen.com/**

Want a fun site to assess computer skills—without doing a "test."
    http://www.funderstanding.com/k12/coaster/

Don't create a lesson plan without first checking here! **http://www.merlot.org**

Microsoft templates: **http://officeupdate.microsoft.com/templategallery/**

Free PowerPoint templates: **http://www.presentersuniversity.com/downloads/index.cfm**

Wonderful online tutorials for Microsoft products. **http://tutorials.beginners.co.uk/index**

All kinds of great tests, some fun some serious. **http://www.queendom.com**

My Faculty Web Page. **http://faculty.fullerton.edu/mstoner**

Interesting online game about health-care policy and medial malpractice. **http://www.**
    takebackillinoisgame.com/play.aspx.

A nursing faculty Web site with very important tutorials for nursing students including APA and PowerPoint.
    http://drgwen.com

Flame warriors. **http://redwing.hutman.net/~mreed/**

Estimate the time you have to live. **http://deathclock.com**

The BEST writing center on the Web—if you have a question you can find the answer here:
    http://owl.english.purdue.edu/

REVIEW QUESTIONS

- Describe how you would prepare each online teaching/learning session for a class in your specialty.
- List ways to decrease technostress for students.
- Develop an introduction for an online class that contains the notion of e-mail etiquette.
- Synthesize the principles of ergonomics to fit your particular students' needs.
- Dialogue about some of the psychomotor, cognitive, and affective considerations you would have during an online lesson format.
- How would you deal with technological failures?
- Explain some gaming techniques that will help the students learn the principles of the content presented (Wargo, 2000).

CRITICAL THINKING EXERCISES

Use Google Scholar to find one answer to a question posed in any chapter in your book.

Review the list of Google labs and use one, provide a two-sentence critique of the lab and tell others if they should or should not use it.

Use Google image search and find the funniest picture or cartoon you can. Select a topic from the textbook. Post the link (NOT the image) online.

Should you allow anonymous postings on a discussion thread?

ANNOTATED RESEARCH SUMMARY

Maag, M. (2005), The potential use of "blogs" in nursing education. *Computers, informatics, nursing, 23*(1), 16–24.

The purpose of this article is to explore and present an innovative method of publishing on the Internet as a motivating learning tool for health-care students in higher-education settings and to look at the tools and the necessary steps used for this burgeoning technology. Web logs, also known as blogs, are an emerging writing tool that are easy to use, are Internet-based, and can enhance health professionals' writing, communication, collaboration, reading, and information-gathering skills. Health-care professionals are expected to be competent in the use of information technology to be able to effectively communicate, manage information, diminish medical error, and support decision-making. However, the use of blogs as an interactive and effective educational method has not been well documented by nurse educators. Nurses and other health-care professionals are required to have effective communication skills. The ability to write clearly is necessary to communicate patients' needs, medical data, and contribute to the body of health profession research. Furthermore, health-care professionals are poised to advocate preventive health-care measures through education. Suggestions for educators who are interested in using Web log technology in their courses are provided.

Alexander, J. G. (2002). Promoting, applying, and evaluating problem-based learning in the undergraduate nursing curriculum. *Nursing Education Perspectives, 23*(5), 248–253.

Since its development in the 1960s, problem-based learning (PBL) has become increasingly prominent in nursing education. In 1998, Stamford University received a grant from the PEW Charitable Trusts to promote, apply, and evaluate PBL in its undergraduate curriculum over 3 years. It has become integrated into the nursing curriculum in clinical and nonclinical courses.

Descriptions of its implementation in specific courses are provided, and its usefulness in nursing education discussed. Evaluations and test scores indicate that PBL has had a positive effect on the students and exceeded the educational expectations.

Beers, G. W. (1995). The effect of teaching method on objective test scores: problem-based learning versus lecture. *Journal of Nursing Education, 44*(7), 305–309.

This study investigated the effect of teaching method on objective test scores of students in a school of nursing. The hypothesis stated that there was a difference between objective test scores of students who were taught content on diabetes using problem-based learning (PBL) and students taught the same content using the traditional lecture method. A pre-test and post-test were administered to both groups of students. Both the pre-test and post-test scores of the two groups were compared using an independent test, and no statistically significant difference was found in the scores of the two groups. The results of this study show no difference in objective test scores based on teaching method.

Browne, M. N., Freeman, K. E., & Williamson, C. L. (2000). The importance of critical thinking for student use of the Internet. *College Student Journal, 34*(4). http://static.highbeam.com/c/collegestudentjournal/september012000 /

Students are increasingly so dependent on the Internet for their information that critical thinking programs that do not address the form and quality of persuasion on that medium are flirting with an anachronistic pedagogy. This paper documents the absorption of postsecondary students with the Internet as a source of "knowledge," spells out the attendant dangers, and suggests the essential first step in applying critical thinking to the Internet.

Burbach, M. E., Matkin, G. S., & Fritz, S. M. (2004). Teaching critical thinking in an introductory leadership course utilizing active learning strategies: A confirmatory study. *College Student Journal, 38*(3). http://static.highbeam.com/c/collegestudentjournal/september012004/

Critical thinking is often seen as a universal goal of higher education but is seldom confirmed as an outcome. This study was conducted to determine whether an introductory level college leadership course that encouraged active learning increased critical thinking skills. A pre- and post-assessment of critical thinking skills were conducted using the Watson-Glaser Critical Thinking Appraisal. Significant increases were found in the Deduction and Interpretation subtests, and total Critical Thinking. Student engagement in active learning techniques within the context of studying interpersonal skills for leadership appeared to increase critical thinking.

Cotton, K. (1988). Classroom Questioning Close-up No. 5. School Improvement Research Series. Portland, OR: Northwest Regional Educational Laboratory.

This study synthesizes findings from 37 research reports on the relationship between teacher classroom questioning behavior and a variety of student outcomes. The study found that when teachers ask higher-cognitive questions, conduct redirection/probing/reinforcement, and/or increase wait time, the cognitive sophistication of student responses increases.

Drummond, T. (2002). *A brief summary of the best practices in teaching: Intended to challenge the professional development of all teachers.* **Seattle, WA: North Seattle Community College. http://northonline.sccd.ctc.edu/eceprog/bstprac.htm**

A thorough summary of best practices in instructional methods.

Fry-Welch, D. K. (2004). Use of threaded discussion to enhance classroom teaching of critical evaluation of the professional literature. *Journal of Physical Therapy Education, 18*(2),48–53.

Reflective thinking is important in developing critical-thinking skills necessary to critically evaluate the professional literature. Use of threaded discussion as an adjunct to in-class teaching engaged the students in reflective discussion before class sessions. This method of instruction allowed the professor to review the threaded discussion and assess student understanding of the discussion topic before class. Lecture then could be used to dispel areas of confusion and misinterpretation by the students. Web-based threaded discussion is a valuable pedagogical tool to use as an adjunct to on-campus courses.

Loving, G. L, & Siow, P. (2005). Use of an online case study template in nursing education. *Journal of Nursing Education, 44*(8), 387–388.

Combining the case study approach and the Internet.

Ogden, W. R. (2003). Reaching all the students: The feedback lecture. *The Journal of Instructional Psychology,* March. From http://www.findarticles.com/p/articles/mi_m0FCG/is_1_30/ai_99983044

The feedback lecture was developed at Oregon State University at a time when questions regarding the changing nature of students seeking higher education came in conflict with existing staff and resources. The method, which involves prelecture activities, short lectures, discussion groups, and postlecture activities, contributes directly to an instructional delivery system. The feedback lecture enables students to learn by their own strengths while providing ample opportunity for developing related strengths in other areas.

Russell, N. (2004). Student expressions: Journaling….A nursing student's perspective. *SNRA Newsbulletin.* http://www.srna.org/communications/newsbulletin.php

This Canadian student shares her frustrations and eventual conversion to journaling as a teaching method. She verifies that the purposes of journaling include one or more of the following: to develop critical thinking, to provide an opportunity for reflection, to give insight into the student's progression in nursing skills and clinical practice, and as a means of dialogue between faculty and student.

Simpson, R. (2002). Virtual reality revolution: Technology changes nursing education. *Nursing Management, 33*(9), 14–15.

Virtual technology can increase nursing students' clinical skills without risking harm to patients and can help prepare nurses for new practices, such as robotic surgery.

vanGelder, T. (2005). Teaching critical thinking: Some lessons from cognitive science. *College Teaching.* From http://www.heldref.org/ct.php.

This article draws six key lessons from cognitive science for teachers of critical thinking. The lessons are: acquiring expertise in critical thinking is hard; practice in critical-thinking skills themselves enhances skills; the transfer of skills must be practiced; some theoretical knowledge is required; diagramming arguments (argument mapping) promotes skill; and students are prone to belief preservation.

Chapter Outline

THE LEARNING RESOURCE CENTER

Pamela Roberts

9

Learning Outcomes

Upon the completion of this chapter, the reader will be able to:

- Describe the various uses for the Learning Resource Center.
- Discuss design considerations for creating a Learning Resource Center.
- Develop organizational considerations for the use of physical space, personnel, activities, and supplies.
- Understand the specific maintenance requirements for the Learning Resource Center.
- Explain how skill competencies may be validated in the Learning Resource Center.
- Describe the documentation requirements for the Learning Resource Center.

Key Terms

Beta testing
Computer-assisted programs
Learning Resource Center (LCR)
Scenario-based testing
Self-directed learning
Simulation laboratories
Skill competencies
Virtual reality

The current nursing education environment must provide a venue for students to build and practice **skill competencies.** Earlier in the history of nursing education, students learned by performing skills on one another, a practice that is no longer recommended. Today these former "Skills Labs," have developed into actual **Learning Resource Centers (LRCs),** whose function is limited only by the creativity of the faculty who use them. This chapter will focus on LRCs, and the role of the faculty in their creation, maintenance, and use.

Definition of the LRC

The LRC is a specific area or room designed for or furnished with equipment that serves the needs of a particular population and enables this population to learn principles and techniques that will be required for their nursing practice. It is a setting in which variables relating to client care can be simulated, manipulated, and controlled to enhance learning. The LRC has various uses, depending upon which model a particular nursing education program chooses. Uses vary according to the particular program, curriculum, and resources (Gaberson & Oermann, 1999). Some programs incorporate an LRC component in only the first clinical course. Some schools require an LRC component in all courses in a program; use of the LRC changes as theory and skill integration progresses. There are also many models in between that include (1) introductory LRC sessions in early courses that do not yet have a clinical component; (2) selected courses where the LRC setting enhances the theory component; or (3) isolated LRC assignments within a clinical course.

More importantly, LRCs are no longer simply the "Skills Laboratories" they once were. In order to become a true resource where learning and critical thinking take place, the nursing LRCs currently are marvels of technology, where mannequins can be programmed to simulate actual client vital signs, pathology, and symptoms. Scenarios can be written to include all of the data nursing students would find on a client's chart. Depending on the objectives of the experience, students may need to collect data, synthesize information, formulate a plan, and implement care to meet the client's needs. LRCs also can provide a place where students come strictly to practice an isolated skill. Nursing instructors work to create actual simulations that require students not only to learn and practice skills, but to assess, plan, and act—where those actions frequently involve the implementation of client care involving the performance of several skills, perhaps modified to fit the situation.

How Programs Integrate LRCs

The LRC could exist solely as a supplement to the curriculum, where students may come to practice on a voluntary basis those things that they determine important to practice. Or, it could be an extremely structured requirement used to implement the curriculum—one in which all students are required to spend a certain number of hours in the laboratory setting. Indeed, the technology exists that will provide simulations that can rival actual clinical settings in challenging students to plan and implement nursing care. Hours students spend in the LRC can be granted recognition in terms of earned credit hours. Whether a program has its own formula for converting LRC hours to credits, or considers LRC experiences equivalent to clinical time in terms of credits is a decision that needs to be made. Those charged with implementation of the curriculum of a program need to be actively involved in the process of determining the purpose and objectives of the LRC.

Who will the internal and external customers be? Who will use and have access to the LRC? Clearly, the LRC is for students and faculty in the nursing program to use. Graduate nursing students in advanced physical assessment courses or nurse practitioner tracks may share the laboratory with undergraduate students, either simultaneously or consecutively. Depending on the objectives, there may be other customers who will have occasion to use the nursing LRC. If the institution hosts other allied health professions, it may be necessary for more than one program to use the LRC. Continuing education courses that may require a hands-on component may also use the LRC. If the program includes student participation with community health, community members may be invited to participate in health education or learning activities. Assessment courses, or formal testing scenarios, may rely on the use of standard patients, actors who are given a specific role to simulate an actual client scenario. Vendors will visit the laboratory, either solicited or soliciting, when new purchases are being considered.

Creating an LRC: An Overview

Programs of nursing education, some of which did not have formal LRCs, are now realizing the importance of a well-equipped and well-staffed LRC, and are working on ways to develop such an area, or refine the laboratory space they have. Programs that had an area set up where students could be introduced to skills and practice those skills as part of demonstration in individual courses now realize that this space needs to be more formal. Creating an LRC—as a resource that exists on its own, with its own staff, supplies, and policies—should take place in a systematic manner. Many schools of nursing have undertaken the task of hiring personnel who will staff the LRC, and of formalizing the area with policies, procedures, and guidelines that will allow it to be used to its fullest advantage. The decision to create an LRC or to expand a "skills lab" into such a center is an undertaking that requires research, planning, and consultation with others. Creators should perform a needs assessment in order to determine what the particular nursing program has to do to create the ideal LRC to support its program and students optimally.

LRC Objectives

Creators should consider the multifaceted uses of the LRC when undertaking the needs assessment. Next, the objectives for the LRC will be determined based upon the needs assessment (Box 9–1).

It would be helpful to consult with other programs that have LRCs, to consider the many possibilities that exist. Consultation with others that have been through the creation process can

Box 9–1 LRC Objectives

The learning resource faculty and staff are committed to:
1. Making learning resources available to faculty and students.
2. Providing consultation and training to enable faculty and students to use the resources.
3. Promoting a supportive and safe environment where faculty and students can interact with these resources and each other.
4. Supporting mastery based–testing and scoring that provides immediate feedback to students.

offer invaluable information as to methods of optimizing the setting to match the objectives of the curriculum. There should be joint input from all of the potential users, to ensure that all of their needs are considered.

Examination of the program objectives reveals where an LRC experience would provide a beneficial learning experience. In each individual course, consideration of individual course objectives would determine more specifically where an experience in the LRC would best enable students to meet their objectives. After examining these individual objectives, potential users and creators of the LRC can arrive upon specific objectives for the LRC. It is also crucial to keep the objectives of the LRC in mind during the planning process. A center that is going to require extensive student involvement during the course of the curriculum requires more space and more resources than does one that students will use for short periods of time.

LRC Space and Resource Considerations

Once the objectives have been determined, it is time to plan the actual space. It is likely that circumstances dictate limitations in time, budget, and space. It is a rare luxury for programs to be able to construct new space, dedicated solely to the development of an LRC. It is more likely that space has been dedicated or reconstituted to form an LRC. Given that space is almost always an issue, those creating the LRC will have to perform a cost-benefit analysis when choosing equipment and supplies that will fit both space constraints and the objectives of the LRC.

The amount of space also depends on the users and number of learning resource materials. The LRC needs to have a warm and inviting atmosphere for learning designed to support visual, auditory, and tactile learning. It needs to be well lit, colorful, and bright. Even surface flooring needs to be considered. If noise is a factor, the room needs to have carpeting that will help absorb the noise. If this is not a major consideration, hard surface flooring may be more appropriate for cleaning and maintenance purposes (Rideout, 2001). Another space area that is sometimes overlooked is the placement of the electrical outlets. The electrical outlets need to be located close to the equipment or the equipment needs to be flexible enough to be moved to the outlets. Rideout (2001) suggests a space minimum of 1000–1500 square meters for a well developed LRC. Take a look at this site in England, which is considered "state of the art" for space and resources for an LRC (www.clinicalskillscentre.ac.uk).

Time and Budget

Another factor to consider when creating an LRC is time. Given an unlimited amount of time, plans for an LRC would be more elaborate, allow for more growth, and allow for greater flexibility in use. Time constraints and deadlines in the planning process, however, usually do not allow for the process to continue indefinitely. Deadlines for initial plans, and revisions to those plans, need to be carefully identified and maintained.

As with any undertaking, budgetary considerations play a large part in the creation of any new space, and particularly so with an LRC. There are many ways to fund these spaces. There are companies that will provide free consultants, to help plan, develop, and furnish an entire high-tech LRC. For those programs with a stricter budget to consider, LRCs can be just as functional, but require a bit more imagination and manipulation to assemble (Box 9–2).

Donations and grant monies can be very helpful at the time of initial planning and throughout the duration of the LRC's existence. Keep in mind that LRC technology is evolving continually and that what a program purchases now may be outdated in several years. A long-term budgetary plan for the LRC will not only keep the program within its cost restraints but will help with future necessary spending to keep up with developing technology.

Box 9–2

165

Creating an LRC: An Overview

Consider these ideas when creating an LRC:
- Forming an alliance with acute care institutions and having items that were opened and not used given to nursing schools (Examples: pleurvacs, redressing kits, Foley catheterization kits).
- Contacting equipment vendors and seeing if "loaners" may be used on a semipermanent basis (Rideout, 2001).
- Considering if vendors provide supplies for purchased equipment (Example: tubing for each intravenous pump purchased).
- Being an "alpha" or "beta" site for testing new equipment before use on the market (Example: virtual reality Foley catheterization simulator).
- Partnering with other disciplines and sharing resources (Example: physician assistant, physical therapy, or residency programs).

Equipment

LRCs use a variety of equipment, such as beds, examination tables, bedside cabinets, overbed tables, medication carts, stretchers, wheel chairs, and so on, to reconstruct and simulate settings. Mannequins and models are used for demonstrations, return demonstrations, and practice. Consumable items and supplies are also needed as well as a storage area, where those supplies that are not in use can be contained.

Equipping the LRC requires careful planning and input with careful analysis of objectives of the curriculum the LRC supports. How a program decides to furnish the LRC depends primarily upon its objectives and its resources. Schools that choose to have dedicated amounts of time devoted exclusively to experiences in the LRC may choose to equip the LRC with a variety of simulation settings—acute care, outpatient, and even simulated apartments. Having these settings in the LRC create a "real lifelike" situation that assists the students in making the transition from the LRC to their clinical settings. Research has demonstrated that these simulated areas help decrease anxiety, provide realistic settings, and promote more effective and satisfied experiences for students (Feingold, Calaluce, Kallen, 2004; Jeffries, Rew, & Cramer, 2002; Jeffries, Woolf, & Linde, 2003; Mole & McLafferty, 2004; Morgan, 2006).

Mannequins that simulate actual patients cost a lot in terms of money and time to learn to program and use them effectively. More traditional mannequins, which are more cost-effective, may achieve the same objectives but are lower tech. Programs also weigh the cost and use of furniture, consumable items, and storage supplies in order to determine LRC needs.

Determining User Numbers

The LRC will need to be spacious enough to accommodate the number of students and faculty who will be using it at one time, and the total number who will be using the LRC throughout the course of the semester. Ideally, the LRC space would be planned allowing for the actual number of students who will be using it and allowing for growth in both numbers of students and instances of use. Unfortunately, in most institutions of higher education, the space is dictated by whatever the size of any unoccupied area may be at the time. The LRC furnishings just have to fit in that area. This usually results in a compromise.

In some nursing programs, students do not even begin to use the LRC until they are starting their nursing courses in either their sophomore or junior year. During this time, students are exposed to a large variety of skill competencies. This usually starts with basic or core competencies (vital signs, interviewing skills, catheterization, tube feedings, etc.) and progresses to higher level skills (arterial lines, pulmonary artery pressures, ECG interpretations, etc.). In addition,, students take more than one nursing course a semester. It is not unusual to have students in either pediatrics or obstetrics currently having at least two clinical days of experiences. This means that the LRC will be used for skills specific to their discipline.

When the LRC is created in such a way that it consists of several rooms (pediatric, nursery, acute care, community health), it allows students from the different nursing courses the ability to work simultaneously on their skill competencies in the LRC. If the LRC is created with the "open classroom" concept (one large room), it will need to be equipped or supplied with components for specific courses in certain areas of the LRC, or have the supplies and mannequins flexible enough so that they may be moved to different portions of the LRC or to other classrooms.

When many students are using the LRC, other things need to be considered; namely times of operation, other LRC assistants, and even specific LRC guidelines to facilitate effective and efficient use of the LRC (see Box 9–3).

Consider Laws and Regulations

Creators of the LRC must consider relevant laws and regulations when planning. The LRC must comply with rules of the Occupational Safety and Health Administration, Center for Disease Control regulations, and federal and local laws (see Box 9–4).

The U.S. Department of Labor, Occupational Safety and Health Administration (OSHA) mandates and ensures that rules and regulations are in place for all the considerations listed in Box 9–4. OSHA addresses and provides guidelines on ways to minimize or eliminate accidental exposures. It is important to ensure that all the necessary precautions specified by OSHA are followed in the LRC. The OSHA Web site is an important resource and is located at www.osha.gov.

Box 9–3 General Directions for LRC

The student is responsible for:
- Signing in at the front of the room for annual statistical reports.
- Bringing required supplies to the laboratory sessions (watch, stethoscope, penlight, paper, pencil/pen).
- Removing shoes when on beds.
- Arranging linens neatly in the linen closet.
- Leaving beds made and neat.
- Keeping tables and chairs clean and in place.
- Bringing NO food and beverages into the laboratory.
- Following the procedure for checking out a book, video, computer diskette, DVD, and/or piece of equipment.
- Completing all required readings, audio-visual media, and other assignments before practice in the laboratory.
- Wearing clothing appropriate for the skill being practiced.
- Practicing activities alone, with a partner, or in a group.
- Bringing the skill competency or validation sheets with them for sign off purposes.
- Replacing all kits in their respective designated storage areas.
- Removing the "cost/replacement" tickets and leaving them in the box provided in the laboratory (this is necessary for replacement purposes).
- Not removing any needles or syringes from the laboratory.

Box 9–4 LRC Regulatory Considerations **167**

- Safety
- Ergonomics
- Handwashing
- Latex allergies
- Electrical hazards
- Universal precautions
- Hazardous materials
- Blood borne pathogens
- Needle and syringe disposal

Source: The U.S. Department of Labor, Occupational Safety and Health Administration (OSHA).

Another component of safety deals with hazardous wastes. This is covered by the use of Material Safety Data Sheet (MSDS). The MSDS is a document that contains information on potential hazards (health, fire, reactivity, and environmental) and how to work safely with chemical products. Such sheets are an essential starting point for the development of a complete health and safety program that governs all LRCs. The MSDS contains information on the use, storage, handling, and emergency procedures all related to the dangers of hazardous materials. An important website for additional information on MSDS may be found at www.ilpi.com/msds.

Organization and Maintenance of the LRC

Organization of an LRC involves many areas: organization of the physical setting, organization of the people who are going to be in the center, organization of the activities that occur, and organization of supplies.

Organization of the Physical Setting

Most LRCs are multifaceted areas where much diverse learning can take place. Effective organization of the LRC is key to optimizing usage to meet the students' needs. Although the setups are different, most contain a simulated client-care area, whether it is a simulated acute care facility wing, room, or a number of client-care components assembled in various designs. The initial planning stages need to include blueprints, where the space is designed and measured. Those programs that have an architect available for this process are fortunate; many times, however, it is the task of the nursing faculty members to complete these designs. The dimensions of the furnishings that are desired for the LRC space need to be considered in terms of the space that is actually available. Design plans are created (see Box 9–5), then amended, then revised, as those involved realize the reality of what the space will allow.

Design plans have to allow for storage, a commodity that is rarely in adequate supply in the LRC setting. There also must be some type of desk or office space for the instructors or staff. LRC spaces need to be flexible, as the need to move objects, models, and furniture is constant. The area in which the student needs to perform client-care needs to be spacious enough to accommodate moving and manipulating equipment. Common areas need to be spacious enough to accommodate the movement of people and equipment, sometimes large pieces of equipment. Tables and desks frequently need to be moved to accommodate group work or discussion, or to be separated when

Box 9–5 Consideration for Physical Space

Disposal units	Simulators
Equipment	Sinks
Mannequins	Skill competency stations
Office space	Storage for supplies and mannequins
Patient care areas	Supplies
Rules and regulations	Technology
Security	Traffic flow
Scheduling	Video cameras
Self-directed learning	Videos, DVDs, and CAIs

students are working on individual projects. Mannequins may need to be placed in or out of the beds, depending on the objectives of the particular experiences. Careful observation of the traffic flow and patterns, and on-going evaluation of use, can result in a workable organizational plan. Good initial planning is helpful in organizations, but LRCs need to be responsive to the demands generated by the patterns of current use, and creative interventions in reorganization can be of great benefit.

Preparing the Laboratory Before Use

Another necessity for allowing students to build skill competencies in the LRC is to prepare the LRC adequately for the sessions that have been planned. Whether the faculty of the particular course or the LRC staff will be preparing the laboratory before scheduled activities, there needs to be a method whereby required equipment is provided and available for student use. Creating a master list of what equipment is required for each experience is a way to accomplish this. All of the equipment needed for a particular laboratory class, or testing session, needs to be set up in advance. Although there may be a system of storing supplies in boxes according to their use in particular tasks, these still need to be procured, and the contents arranged appropriately. Adaptations to the mannequins may need to be made, depending on the requirements of the scheduled client care scenario. Specific information pertaining to the requirements involved in setting up the LRC needs to be logged, and kept in an area that is readily accessible. In situations where work-study students and graduate assistants who may be employed in the center are not familiar with the names of all the equipment, taking pictures of the specific laboratory setups is a valuable tool. These pictures can be taken with a digital camera, and not only kept available for referral for laboratory setups, but also distributed, before the session, to all of the instructors responsible for teaching various sections in a course.

Organization of the People in the Laboratory

In order for the LRC to meet its objectives, the organization of the people who are going to be in the space is also of utmost importance. This aspect of organization is a challenge because there are so many people who need to use the LRC, and so many reasons various people may need to be in the same space at the same time. It becomes important for the flow of activity to ensure that everyone in the center is able to accomplish their objectives in as efficient a manner as possible. Of the various people who need to be in the LRC, students and instructors are probably the most prevalent users. Whether the LRC is assigned its own unique staff is dependent on the objectives

Box 9–6 Job Description for Coordinator of LRC **169**

- Manage day-to-day operations of the LRC.
- Prepare annual budgetary requirements.
- Provide orientation program for students and faculty.
- Design implementation strategies for use of the LRC.
- Create documentation guidelines for skill competency.
- Develop policies and procedures for use in the LRC.
- Facilitate the LRC as an area to enhance student learning.
- Perform daily, monthly, and annual maintenance requirements.
- Follow external agency rules and regulations that govern the use of the LRC.
- Evaluate new technology that enhances the LRC activities.

Organization and Maintenance of the LRC

and resources of the program. Ideally, it is helpful to have a full-time director, manager, coordinator, or supervisor, to oversee the day-to-day operation of the LRC (see Box 9–6). It is also helpful to have instructional and support staff; many institutions use work-study students or graduate assistants as staff.

LRC Staff

When the objectives and numbers of students support a number of LRC staff, staffing patterns need to be established carefully to ensure adequate staffing is available at the times students prefer. Optimal staffing would allow student needs to be met in a timely manner, and would allow staff sufficient time to arrange the equipment and scenarios necessitated by the activities taking place. Once again, tracking patterns of student use is vital. Having students make appointments is one way of ensuring that all students can be accommodated according to their needs. These appointment patterns can be studied, and staffing needs can be adjusted to have staff available at times when most appointments are scheduled. Having students sign in when they enter the LRC will also yield information as to the patterns of use.

The LRC staff members act as instructors, evaluators, role models, mentors, tutors, counselors, advisors, conservationists, trash persons, repair persons, movers, and clerks. It is necessary to know the objectives of all of the students and groups who are using the center, whatever the course or program. Once an LRC staff member has been hired, he must be given an adequate orientation. Course outlines, skills checklists, supply lists, scheduling information, and client scenarios all need to be available to staff and course instructors. Even with the most detailed orientation, there will always be new situations to contend with, and there will always be new learning experiences for the staff. Students who work in the LRC as work-study students or graduate assistants need to have a specific job description and clear guidelines as to what their responsibilities are. They need to have a clear understanding of confidentiality rules, when their role involves interactions with other students. Managing staff is also necessary to ensure smooth functioning and allowing students to meet their objectives. If the role of the LRC staff involves testing students on the performance of an aspect of client care, the staff needs to be consistent in its grading criteria. This may be accomplished by using checklists with specific directions; procedural steps; critical factors (statements) that students must perform (example: wash hands before starting the procedure, identify the patient by asking her name, maintaining sterile technique); priority sequences (step one before step two); and time factors (example: start CPR within 1 minute after finding the client lifeless). Finally, staff meetings, where issues such as consistency are addressed, are a necessary component of the role.

Nursing Faculty

Nursing faculty members in individual courses also use the LRC, and their needs must be accommodated as well. Nursing faculty members need to communicate as far in advance as possible when their courses require use of the laboratory setting. In some programs, this is built into the course schedule, and is done well before the beginning of the semester. In other programs, it is up to the individual instructors to integrate the LRC experience as they see the need. An optimal LRC setting would be one in which all students who needed to use the LRC at the same time would have all of the equipment and space they needed to be able to meet their objectives. The optimal situation is not always possible. Many times, students need to share equipment and space in order to accommodate the number of students who need experiences with the resources available. It may be necessary to restrict times when students can come in for independent practice, if it conflicts with the needs of a class that is scheduled for a learning experience at a given time. If there is not staff dedicated solely to the LRC, then the instructors who are in the laboratory need to be accountable to their students and take actions to enhance its operation. They need to be oriented to the center before using it, to be knowledgeable in the operation of required equipment, and to obtain needed supplies to ensure that the students' needs are met. Students, too, need to have clear guidelines as to their roles and expectations when using the LRC. Published guidelines of hours, programs, activities, rules, and regulations need to be distributed to students, so that this information is clear to all. An initial orientation will also enable students to be familiar with what the LRC offers, and will help them to meet their objectives.

Other Users

Depending on the program, members of the community may also be using the LRC. Programs that invite community members in for various health screenings and health education activities frequently conduct these activities in the LRC. This can become a valuable learning experience, but it is important to ensure the safety of the community members during their visit.

Depending on the parent institution and the types of health programs offered, there may be other disciplines that need to share space in the LRC. Students in other programs, such as Physical Therapy, Occupational Therapy, Physician's Assistant, Respiratory Therapy, EMT, and Medicine may have a portion of their educational experiences occur in the LRC. Scheduling then needs to occur according to the dictates of the parent institution, and the objectives of the other disciplines. Blocks of time may be set aside for use by another discipline, or students from different disciplines may be sharing the space at the same time. As long as the learners have clear objectives and guidelines, the learning experiences should not be compromised.

IT Staff

To use the technology that is available in the LRC to its fullest potential, it is necessary to work cooperatively with the Information Technology (IT) staff of the institution. Information Technology staff members will need to work collaboratively with the center staff to ensure that the technology tools in the LRC are properly installed. Simulation mannequins and **virtual reality** programs also may require trouble-shooting, at times, and the Information Technology staff can be very helpful in ensuring smooth functioning of this equipment. To ensure easy access to problem-solving technology, easy-to-follow directions should be posted adjacent to the technology, with direct line numbers for IT personnel.

Organization of Activities That Occur in the Laboratory

Because of the variety of learners and learning experiences that take place in the LRC, scheduling and organizing activities are extremely important. LRC calendars, or schedules, need to be carefully developed with all of the planned activities well identified. Confusion and conflict can be prevented by a clearly labeled schedule. It is advisable to have an overall calendar identifying all of the activities planned for a semester, and then publishing a weekly, and/or daily activity schedule, to guide staff, faculty, and students in the activities that have been scheduled during a given time frame. Some institutions have placed these schedules on a computerized platform, such as Blackboard, which provides easy and quick visualization of all the LRC activities.

There are laboratory sessions scheduled as components of courses; there are scheduled times students may come in and practice; there may be scheduled testing sessions, or informal learning activities planned. Whatever activity needs to take place, there needs to be adequate space and equipment to accommodate the needs of the participants. Many times, various activities can supplement and complement one another, as students from various disciplines, programs, and courses can work alongside each other, sharing information while each accomplishes their own objectives. In this manner, students may actually enhance their learning while contributing to the learning experience of others. At other times, too much activity will impede the students' ability to concentrate, perform, and learn.

Multiple requests for experiences need to be considered carefully. Although the inclination would be to grant all requests for experiences in the LRC, there has to be a balance in order that optimal experiences can take place. There needs to be sufficient time between scheduled activities to allow for cleaning up from one experience and preparing equipment for the next. Back to back scheduling that does not allow time for adequate preparation of an area will not be conducive to the efficient accomplishment of learning objectives. Scheduling too many activities in a short period of time may become overwhelming to the LRC staff, and to the students.

Organization of the Laboratory Supplies

Consumable equipment and other supplies in the LRC must be organized, in order to be able to find what is needed when it is needed. This is one of the most time-consuming efforts; the equipment required for each experience may change, the amount of equipment required from experience to experience may change, and the need for certain equipment may overlap. Over time, the equipment itself may change, necessitating continuous updating and reorganization. Although it is possible to store materials in many ways, one organized way of doing so would be to store each piece of equipment in its own particular space, according to alphabetical order. But alphabetical order may not be efficient when preparing equipment necessary for particular learning experiences or practice sessions. It may be more efficient to store materials in storage bins clearly labeled with the title of the laboratory session during which they are to be used. For example, if students are going to be learning to start a peripheral intravenous line, if all of the Angiocaths, tourniquets, 2×2s, alcohol swabs, Betadine wipes, and saline locks are all stored together, simply locating and pulling out the bin marked "Peripheral Intravenous Start Equipment" saves the person setting up from having to obtain all of the individual components from the areas in which they are stored. Several boxes stored together and labeled "1 of 2" and "2 of 2," is one solution if one box cannot contain all of the materials needed. Occasionally, attaching an item to the outside of a storage box may be necessary if the item is particularly large or oddly shaped. Storing supplies in boxes allows for neat stacking and organization according to course, frequency of use, or program, depending on the purpose and use of the LRC.

If more than one group of students, or a large group of students is going to be working together learning or practicing the same specific skill, or implementing the same components of care for a client in a simulation, it may be necessary to have several boxes containing identical equipment. Another aspect of organizing supplies is to encourage students to use supplies in a professional manner, and to replace what has been used, and put back what has been taken out, so that subsequent students will have the supplies readily available. In terms of conservation of consumable supplies, always a priority in terms of budgeting, it is quite useful for students to learn to rewrap sterile packages that they have used, so that a subsequent student can reuse the same supplies without compromising the learning experience. If mannequins are going to be used in the implementation of the procedure, the fact that the supplies are no longer sterile does not matter.

Along the same lines, another helpful lesson that students can learn in the LRC is the cost of individual supplies. This is an area that has been neglected greatly in nursing education, and in these times of health-care funding inadequacies, knowledge of what supplies cost could be helpful in reducing waste in health-care facilities. Students who are cognizant of the cost of supplies can aid in reducing costs by learning to implement nursing care in an organized and efficient manner.

Maintenance

The maintenance of equipment, supplies, and space in the LRC coordinates well with the organization of the equipment. Ensuring that the equipment in the LRC is organized can contribute to creating a schedule for its maintenance. There is a constant need to track and implement maintenance for a variety of items, in many different areas. In order to enable the mannequins to continue to be used for skills, such as inserting tubes and infusing fluids, there are regular and routine maintenance tasks that need to be done. Regularly lubricating areas, cleaning and drying tubing through which fluids are infused, and generally cleansing parts is a necessary part of maintenance. Despite this routine care, the mannequins do suffer from the wear and tear of the frequent use they receive. Caring for other equipment used in the LRC also needs to be scheduled on a regular basis. There is a large assortment of support equipment used in the teaching and implementation of client-care procedures that requires maintenance: pumps, aspirators; devices for measuring vital signs— sphygmomanometers, electronic blood pressure machines, pulse oximeters, electronic thermometers, otoscopes, ophthalmoscopes, audiometers, to name a few. These tools need to be inspected on a routine basis, and interventions need to be performed when indicated. Even tasks such as the replacement of batteries, bulbs, and tubing need to be performed regularly, in order to maintain optimal functioning. One method of ensuring these tasks are routinely implemented is to assign a staff member, or instructor, to perform checks on a recurring basis, perhaps once a month. All of the durable medical equipment needs to be maintained; some of it may be under warranty and the cost and schedule for repairs and preventive maintenance are covered. Other equipment may need routine servicing, which would need to be factored into the budget so that funding is available when required. Simpler maintenance tasks, such as bed-making, and keeping the linens for the beds and examination tables clean and organized, can also be tracked by means of a schedule.

Skill Competencies

The primary reasons that LRCs exist are for nursing students to have a setting where they can develop and master proficiency in the implementation of client care. Whether isolated, or combined in a scenario, there needs to be a decision as to specifics regarding skill competencies. Skill competencies are a listing of all the required skills or procedures that a student needs to acquire over the course of his education. The skills may be listed in a variety of ways: (1) in alphabetical order, (2) by course requirements, or (3) by level of student (sophomore to senior). A variety of elements are required to be completed for the student to pass the skill competencies successfully. These elements include the theoretical information necessary to understand the skill or procedure;

critical elements or those things that need to be performed so that no injury or harm occurs to the clients (example: maintaining sterile technique); and time frames when it affects the outcome of the skill/procedure that is performed (example: CPR). Other components that may be found on a skill competency checklist are validation areas for skill performance in the lab or clinical area, with areas for documentation by the faculty (see Box 9–7).

Those creating the LRC need to decide which skill competencies will be developed in the LRC, how they will be developed, and which skills competencies will be considered necessary to include for proficient performance of a particular skill. A curriculum committee meeting is an ideal place for this planning process to begin, as skill competencies cross the curriculum, and all courses and learning objectives need to be considered. The curriculum committee, considering the objectives of the program, then decides what portion of the program requires LRC components, and which skills, and skill competencies, need to be included in each course. Once it has been determined which competencies need to be introduced, the committee determines which skills need to

Box 9–7 DeSales University Skills Checklist, Department of Nursing and Health

Name: _____ Date:_____

Seniors

Skills	Clin Exp	Date	Lab Comp	Date	Clin Comp	Date
Arterial lines: care of						
Dressings: complex						
Electrocardiogram: Diagnose						
Monitoring						
Initiating						
Emergency equipment						
Endotracheal tubes: care of						
Intravenous: starting						
Pulmonary arterial line (PAL) Care of Measurement of pulmonary capillary wedge pressure (PCWP)						
Specimen collection: arterial blood sample						
Sengstaken-Blakemore tube: care of						
Suctioning: endotracheal						
Telemetry						
Venipuncture						

be mastered. These can be detailed in a Competencies Master Plan. Not all skills involve intense instruction and time investment to achieve mastery. The LRC can be used to focus on those skills that are best learned and mastered in that environment. For example, therapeutic communication techniques can be introduced and practiced in an LRC setting, particularly if there is emphasis on using these techniques in interactions with clients in health-care settings, but they can be just as easily introduced and mastered in a setting other than the LRC. Time constraints also guide which competencies need to be mastered in the laboratory session, as the time spent in the LRC competes with student time spent in theory-building activities, as well as in the clinical setting.

After the faculty has made a decision about which competencies will be introduced and mastered in the LRC setting, planning on how best to implement the process begins. Instructors should carefully delineate the specific objectives that are to be met in each laboratory session. Again, there should be a planning session in which this information is decided by a dedicated group of people. A curriculum committee may be charged with this task, or a task force set up for this purpose.

Further decisions need to be made about how the skills will be introduced, mastered, and evaluated. Generally, it is necessary for each program to have internal consistency. Policies regarding skill competencies need to be established throughout the entire program. Every course does not need to be cookie-cutter identical, but there does need to be congruency in what is presented in the LRC, and how it will be evaluated throughout the program. The activities that take place in the LRC can vary greatly from course to course and program to program. Many programs choose to introduce selected skills in a formal manner, with identified objectives and skill checklists. A nursing faculty member in the course is assigned to present the content to the students, and the students practice with supervision and guidance. This may be the extent to which some skills are introduced, or there may be a requirement to complete a formal testing process to determine competency.

Testing

There is also the question of how to decide if an individual, or group of students, has achieved competency in a particular skill or skills. This decision has many prongs. The amount of time that will be spent learning the skill will need to increase if there is going to be testing for competency achievement. How will the testing be carried out? Who will do the testing? And it is possible that skill competency could be evaluated in various ways. It depends on the skill, the curriculum, the faculty, and the philosophy.

This testing process could be accomplished in a variety of ways. In some cases, the course instructor may be able to validate that the students are competent following a return demonstration of a newly introduced skill. In other cases, the students separate LRC learning sessions from testing sessions. Testing is completed in a formal manner, with a student using the laboratory specifically for a testing scenario, and needing to be evaluated according to preset criteria. Students may be prepared to test on a specific, predetermined skill, or they may be presented with an unknown scenario upon arrival, which requires them to identify and correctly perform one or several skills. These decisions are usually determined by the faculty to best meet the educational objectives of the particular program. Teaching and testing can be accomplished in a variety of creative ways of which simulation scenarios are just one.

In addition to determining what needs to be taught and tested, the faculty needs to come to an agreement on the method of evaluation to use in the LRC, if evaluation is to be done. Grades can be assigned to the performance of a skill, with grading from "Pass/Fail" to any of a variety of number or letter grades. As is usually the case, this area is one of concern for students and faculty alike. On one hand, students who feel that they are very good at the psychomotor domain and wish to have that reflected in a numerical grade, conflict with those students who feel that a numerical ranking system increases the level of anxiety over the performance to a greater degree than would a pass/fail grade. Testing faculty members understand the subjectivity inherent in assigning a grade to a return demonstration session, and may prefer to reduce that subjectivity by using a pass/fail grading system. This subjectivity is readily apparent when decisions are being made as to what behaviors are needed to perform a task in a competent manner. Some faculty members feel strongly that certain steps need to be performed in a certain order, whereas others argue that those particular steps could be accomplished in a variety of approaches. Faculty members have to come to an agreement on the development of the testing and grading methods used, and need to be as specific as possible in the grading criteria. Some schools have chosen a proficiency system, where a grade of "P" is given when a student is proficient in a skill, followed by a number, or series of numbers, which indicates a degree of proficiency. For example "P.4" may be the most proficient, and "P.3.1" may indicate that a student was proficient enough to be considered competent, but did not perform the procedure during the test as proficiently as possible. There is a cut off, determined by the faculty, below which the student cannot be considered competent or proficient, and therefore is not considered safe in the performance of that particular skill. Again, faculty philosophy, creativity, and objectives dictate the manner in which the evaluation is graded.

After that decision has been made, it needs to be followed by a consequence for not achieving a passing grade in a testing situation. The least punitive consequence is that a student continues to practice and repeat the performance of the skill in a subsequent testing situation. The most punitive consequence is receiving a failing grade, either in a number grade that is factored into their course average or in a "Pass/Fail" grading system in which a failure in a laboratory testing situation is known in advance to the student to result in a failure in the particular course. And there are an infinite number of variations in between—from a student being able to repeat a test only a certain number of times without penalty, to a student who will receive an LRC warning that may result in a grading penalty if repeated within a certain designated time frame. Consequences may also affect a student's ability to implement client care during a clinical component of a course. Policies may dictate that students not be allowed to perform any skills that require LRC testing on clients in the clinical area, until those tests have been completed successfully.

Psychomotor Skill Development

"I hear and I forget. I see and I remember. I do and I understand." In his quotation, Confucius captures the essence of the value of the LRC. Promoting psychomotor skill development in students is one of the many essential functions of the laboratory setting. The LRC provides an excellent venue for students to conceptualize and put into practice, skills that they have read about or seen demonstrated in audio-visual materials. Many nursing students state that their preferred mode of learning is centered in the psychomotor domain, and the LRC is the perfect match for students who learn best in that manner. Allowing students to view and handle the equipment; watch demonstrations, either live or audio-visual; and practice on nonthreatening models or mannequins until they feel comfortable with the procedure proves invaluable. Having personnel available to guide and answer questions and to cue the student, further encourages the development of psychomotor skills. There is a long tradition in nursing that practicing skills in this manner does lead to mastery over time.

The variable that changes when implementing the procedure for the first time on a live client is the client response. Whereas the mannequins are quite happy to go along with any procedure the nursing student has planned, clients are not always as cooperative. Actual clients have differences in anatomical structures, responses to stimuli, mobility, vital signs, and pathological conditions. These are all variables that can come up in the laboratory setting. Students are expected to apply on-the-spot decision-making, and alter procedures according to variables they have assessed. Client scenarios, frequently resembling actual client charts and flow sheets, are prepared before the learning experience, and a student may find it necessary to change the traditional way a procedure is performed in order to fit the situation. Whether the client has a condition that makes him unable to assume the traditional posture that is the norm for implementing a certain procedure, or the client is allergic to a material that is usually used, it is possible to manipulate the circumstances to mimic real-life situations, requiring students to plan, consider alternatives, and make decisions to alter traditional implementations in skill performance.

Instructors have been working on creative ways to simulate reality closely, even while working with static mannequins and equipment. Mannequins have become more and more realistic. They come supplied with interchangeable parts that contain, for example, realistic, deep wounds, as well as gangrenous toes and amputated limbs. These mannequins allow students to practice wound care that simulates a client's real wounds. Instead of enabling students to practice just the procedure of performing wound care, the use of these mannequins allows students to measure, assess, and describe the wound. The latest generations of mannequins are simulators that can breathe, have heart rhythms, and show response to interventions by having those changes become apparent on a monitor, through computer programming. These mannequins can allow for scenarios that simulate trauma, burns, and even active hemorrhage. Students not only have the opportunity to implement all types of hands-on psychomotor skills, they have to develop strategies to perfect assessment skills, set priorities, and act—all in a matter of minutes. Failure to do so can actually result in the "death" of the simulated client. These simulators challenge instructors to develop realistic scenarios that will reflect actual client situations.

The LRC, therefore, becomes not only a domain where psychomotor skills are learned, practiced, and tested, but it becomes one in which critical thinking, prioritizing, and decision-making can also be practiced and refined. The direction in which the LRC is heading is one in which clinical assessment skills, integration of theory and evidence-based research; critical thinking, decision-making, and prioritizing are all combined in **scenario-based testing.** At this time, students are given a set of data, the simulated model is programmed with certain variables, and students respond to these variables in the assessment of the model, by making decisions about the required interventions, and implementing care for the client. Following the implementation and documentation of care, instructors meet with students in debriefing sessions, to review the salient points that have been learned through this experience. This technology can be applied to all levels of learning—beginning students can assess a preprogrammed blood pressure in a model's technological arm, decide if the level of blood pressure is within normal limits to proceed with medication administration, and go on to carry out those procedures, for example. This situation can be adapted in many ways—it can be used as an initial learning experience in which students are introduced to skills, and expected to bring some theoretical knowledge to apply to the situation; it can be used for competency testing—either directly observed or videotaped for review; or it can be a practice situation in which students come to learn skills independently that they may not encounter in the clinical area or may not have time to have practiced in a traditional laboratory classroom time block. It will be possible to create entire simulated clinical experiences for client conditions that a student would not normally encounter in live clinical settings—clients who are in the middle of hypoxic episodes, myocardial ischemic events, or trauma situations, such as burns and hemorrhages. This is especially important in a time when clinical rotation experiences may be difficult to find. Changes in available regional clinical experiences, including increases in acuity level of hospitalized patients, specialized care, shortened hospital stays, and an increase in

A relatively recent challenge for instructors, and one that will be ongoing, is learning to use the amazing technology that exists. The companies that manufacture these complex simulators do provide orientation sessions. Group sessions are sponsored by these companies, in which users can come together to share experiences, ideas, and scenarios. It is a time-consuming endeavor to construct scenarios that will provide students with enough information to guide them through a simulation experience, without providing too much information to impair the critical thinking process. And students will pick up inconsistencies, which may occur with any instructor-developed tool. So time needs to be spent devising scenarios, **beta testing** these scenarios with students, and then revising them. Learning to manipulate and operate the simulators is also an ongoing process; there are such a variety of capabilities, it takes practice and patience to learn them all.

the number of outpatient facilities, have decreased the availability of in-patient experiences for nursing education. Clinical simulations provide an acceptable alternative for a variety of hands-on client scenarios that were previously offered only in the clinical setting. Box 9–8 discusses the use of simulators and scenarios in teaching.

Self-Directed Learning

The LRC is also a valued resource for **self-directed learning,** which is: "a process in which students take the initiative to diagnose their learning needs, formulate learning goals, identify resources for learning, select and implement learning strategies, and evaluate learning outcomes" (www.netnet.org/students/student%20glossary.htm).

In addition to an arena for learning techniques for client care and psychomotor skills, LRCs also house computers, audio-visual equipment, and a collection of books and printed materials. Students are free to use these resources in meeting their identified needs. Students who are visual learners can reap benefits from this type of opportunity. Becoming more available and popular are self-directed **computer-assisted programs,** which are also available in a variety of topics, ranging from medication calculations to arterial blood gas interpretation. These are programmed instructions in which the students progress through didactic presentations, answer questions, and are given immediate feedback as to whether their answer is correct or not. If correct, the students are able to progress to the next self-directed program or lesson. If incorrect, students are able to remediate, and continue to progress through information that reinforces rationales for the correct answer. Self-directed computer-assisted programs are usually interspersed with attention-getting graphics and animation, and are generally a fun way to acquire or reinforce learning.

Virtual reality is another tool available in LRCs, and is an area that is likely to grow in future years. Virtual reality is the simulation of a real or imaginary environment visually in the three dimensions of width, height, and depth that may provide an interactive experience visually in real time with sound, tactile responses, or other forms of feedback. The virtual reality simulators may be used individually for self-directed learning, with groups for instructor-directed learning, and even for testing purposes. Currently available virtual reality computer programs involve phlebotomy and initiating intravenous therapy, peripherally and centrally. Students can, for example, select an appropriate vein, apply a tourniquet, and actually complete the steps to initiate an intravenous line, including retracting the skin and virtually inserting the correct size needle, all accomplished by means of a computer. A student can be debriefed afterward, and learn whether the procedure was successful, whether or not it was painful, and other helpful information. These learning tools are invaluable in allowing the students to be independent learners, to come into the LRC and independently initiate the activity and complete it at their own pace. Students are free to repeat activities to enhance their understanding; and to skip sections that they may feel are not needed at the time. These learning resources are also nice for instructors; the students do not necessarily need their assistance or guidance to complete the activity.

Nevertheless, the initial acquisition of the hardware and software for these independent study programs is quite an expense, and continued upgrading and acquisition of new materials is an ongoing challenge, in terms of funding and previewing new materials. Although the students use these resources independently, it may still be necessary to create a system in which students can self-schedule appointments, particularly with required or popular programs. In these cases, it may also be necessary to limit the amount of time any one student may use the resource at each session in order to accommodate the needs of all the students in the course or program. The LRC is a place where self-directed learning has traditionally been enabled and encouraged. In the future, the LRC may be where the learning materials originate, but the actual learning could take place anywhere.

Documentation

As in any area of nursing education, the LRC requires that users document activities that take place. Policies and procedures, job descriptions, evaluations, information sheets, annual reports, and grant reports are some of the areas that require documentation.

Policies and procedures need to be developed and made available to students, faculty, and staff. The need for, and format of, these policies will most likely be dictated by the policies of the institution. Job descriptions for all personnel and work-study students who work in the laboratory need to be developed and available, according to the requirements of the educational institution. Information regarding the operation of the LRC—guidelines for use, calendars, schedules of activities, operating hours, etc., needs to be compiled and disseminated in some fashion.

If there is going to be evaluation of student performance in implementing an aspect or aspects of client care, there needs to be an evaluation form specific to the particular aspect evaluated. This form would commonly be generated by the instructors in the specific course or program, often in conjunction or consultation with the LRC personnel. The LRC staff, or course instructors, would need to be familiar with the evaluation tool before the evaluation process takes place. It is helpful if all of the evaluation tools are kept available for reference in the LRC. There needs to be some type of record kept in the LRC, detailing who has successfully completed evaluations, in order to facilitate tracking and scheduling students.

Another aspect of documentation that needs to be completed is an annual report, in a format designated by the institution or program. This report is needed to document the activities that took place in the LRC, acquisition of supplies and equipment, evaluation of the implementation of programs, and overall appraisal of the operations of the learning laboratory over the previous year. If there have been grant monies awarded, there may be documentation and reports regarding the implementation of the funding, the contents of which would be specified by the grantor.

Summary

The LRC is one component of a nursing program that interfaces with the administration, instructors, and students in all courses, and possibly with other programs. It is a setting that frequently hosts the community, visitors, and prospective students, as well as a variety of other personnel from the educational institution. Although it may be called by names other than the LRC, depending on the philosophy and objectives that guide its function, it serves as a vital, dynamic support to the nursing education program. The LRC requires that careful detail be given to organization, maintenance, and documentation for all the activities that occur in this setting. It entails not only psychomotor skill development but a variety of other strategies, such as computer-based and self-directed learning, virtual reality, and simulated learning with a variety of mannequins, auditory teaching devices, and even simulated patients. Ensuring optimal function of an LRC can be challenging, frustrating, and tiring—but it is always exciting and rewarding.

R e f e r e n c e s

CETL—Centre for Excellence in Teaching and Learning. Retrieved August 25, 2006 from **http://www. clinicalskillscentre.ac.uk/index.htm**

Feingold, C. E., Calaluce, M., & Kallen, M. A. (2004). Computerized patient model and simulated clinical experiences: Evaluation with baccalaureate nursing students. *Journal of Nursing Education, 43*(4), 156–163.

Gaberson, K. B., & Oermann, M. H. (1999). *Clinical teaching strategies in nursing.* New York: Springer Publishing.

Jeffries, P. R., Rew, S., & Cramer, J. M. (2002). A comparison of student-centered versus traditional methods of teaching basic nursing skills in a learning laboratory. *Nursing Education Perspectives, 23*(1), 14–19.

Jeffries, P. R., Woolf, S., & Linde, B. (2003). Technology-based vs. traditional instruction: A comparison of two methods for teaching the skill of performing a 12-lead ECG. *Nursing Education Perspectives, 24*(2), 70–74.

MSDS online. Retrieve August 25, 2006 at **http://www.ilpi.com/msds/**

Mole, L. J., & McLafferty, I. H. R. (2004). Evaluating a simulated ward exercise for third year student nurses. *Nurse Education in Practice, 4*(2), 91–99.

Morgan R. (2006). Using skills laboratories to promote theory-practice integration during first practice placement: An Irish perspective. *Journal of Clinical Nursing, 15*(2), 155–161.

Rideout, E. (2001). *Transforming nursing education through problem-based learning.* Sudbury, MA: Jones and Bartlett Publishers.

Self-directed learning definition. Retrieved August 30, 2006 from **http://www.netnet.org/students/ student%20glossary.htm**

U.S. Department of Labor, Occupational Safety & Health Administration. Retrieve August 25, 2006, from **http://www.osha.gov**

REVIEW QUESTIONS

- Explain how the LRC could shift its focus from teacher-directed learning to self-directed learning.
- Discuss the learning needs of the various users of the LRC.
- Develop strategies to enhance testing for skill competencies using audio and visual capturing capabilities.
- Describe the impact of technology on concept and skill development in the LRC.
- Search the Internet to determine "virtual" learning experiences that may be used in the LRC.
- Create evaluation strategies for learning in the LRC.

CRITICAL THINKING EXERCISE

Redesign a center for learning with access to and connectivity to resources (internal and external) in your nursing department. The focus of the redesign is centered on the following:

◗ Philosophy and mission of the LRC

◗ Curriculum needs, space, equipment, and staff of the LRC

ANNOTATED RESEARCH SUMMARY

Haskvitz, L. M., & Koop, E. C. (2004). Educational innovations. Students struggling in clinical? A new role for the patient simulator. *Journal of Nursing Education,* *43*(4), 181–184.

Our students trust that we will provide them with information and opportunities to practice what they have learned in the classroom. When students are not meeting established objectives in the clinical environment, the possibility for error increases, frustration and the students' stress levels escalate, and patient safety is jeopardized. Traditional remediation methods may reduce students' already low levels of confidence, putting more stress on the students and creating an environment prone to errors. We devised a remediation plan using the human patient simulator to meet the needs of such students and their clinical preceptors, while preserving patient safety. The **simulation laboratory** is a safe place to practice skills until a specified level of proficiency is reached. In this environment, students gain back confidence in their abilities. By using the simulator in this novel way, student learning is enhanced, while patient care and safety is optimized.

Winslow, S., Dunn, P., & Rowlands, A. (2005). Establishment of a hospital-based simulation skills laboratory. *Journal for Nurses in Staff Development, 21*(2), 62–65.

Today's health-care environment requires that nurses be prepared for increasingly complex patient populations. Simultaneously, managers and educators are challenged to provide competency verification programs and continuing education opportunities with fewer resources. Hospital clinical educators share a staff development initiative of launching a unique simulation skills laboratory. The laboratory is designed to ensure that nurses can meet the needs of patients in today's health-care arena.

Van Sell, S., Johnson-Russell, J., & Kindred, C. (2006). **The teaching power of high-tech dummies.** *RN, 69*(4) 30–35.

If the thought of a teaching mannequin calls to mind an image of a "dummy" with rubbery body parts, think again. Nursing students are now practicing on lifelike mannequins that can speak and respond to pharmacological interventions.

Morgan, R. (2006). Using clinical skills laboratories to promote theory-practice integration during first practice placement: An Irish perspective. *Journal of Clinical Nursing, 15*(2), 155–161.

The aim of this study was designed to investigate how a select cohort of nursing students experienced its first practice placement in a large Irish teaching hospital. The objectives of this study were to investigate who students learn from, what skills they learn during their first practice placement, and if the use of clinical skills laboratories before their first practice placement helped students relate theory to practice during their first practice placement. Interviews were conducted using a semistructured interview schedule. The participants identified that sessions taught in the clinical skills laboratory before the first practice placement, which they identified as "basic nursing skills" such as taking and recording vital signs and hygiene needs of patients, were useful and helped them to integrate theory to practice during their first practice placement. Clinical skills laboratories are essential to help students develop the collaborative skills required for a profession like nursing. It is essential that students are adequately prepared to carry out clinical skills during their first practice placement, and have the ability to link theory to practice.

Chapter Outline

INSTRUCTIONAL METHODS 10

Lucille A. Joel

Learning Outcomes

After completing this chapter, the student will be able to:

- Choose the instructional strategy that best suits the educational objectives, the predisposition of the students, and the talents of the teacher.
- Construct an instructional strategy that mixes varied methods of teaching and learning.
- Be confident to try a variety of traditional and nontraditional instructional methods.

Key Terms

Case method	Lecture
Concept mapping	Problem-based learning
Debate	Question and answer teaching
Group discussion	Recitation
Instructional methods	Reflective practice groups
Instructional strategy	Role playing
Jigsaw	Seminar
Journaling	Simulations

The strategy for teaching must be modeled after the environment in which students find themselves. To be out of step with the realities of life is a sure prescription for failure. Thirty years ago, formal **lecture** and discussion prevailed as the strategies of choice in teaching. And students looked to the teacher for the ultimate word on knowledge and the guidance to apply that knowledge to life. But things have changed. We are caught in a fast-paced environment, where knowledge and technology continue to grow and multiply with breakneck speed. We are overwhelmed by the amount of information available to the student, and faculty members often find it difficult to sort out what is necessary from what is interesting. Students expect the same fast pace in learning as they experience in living, and they assume they will be prepared for an occupational role.

These observations of today's environment provide strong direction for building **instructional strategy** or the broad plan for the learning experience. The strategy consists of a host of variables that ultimately drive the selection of the best instructional method or teaching technique for each occasion; or better yet, several methods that are integrated into a new and creative whole.

Instructional Strategy

Choosing an appropriate teaching method is an art form in itself. Choice is driven by the objectives to be achieved, the talent of the teacher, the environment, and the learning style of the student. All of these variables are part of strategic choice. In other times, the style favored by the teacher prevailed over any other, and most assuredly weighed more than the students' choice and even environmental factors.

Domains of Learning

The most fundamental understanding necessary to make instructional strategic choices are the domains of learning. Although covered more thoroughly elsewhere in this text, they are presented here to put strategic decisions in perspective. Objectives target learning in the cognitive (thinking), affective (feeling), or psychomotor (skill) domains (Bloom, 1956). And there are teaching strategies that work better with one domain than another, though assuming any exclusive relationship is naïve. For example, though lecture is most directed toward the cognitive domain, the creative teacher can include an affective component, purposefully churning up feelings and attitudes about the subject under consideration. In a similar manner, **group discussion** and **role playing** are labeled as affective domain techniques, but there is great potential to address cognitive learning. Unless the group is exclusively process-oriented, there must be an area of content to give the discussion substance. The secret is in the creativity of the teacher.

Learning Styles

Today we also know much more about learning styles, and how personal style influences the choice of a teaching strategy. Learning style refers to the ways individuals process information. No learning style is any better or worse than any other, but they do differ among individuals and they are measurable. The right-brain/left-brain dichotomy is one construct in style. One needs structure, the other room for creativity and innovation, but both have to be helped toward a whole brain way of thinking and learning. Field-independent/field-dependence is important to consider in determining whether a person sees the whole first (field-independence) or specific parts (field-dependence). This is no idle issue: the field-independent learner will need an overview first, with clarity on the end results of the learning experience; the field-dependent learner needs attention to the detail of the parts before assembling the whole.

In the Productivity Environmental Preference Survey (PEPS), Dunn and Dunn (1978) identify 21 characteristics that influence the learning of individuals. Some include: the best time of the day for learning; whether one learns better from peers, from an authority figure (teacher), or by oneself; and whether one is analytical or impulsive. Other inventories reveal if we learn best using all of our senses; or are better served using sound, or taste, or another sense exclusively. Is locus of control an issue—are you externally or internally driven, self-directed or more comfortably directed by others? It is obviously impossible to characterize each of these qualities for every student, but the teacher has a responsibility to be well versed in their existence and alert to their manifestations. Always allow learners to say when a teaching method is not working for them, and encourage them to expand their style range rather than seek comfort. Provide a choice among teaching strategies where possible. One student may choose learning from case discussions in a study group; others may prefer a large lecture session. Another may like to search out his own resources using the Internet, while a classmate may want clear direction as to what the teacher sees as the best resources.

Instructional Methods

Instructional methods have customarily been organized according to:

- The degree of *control maintained by the teacher.*
- The extent to which the *learner is active* or *passive.*
- Whether the technique is *student-centered* or *teacher-centered.*
- If the focus is *content or process.*

These distinctions are embedded in the nature of the method, although adjustments can be made easily. The lecture is teacher-centered, but the artful teacher can incorporate questions and discussion that allow some of that control to flow to the student. The group discussion can be minimally active for the student if it is led by the teacher, and proceeds according to her or his agenda; or active and process-oriented if it is a student-led group focusing on the interpersonal dynamics before them. No class session should depend exclusively on one or another method. Methods are mixed and matched to maintain attention and maximize learning. And the teaching method should be selected primarily to support the nature of the learner and the behavioral objectives to be accomplished. The preference of the teacher is also important, but should not be the exclusive concern. In addition, resources are always a consideration: time, space, budget, and numbers of students.

No writing on instructional methods would be complete without a comment about computers and today's educational scene. Every student experience should be computer-enhanced, through written material, or the provision of a mechanism for threaded discussion. The teacher can initiate these discussions by proposing a controversial question, and the student will follow with responses. The threaded discussion is also a valuable tool for evaluation. You can easily tell if students are conversant in the material that has been taught, and can determine if they are able to manipulate the content cognitively.

Creating Set

An important concept in teaching, regardless of the strategy, is *"creating set."* The term refers to the response in the individual that predisposes that person to learn. The process that the teacher institutes to create set is called *set induction*. DeCecco and Crawford have identified three stages for set induction: arousal, expectancy, and incentives (1974). This is a preinstructional process, which clarifies the goals of instruction, motivates the student to learn, and helps them to see the relevance of the learning to real life. At the beginning of a class, the teacher will create some excitement, and even anticipation, about the content and processes that will be introduced (arousal). The expectation is established that this will be a part of their day-to-day practice, thus critical to master (expectancy). Then the objectives are discussed, and reiterated in clear language that leaves no doubt about what is to be achieved. Finally, the students are reassured that they will succeed, and that the teacher is there to guide their progress, provide feedback, and institute course corrections as necessary (incentive). This is also an excellent opportunity to connect to earlier educational experiences, showing how the parts contribute to the whole (deTornyay & Thompson, 1982). In other words, (tell students how) that knowledge mastered at an earlier stage of their program is a critical foundation for these new challenges.

Traditional Methods of Instruction

The lecture and discussion constitute the backbone of instructional methods. This is in no way meant to stifle the spirit of adventure that should accompany every day of teaching. Each of these methods can be varied in countless ways to make them new and different, but the core is still lecture and discussion.

Lecture

The lecture is a common technique in teaching, probably because most teachers were taught in this mode; and we teach as we were taught. The lecture is suited to large groups, and may take several forms. The formal lecture uses a very tight and polished format; it provides for only minimal exchange between student and teacher. The lecture is an efficient, cost-effective way of disseminating content to a large number of people in a reasonable time frame. It is most effective in the cognitive domain. This domain refers to the acquisition of information and the learner's intellectual abilities. The lecturer does not just present information, but also demonstrates patterns, highlights main ideas, and generally presents a unique way of viewing the topic. The masterful lecturer uses the occasion to role model problem-solving and critical and creative thinking. Good teaching requires self-awareness and "split-consciousness." "Split-consciousness" is the ability to pay attention concurrently to both the content of the speech and its delivery. In fact, these qualities lie at the very heart of all types of truly effective teaching.

Often lecture is combined with ***recitations*** that involve smaller numbers of students. In recitation, points made in the lecture are explicated and students are given an opportunity to question or present their own ideas on the subject material, thus providing affective domain learning. The affective domain is known as the "feeling" domain, and involves the depth of a person's emotional response to the subject matter in terms of attitudes, beliefs, and values.

Though the lecture is largely teacher-centered, more active involvement of students is possible. The teacher can encourage student participation during lecture, by using controversial questions or "devil's advocate" positions to engage and provoke the learner. In a lecture with a relatively manageable number of students, the tool presented in Box 10–1 may be useful to award a grade for class participation.

Whether a relatively passive or more active process, lecture takes considerable preparation time on the part of the teacher, and requires mastery of the topic. The lecture format does not presume that teachers know it all, and they should be open to admitting when there are points about which they are not conversant.

Every lecture should be approached inductively, sharing with students the objectives, outcomes, and expectations of the session. This occurs in the *introductory phase*, and typically should

Box 10–1 Criteria for Participation in Discussions **187**

Participation in class/Internet discussions is evaluated according to the following scale for _____% of your grade:

A   Initiates relevant and thought provoking discussion; raises issues and concerns that have not been proposed before; articulates alternative points of view; proposes additional readings or other scholarly resources.

B+   Active participation in discussions: applies content to related situations, asks thought-provoking questions.

B   Participates in discussion: comments limited to assigned readings or specifics of the discussion.

C+   Responds to questions; no additional participation.

C   No involvement in Internet discussions (where the Internet is used); but participates in face-to-face discussion.

F   No substantial participation at any time.

be no more than 5 minutes. A brief overview of the content is helpful, in addition to some idea of how this material is essential to their professional life, and the assurance that they can learn what is necessary. The reader is referred to the comments on *set induction* earlier in this chapter.

The *body of the lecture* should be well organized. Transition from one topic or subtopic to another should be seamless. In nursing, it is impossible to introduce students to all the content that is necessary to practice. That being the case, reading and library research assignments should have been completed before any lecture. The lecture should be used to tease out and clarify the fine points, and to demonstrate evidence-based, critical, and creative thinking. The teacher should serve as a role model, provoking the students to question and challenge their thinking. This is antithetical to the usual formal lecture, but much more productive with students preparing for professional practice. In other words, material assigned for out-of-class reading may be taught through application and demonstration. Case material is often stimulating and makes content "live." Process becomes content. See Box 10–2 for examples of techniques that enhance critical thinking and supplement the traditional lecture.

In lecturing, notes are helpful and often necessary. Make them brief and unobtrusive. Reading notes verbatim is not acceptable. The session should appear effortless. The lecturer should make each individual in an audience of hundreds feel as if she or he is the only student. Make eye contact with a student in each of the far corners of the room. Use creative movements and avoid using a podium. Move around the room if possible, and put your notes on index cards, overheads, or PowerPoint. Keep these notes to a minimum. Introduce a change of pace periodically. Woodring reminds us that an individual's optimum attention span is "roughly one-minute per year of age up to the approximate age of 45" (2001). Plan changes of pace or breaks accordingly.

The lecture session closes with a definite *conclusion* of no more than 5 minutes. The teacher should take this opportunity to summarize key points from the lecture; reiterate the objectives, outcomes, and expectations stated in the introduction; and build a case for the essentiality of the content, not necessarily in that order.

In research on what makes lectures and lecturers unsuccessful, the criticisms have focused on the teacher, not the method. Comments speak to a lack of organization, poor quality or absence of visual aides, lack of enthusiasm in delivery, too great a dependency on notes, inadequate knowledge of a subject, obliviousness to learners' need for breaks, and no acknowledge-

- Muddiest Points: At the end or beginning of class, have students write down the points about which they have the most confusion and then anonymously hand in their response; the teacher discusses these points at the beginning of the next class (Angelo & Cross, 2005).
- Concept Mapping: Have students construct a concept map showing ideas and connections about what went on in class. Best done simultaneously with the class and handed in immediately. Can also be used diagnostically. Helpful to provide an outline of class material to reduce the need for note taking during this process.
- Students generate test questions; require them to be at a higher level of cognition.
- Minute Paper: At the end of a teaching session students are asked to take 1 or 2 minutes and answer the question: "What was the most important thing you learned here today?" or "What are you most curious to learn some more about?" (Angelo & Cross, 1993).
- Have students consider something written for the lay public; editorials are good. Critically analyze the piece: is adequate information given; is the information reliable; is the piece biased, and if so what is the other point of view; if a problem is presented, what are the alternative conclusions/solutions; what outcomes would be best, most realistic, and how do you know if they are possible?
- Brainstorm for answers to a question or a case study. Encourage students to augment their thinking with hunches, and the use of intuition.
- Encourage students to identify the principle at the heart of a situation.
- Produce as much ambiguity in the classroom as possible. Don't give students clear-cut material. Give them conflicting information that they must think their way through (Strohm & Baukus, 1995).
- Use higher-order questions, and allow time for thinking before entertaining an answer.

ment that adult learners like to participate (Woodring, 1997). Though this study is 9 years old, the criticisms still ring true.

From the perspective of the teacher, many criticize that students are so completely occupied with note taking that they miss the central message of the lecture. Providing students with an outline of the content or printout of a PowerPoint presentation may eliminate the need to take copious notes. For many, however, taking notes is a big part of the learning process and even if an outline is provided, they will still choose to take notes. Using the computer, it is easy and necessary to provide outlines and other supplementary class material to students.

Discussion/Questions and Answers As an Adjunct to Lecture

Discussion and questions and answers are frequently used as an adjunct to lecture. Most educators agree that lecture should be accompanied by some opportunity for student expression or reaction. Although this does not automatically produce effective teaching, adequate incorporation of active student involvement will greatly facilitate communication. Along with satisfying the need for involvement, this approach to teaching also provides feedback for the teacher on how the content is being received and whether students understand what we are teaching. Inviting students to participate by asking questions or prompting discussion also conveys the message that it is their class rather than the teacher's class. Such identification with the teaching-learning experience may well motivate students and increase their learning level. The advantages of offering these techniques are discussed further under group discussion.

The use of questions and answers in class is a perfectly legitimate approach to teaching, but a distinction should be made with discussion. Perhaps the best way to show a difference is to emphasize the kind of question involved. **Question and answer teaching** almost always deals with factual data and objective responses, the lower level of the cognitive domain. Very often it is a review of material previously studied by the students, or just covered in a lecture. Although thought questions can certainly be used in this approach to teaching, there is a tendency for a thought question to lapse into discussion. Both of these techniques are appropriate, but teachers should be able to identify when they are using discussion as opposed to questions and answers. In higher education, the use of question and answer in the traditional sense is rare; and teachers should model their outreach for class interaction on higher levels of the cognitive domain, which should easily initiate discussion. The reader is referred to Box 10–3.

It is important for the teacher to direct any question to the whole class before specifying a student to answer. Challenge will soon be extinguished when students know that questions are coming in a certain definable pattern, or if the name of a student is always attached right at the outset. Never be negative toward a student's response. Even when the wrong answer is given, the good teacher will find some element of truth or commendation to reinforce the response.

Group Discussion

Group discussion is learner-centered with the teacher assuming the role of facilitator and content resource. Group is active learning for both the affective and cognitive domains. The primary benefit of discussion is its emphasis on individual thinking skills, the opportunity for students to

Box 10–3 Questions of a Higher Cognitive Order, Meant to Initiate Discussion and Critical Thinking

1. Questions of clarification:
   Could you give me an example?
   Is your basic point _____ or _____?
2. Questions that probe assumptions:
   You seem to be assuming _____.
   How would you justify taking this for granted?
   Is this always the case?
3. Questions that probe reasons and evidence:
   How could we go about finding whether that is true?
   Is there reason to doubt that evidence?
4. Questions about viewpoints or perspectives:
   How would other groups or types of people respond? Why? What would influence them?
   How would people who disagree with this viewpoint argue their case?
5. Questions that probe implications and consequences:
   What effect would that have?
   If this and this are the case, then what else must also be true?
6. Questions about the question:
   To answer this question what questions would we have to answer first?
   Is this the same issue as _____?

   Although these types of questions may be more the responsibility of the teacher in the beginning of the school year, with consistent modeling and encouragement students should increasingly take responsibility for asking these questions of themselves and their peers.

> Establish the habit of bringing up issues from the local, regional, or national press/media at the beginning of each class. Make sure the topics are related to the course content, and try to be controversial. Contacting the Web site of the newspaper or any media service, and searching categorically can easily accomplish this. Encourage personal opinions, analysis, and the introduction of other topics in the public eye. Gradually reinforce the behavior of those students who begin to contribute their own news interests. Use the scale in Box 10–1 to measure change.

translate information into their own words in a public arena, and reflect upon their own learning and reaction. Thus, good discussion sessions must engage all students in a dialogue and be facilitated closely by the teacher.

The group can be a rich venue for exchange of information, as well as feelings, values, and opinions. It is crucial to have clear and well-developed objectives that are shared at the beginning of every group session, and reviewed periodically. This will keep the group from becoming aimless. In fact, two sets of objectives are in order, one for content and the other for the process of the group experience. The discussion method may prove especially difficult for the novice teacher, so the need for objectives focused on process is especially strategic.

It becomes the role of the teacher to keep the discussion on track, tie points together, transition between topics, and maintain an environment of trust. Respectful attention and tolerance must be the operational rule, and should be modeled by the teacher. The teacher must be well versed in the subject matter, and the students must have some working knowledge; "otherwise, the discussion will be based on pooled ignorance" (Fitzgerald, 2003). In the role of expert, the teacher must be alert in case any group member interprets information incorrectly. The teacher assumes the role of facilitator and the content evolves from the work of group members, creating the potential for erroneous facts or misinterpretation. In addition, because students characteristically defer to faculty, it has to be made clear to students that their opinions are the most important in this learning process. Just getting people to talk does not guarantee that a genuine learning-by-discussion situation is in effect. The teacher is responsible for the quality of the discussion and the achievement of the learning products.

Teaching by discussion uses one of the best principles of the learning process, namely, active student involvement in the experience. A good discussion will help students to think and think about thinking. This is what is characteristically defined as critical thinking. It allows students to share ideas, receiving peer support, and developing a tolerance for those with whom they may disagree. The feeling of belonging that can be created is experiential (part of the experience), and contributes to reinforcing and retaining previous and current learning. The group milieu, if it is nurtured correctly, gives students an opportunity to correct earlier misconceptions and gain a sense of direction. Critical and creative thinking can be developed and skills of verbal expression stimulated. Teaching by discussion is also a motivational technique that encourages a student to think through concepts that have been hazy. Wrong conclusions may be corrected through the influence of the group rather than through the unilateral actions of the teacher. Problem-solving techniques are learned and can be applied not only in the search for knowledge, but also in all aspects of life.

In determining the best group size, one must consider the need for diversity of ideas, and the degree of interaction that is possible. Arnold and Boggs recommend that a group of six to eight individuals is ideal (2003). Others believe that closer to ten is better, with the teacher work-ing to regulate the dynamics of the group, and aiming for participation that is universal and equal. In either case, the goal is to provide enough students for rich interaction, yet not so many that the discussion becomes unruly.

The teacher should also be attuned to cultural factors, realizing that some students will find it difficult to participate actively in the group because of their background. This is most observ-able with students who are recent immigrants to this country. Adult students are particularly com-fortable in discussion groups, since they often come to the educational experience with highly developed communication skills and some group experience already. For the less sophisticated learner, these skills will be one of the goals of this method. This should be a consideration in decisions on group composition. Does heterogeneity in group help some students to develop at the expense of others?

The group discussion may take many forms. Planned *debate* between groups or within groups helps to expand the thought process, and sharpen reasoning. In the **seminar**, each member completes assigned readings before the meeting, allowing an active discussion. The ***case method or problem-based approach*** is best used in conjunction with clinical application courses, and offers the opportunity to apply the standard of evidence-based practice, and develop critical and creative thinking skills through the consideration of case **simulations** or actual clinical material (Bentley, 2002). **Problem-based learning** is particularly effective with adult learners whose pri-ority is the practical application of what they have learned. *Recitation* groups allow for guided study and further explication of content that has been presented in larger lecture sessions. These are usually breakout groups from a larger lecture session. ***Reflective practice groups*** encourage the examination of nursing care to expose the contradictions in one's own practice, and are best positioned as part of the pre- and post-clinical conference experience. The greatest problem with reflective practice groups is the need to have a safe environment for disclosure. Absent a cohesive group, full disclosure is difficult or impossible (Noveletsky-Rosenthal, 2001). Discussion groups may also be exclusively *process oriented*, aiming to give students some insight into their interper-sonal skills, and develop options for productive social and professional living.

Less Traditional Methods of Instruction

The imagination knows no bounds where instructional methods are concerned. More traditional methods may be augmented with new techniques. Novel and creative approaches to teaching are made possible through evolving technology. Whatever seems to work to facilitate learning is wor-thy of a trial, evaluation, and serious exposure to the research process.

The Jigsaw

Jigsaw is a cooperative strategy that involves group learning. The name "Jigsaw" is given for the structure of the activity within the group. A group is given a task or problem with a packet of information sufficient to allow creative and critical thinking about a solution or mastery of the task. Within the group, each member is given one part of the packet (a "piece of a puzzle") to work with. Each member then shares what they have learned with other group members—the goal is that all group members eventually learn all the information within the packet, but with the help of each other. The group depends on each individual in order to accomplish the task.

In a variation of this first approach, a large class is broken up into small groups. The same packet of materials is given to each group, and parts assigned to individual members. Then, however, the students who are responsible for the same section in the various "home" groups join together and form a new, temporary focus group whose purpose is for the students to:

• Master the material in their section.
• Enrich their thinking and enlarge their perspective through "groupthink."
• Develop a strategy for teaching what they have learned to the other students in their original "home" learning group.

First introduced by Aronson, Blaney, Stephan, Sikes, and Snapp (1978), the jigsaw structure of group discussion promotes positive interdependence and also provides a simple method to ensure individual accountability. The preparation of group packets is time intensive for the teacher. Sections of the packet must be equitable, complete, and contain the best resources. Students may be initially unhappy with this strategy, feeling that they are doing all the work, because this role is traditionally assigned to the teacher. Teachers may be anxious about not covering the expected content. These student and teacher assertions are common toward many of the more nontraditional instructional methods.

Debate

Debate is a procedure in which two or more people compete in trying to persuade others to accept or reject a proposition as the foundation for a belief or behavior. Debate was already mentioned as one technique well suited to group discussion. It is included again here to highlight the academic rigor that the technique demands, and the fact that debate is a hybrid, and differs from discussion in several ways:

• Debate is a presentation of the result rather than the airing of the process.
• Debate is basically competitive whereas discussion should be cooperative.
• Debate centers on an issue that is already defined, whereas a discussion generally is an attempt to delineate factors and define a position.

One of the major difficulties in structuring debates is the clarification of a good resolved. The subject of the debate must also be controversial in nature. The resolved should always be an affirmative statement presenting an issue that is clear not only to the debate participants, but also to the larger audience. The issue should also be debatable, offering an opportunity for both sides to construct substantive arguments. When the negative is blatantly wrong, the debate is sacrificed.

Speakers should be encouraged to attack the primary issues and not waste the limited time wandering down bypaths. In formal parliamentary debate, it is proper to take a vote from the assembly after the debaters have concluded to see which side won. That is probably not a good technique to use when you are employing the debate as a teaching method. The object is to get the issues on the floor, not to establish a winner. No doubt there will be a subjective decision formed in the minds of your students as to which side really has presented the better argument. But there seems to be no value in embarrassing any of the participants by taking a win-lose vote. See Box 10–4 for examples of debate resolves.

Journaling

Writing or **journaling** is a very beneficial technique of instruction that is best applied to the individual, and suitable for learning in both the cognitive and affective domains. Students can write about their knowledge, or their opinions, values, attitudes, and emotions with equal freedom and candor. Later, products generated here can be used with the class, according to student and teacher discretion. Students may be required to journal periodically about topics assigned by the

Box 10–4 The Debate: Be It Resolved   **193**

Resolved: Health care, except in emergency situations, should not be available to illegal aliens without cost.

Resolved: Early childhood vaccinations should be mandatory for every child, other than in instances of medical contraindication.

Resolved: Conventional teaching (lecture, discussion) contributes more to student learning than nontraditional techniques (simulations, computer-enhanced instruction, problem-based/case method of instruction).

Resolved: Sedation is often accompanied by a decline in cognitive function, and patients should be apprised of this side effect before being sedated.

Resolved: The benefits of stem cell research justify the use of human embryos.

Resolved: Developing countries should be able to benefit from AIDS research when their citizens serve as research subjects.

Resolved: Direct-to-consumer advertising causes patients to request newer, more expensive medications that work no better than less expensive therapies.

teacher, or more broadly about a variety of course-related topics, such as: How would you describe the nature of nursing? Describe one incident in your practice during the past week, and the scientific justification for your intervention. What do you have difficulty understanding about this course? Journals may be "stream of consciousness," reflective, or highly analytical; or may be expected to develop from one to another over time. An idea generated as an idle thought may later take on significant meaning, and become the cornerstone of serious critical thinking.

In any event, journaling should provide an opportunity for creative writing, and the most significant value that this holds should be the exploration into self. When individuals articulate feelings or ideas about a certain matter on paper, they tend to discipline their minds into orderly thinking about that subject. That is why teachers so frequently assign term papers and other writing projects that call for the discipline of organized thought processes. This explicates three values of this technique: insight into self, discipline, and organization of one's thinking.

A beginning writer may discover keeping a journal to be awkward, clumsy, uncomfortable, and even too revealing (Hodges, Kelley, & Wilkes, 1996). A major influence on the reactions of students to a journaling assignment is their familiarity with the recording activity. They may have kept a personal diary themselves or read diary-based accounts in literature. Some may have been exposed to the works of scientists, many of whom used diaries in the acquisition of insights and the formation of their theories. Students may have been required to keep journals in other courses. The quality and quantity of any of these experiences may vary but all provide background on which students can draw, thus predisposing them toward the openness, reflection, and organization critical to the journaling activity (Hancock, Mikhail, Santos, Nguyen et al., 1999). And if they bring no history in journaling, and are reticent, require more frequent journaling and shape their entries with sensitive and guiding comments.

Diversity among students in knowledge and attitudes about journals requires faculty to be clear about their journaling expectations. Students need explicit criteria for the form and function of the journal. If it is the expectation that both objective and subjective entries and reflection and analysis be included in journaling, then faculty must emphasize this at the beginning so that students can strive for them from the outset. If a process of development is expected, say so. The student may be told that their initial journals should support a stream-of-consciousness, with the aim of getting their thoughts down on paper, and subsequently become more organized and analytical.

But the standard must be clear. Thus, observations on the quality or characteristics of a student's journal may reflect as much upon the faculty's preparation of the student as on the student herself.

Decisions on journaling are made within the context of the instructional strategy for the course. Faculty members need to ask themselves some salient questions:

• What are the preconditions for successful journaling?
• When and how does the student learn from it?
• What are its risks and benefits?
• Which aspect of the assignment is more important: the process of writing it, the thinking involved, or the final product?
• Is journaling congruent with the faculty's philosophy of teaching and learning?
• Will journals be graded?
• Is the evaluation to be formative or summative?

Answers to and reflections on these questions can clarify the real reasons for journaling and result in a well-articulated and defensible description of the assignment. Journaling is particularly effective in shaping the quality of the student's creative and critical thinking. Moving students along this road involves tedious work for the teacher, patience, and the extensive use of formative evaluation. Summative evaluation is only appropriate at the end of the process.The goal is the same for all students in a course; journaling allows the teacher to personalize the means to that end.

Role Playing and Simulations

Role playing and simulations promote the use of imagination to have students stretch their thinking (Lowenstein & Bradshaw, 2001). Though both simulation and role playing are part of the same category of techniques, there are differences. Role playing "... is a method by which learners participate in an unrehearsed dramatization" (Bastable, 2003, p. 370). Simulation, in contrast to role playing, finds the learner "... rehearsing behaviors or roles that they will need to master and apply in real life" (Bastable, 2003, p. 370). An experience is created that reflects real-life conditions but without the consequences of failure. Today, with health-care provider requirements for increased productivity and patients who are in the delivery system for very short periods of time, real-life experiences are at a premium. While using simulations and role playing, students may try out behaviors and solutions in the safety of the laboratory before they apply them to the real world. In other words, role play and simulation afford students an opportunity to experiment without risk. The reader is referred to Chapter 9 for more discussion of learning laboratories.

Role Playing

Role playing is particularly effective in the affective domain and in developing decision-making and problem-solving abilities. This instructional method is primarily used to arouse feelings and elicit emotional responses in the learner. It is unscripted and improvised. The learner is not mastering a role with plans to use it, but to develop an understanding of other people in the situation. The role players respond to each other—not to the audience—as characters in the scenario. Members of the class not involved in the drama are observers and contribute to the analysis after the dramatization (peer review). The teacher role here is passive, facilitating, and gently guiding, rather than directing.

Many people have had unpleasant experiences with role playing because the teacher failed to warm up the class. Warm-up is necessary for role play. See Box 10–5. Further, those assigned to specific parts of the drama need to be acquainted with their roles. Simply saying, "You're a dying patient and you are her daughter who is afraid to admit her impending death—go to it!" isn't enough information, and those thrown into such a situation will feel as if they have been deserted. The teacher as coach needs to talk to each of the players, interview them "in role," draw out their thoughts regarding the role and role playing, and gently involve them imaginatively in the situation. Roles need to be explained briefly both to the players and the observers before start of the session. There should be enough explanation to allow their participation but not so much that it affects their role taking or later analysis. Students need to know the objectives of the exercise, the story line, how the characters participate, and the role of the observers.

Students report increased learning and better retention using role playing over traditional lecturing (DeNeve & Hepner, 1997). This is not surprising given the active role of students, both actors and observers, with this technique. This comparison, however, is not entirely fair. Role playing meets different pedagogic needs, being structured chiefly for learning in the affective domain, targeting interpersonal behaviors as they reveal attitudes and values. Role playing is particularly useful for practicing therapeutic communication skills and dealing with conflict. But there are disadvantages, too. Development of appropriate role-playing scenarios can be time intensive. Some students are reluctant to participate, because the role playing is done in front of a group of students. Role playing may reinforce stereotypical behavior among students. There are also economic considerations; the method is best accomplished with a small group of students, no more than ten.

Simulation

Simulation allows anticipatory learning (Bastable, 2003). There are a number of types of simulation: written simulation, audio-visual simulation, simulation using models, and computer simulation. Simulation activities involve controlled representations of actual clinical events. This methodology allows the learner to experience "real world" patient situations without risk. Learners are required to assess and interpret the situation, and make decisions based on information provided. Usually conducted in a laboratory setting, simulation learning allows students to execute a variety of skills, including assessment, psychomotor skills, and decision-making. Simulated cases or problem situations can be used for either teaching or evaluation. Both psychomotor skills and cognitive decisions can be incorporated into computer simulation. Cases are presented, information given and requested by the student, decisions made, and feedback supplied.

Both models and live subjects can be used for simulation. Computers have been combined with lifelike models to provide the ultimate in realism and customization of student experiences.

Box 10–5 Warm-Up Exercises for Role Playing

Role playing can be very threatening for those who are unaccustomed to speaking in front of a group, or even for those who are. Warm-up exercises aim to increase bonding among group members and create a climate of comfort and relaxation. (Explain how these work to warm up the class.)

- The group members are guests at a holiday party who have never met each other before. Circulate as you would in a similar social situation, and get to know one another.
- Two volunteers, one plays the sales person for time-share properties in Florida, and the other plays someone who has just answered the phone and wants to be courteous to his efforts.
- A student with a failing grade who is pleading his or her case, and the instructor who is listening and responding.
- A fellow student that you have just met, and want to cultivate a friendship with.
- You have just won the lottery and are sharing your good luck with a friend.

> Role playing is built on the foundation of psychodrama that was brought to the United States as a psychotherapeutic technique in 1924 by Moreno. Some of the methods of psychodrama may prove useful here. One such technique is the role of *"alter ego."* One participant assumes a position behind another of the players, and whispers directions for interaction as she or he would play the role. It becomes optional whether the alter ego's suggestions are heeded. This can be a very supportive technique for a student who is ill at ease with the role or role playing. Another dramatic device has the players make *"asides,"* comments to the audience that the other characters have to pretend they haven't heard. This allows the player to reveal what she or he thinks, but is not able to say. Role reversal is also useful, and involves players changing parts so they can begin to empathize with the other's point of view, even if they don't agree. Speaking from different roles helps people become more conscious of their ambivalence.

The most sophisticated of these are called *high-fidelity simulators*. They are whole-body, computer operator controlled models that reproduce in a lifelike manner the functioning of all body systems, and even have the ability to respond to certain drugs (Bastable, 2003). *Mid-fidelity* does not have the aforementioned capabilities, but permits rapid vital sign and heart/breath sound changes in response to assessment/interventions. *Low-fidelity* includes traditional mannequins, or other noninteractive simulators. These simulators allow students to practice repetitive and high-risk procedures under the supervision of clinical faculty. The use of high-fidelity simulators to educate students for the workplace environment is recommended in the Institute of Medicine report "Keeping Patients Safe: Transforming the Work Environment of Nurses" (2003).

High-fidelity simulation was first used in nurse anesthesia education (Farnsworth, Egan, Johnson, & Westenskow, 2000). Since September 11, 2001 these simulators have become the backbone of Air Force Nursing Education at the Joint Trauma Training Center and the Warskills Simulation Laboratory (Bruce, Bridges, & Holcomb, 2003). Recent availability of SimMan™ (by Laerdal) now affords undergraduate students opportunities to experience and learn via high-fidelity simulation. SimMan scenarios include a teenage asthmatic, middle-age CHF, and multiple-complex critical and anesthesia focused patients. These situations progress from simple to complex, incorporating a range of complications and crisis events, and expecting nursing management in real-time. High-fidelity simulators allow students to practice repetitive and/or high-risk procedures under the supervision of clinical faculty. Studies have shown that high-fidelity simulation is particularly effective with the adult learner (Yaeger et al., 2004). The reader is referred to Box 10–6 for an example of use of simulation with registered nurses.

Simulation, particularly high-fidelity, is expensive, and justification of its use essential. Ravert conducted a meta-analysis of quantitative studies related to computer-based simulations and their effect on education and learning in the health care disciplines (2002). This review indicates that a significant number of these studies reveal positive effects of simulation on skill and/or knowledge acquisition. The potential of computer-based simulation for educational augmentation is enormous, but more research is needed to determine cost effective and successful uses of high-fidelity simulations for nursing education (Ravert, 2002).

A growing trend associated with simulation, especially simulation of the higher order is the learning laboratory. State-of-the-art laboratories are equipped with mannequins; simulators; bedside computers, with Internet access; digitalized video; computer-assisted instructional software;

One hospital whose nursing staff is recognized according to Benner's model of competency describes a three-tiered system to meet the educational objectives of learners. The first tier targets the advanced beginner-competent, and includes introductory offerings that facilitate development of critical thinking, skills, and recognition of deterioration. Low- and mid-fidelity simulation are used at this level. The second tier focuses on the competent-proficient. Offerings center on evidence-based practice and ethical decision-making. Mid- and high-fidelity simulation are used at this level. The third tier targets the proficient-expert. High-fidelity simulation is used almost exclusively at this level. Learners respond to the "patient" and are evaluated in real time, followed by debriefing. The success of mid-/high-fidelity simulation in this setting is such that it is used by most health-care disciplines, and simulation has been required for the annual testing of nursing competencies.

Source: From: Beeman, L. Appropriate Application of Human Simulation Technology Utilizing Benner's Model of Novice to Expert. *Clinical Simulation in Education.* Sigma Theta Tau International, 38th Biennial Convention—Clinical Sessions, November 12–13, 2005, Indianapolis, IN. http://stti.confex.com/stti/bcclinical38/techprogram/meeting_bcclinical38.htm. Retrieved July 20, 2005.

and other interactive software. The laboratories are designed to replicate realistic practice settings, including the basic hospital unit, critical care, pediatrics, neonatal nursery, maternity, home care, and the diagnostic laboratory.

Another type of simulation is the *simulation game*. These games are generally interactive in a problem situation, operated according to set rules, and competitive. Examples of such games are "Mental Hospital," "Into Aging," "The Disaster Game," and "Bafa Bafa." The first two of these games aim to sensitize students to unique physical disabilities that accompany aging and the social disenfranchisement suffered by the mentally ill. The third simulates citizens' roles under disaster conditions and encourages players to cooperate, organize, and plan. "Bafa Bafa" introduces students to the stereotyping experienced by a foreigner in a strange culture.

Simulations (whether written, on computer, as a game, practiced on mannequins, high- or low-fidelity) bring clinically related experiences into the school, and are a more efficient and safer method of providing clinical experiences. It is apparent that many schools of nursing are using simulation teaching and evaluation as a complement to patient-contact experiences. Simulations are being used with a variety of subjects and concepts and with a wide range of student abilities. They have proven to be efficient and effective in these days of tight time schedules, "full" curricula, and crowded clinical facilities.

Case Method and Problem-Based Learning

Case method and problem-based learning (PBL) are variations on a theme. Both use case material or problem scenarios as a vehicle for analysis and/or decision-making. In case method, these scenarios demonstrate how previously acquired knowledge applies to clinical practice. The *knowledge precedes the problem*. Often a step-by-step analysis by the teacher models the critical thinking process, followed by student discussion. In contrast, PBL is not dependent on earlier learning; *the problem comes first*. The problem is posed so that the students discover that they need to acquire some new knowledge before they can understand or solve the problem. Information necessary to devise a solution is not included in the case, and the scenario is open-ended and purposefully "ill-structured."

Problem-Based Learning

An essential component of problem-based learning (PBL) is that content is introduced in the context of complex real-world problems. PBL uses an inquiry model. In PBL, students working in small groups (ideally five or six) or independently; must identify what they know; and most importantly, what they don't know. After asking critical questions and searching for the relevant information, the goal is to solve the problem or at least shed some light on an unclear situation. Posing the problem before learning the associated content tends to motivate students. They know why they are learning the new knowledge. Learning in the context of the need-to-solve-or-understand-a-problem also tends to store the knowledge in memory patterns that facilitate later recall. Before entering into PBL, students should be skilled problem solvers. PBL does not develop problem-solving skills without explicit interventions on the part of the teacher. In some academic situations, a workshop on problem solving precedes the use of PBL.

PBL teaching materials are designed to be "ill-structured" and to imitate the complexity of real-life situations. There is never a simple answer. PBL assignments vary widely in scope and sophistication, and one case may provide the focus for many weeks of inquiry. Students must go beyond their textbooks to pursue knowledge in other resources in between their group meetings. One such resource may be expert opinion. They then reconvene to share and summarize their new knowledge. Students may present their conclusions, and there may or may not be an end product. Again, students ideally have adequate time for reflection and self-evaluation. All problem-based learning approaches rely on a problem as their driving forces, but may focus on the solution to varying degrees. Some PBL approaches intend for students to clearly define the problem, develop hypotheses, gather information, and arrive at clearly stated solutions. Others engage students with problems that have no solution, but are meant for learning and information gathering (Burch, 1997). The primary role of the instructor is to facilitate group process and learning, not to provide easy answers.

The model for PBL was developed more than 25 years ago at McMaster University in Canada. PBL has since become a preferred methodology in business, law, and several medical schools. Interest grew from questions about how well traditional courses educated students to be problem-solvers and lifelong learners. Information-dense lectures, presented by a series of experts to large student audiences, seemed disconnected from the application of content to real life, which requires integration of knowledge, decision-making, and working and communicating with others. The reader is referred to Table 10–1 and Box 10–7 for a summary of the characteristics of PBL and an example of case material.

Case Method

The case method differs somewhat from PBL. The materials used in the case method are more extensive and complete, assuming that previous learning is integrated in the scenario. Case method and the problem-based method both use narratives, situations, select data samplings, or statements that present unresolved or provocative issues, situations, or questions. As a teaching/learning tool, this material challenges participants to analyze, critique, make judgments, speculate, and express reasoned opinions. Above all, although information can be real or invented, the situations presented must be realistic and believable. The information included must be rich enough to make the situation credible, but not so complete as to close off discussion or exploration. Material may be short for brief classroom discussions, or long and elaborate for semester-long projects. The intent is to bring real world problems into the safe and secure world of the classroom. They are "rehearsal for life" (Herreid, 1994).

Both of these techniques place the student in the role of decision-maker, and provide a story or scenario that needs to be made sense of, solved, or resolved. The faculty role is to guide

What:	How?	Why?
Student-centered and experiential	Select authentic assignments from the discipline, preferably those that would be relevant and meaningful to student interests. Students also are responsible for locating and evaluating various resources in the field.	Relevance is one of the primary student motivators to be a more self-directed learner.
Inductive	Introduce content through the process of problem solving, rather than problem solving after introduction to content.	Research indicates that "deeper" learning takes place when information is introduced within a meaningful context.
Builds on/challenges prior learning	If the case has some relevance to students, then they are required to call on what they already know or think they know. By focusing on their prior learning, students can test assumptions, prior learning strategies, and facts.	The literature suggests that learning takes place when there is a conflict between prior learning and new information.
Context-specific	Choose real or contrived case, the content is grounded in the kinds of challenges faced by practitioners in the field.	Again, context-specific information tends to be learned at a deeper level and retained longer.
Problems are complex and ambiguous, and require meta-cognition	Select actual examples from the "real life" of the discipline. Require students to analyze their own problem-solving strategies	Requires the ability to use higher order thinking skills such as analysis, synthesis, evaluation, and creation of new knowledge.
Creates cognitive conflict	Select cases with information that makes simple solutions difficult: while the solution may address one part of a problem, it may create another problem. Challenges prior learning as previously noted.	The literature suggests that learning takes place when there is a conflict between prior learning and new information.
Collaborative and interdependent	Have students work in small groups in order to address the presented case.	By collaborating, students see other kinds of problem-solving strategies used, they discuss the case using their collective information, and they need to take responsibility for their own learning, as well as their classmates'.

Source: Gallow, D., & Grant, H. What is problem-based learning? University of California, Irvine: Problem-Based Learning Faculty Institute. With permission. http://www.pbl.uci.edu/whatispbl.html. Retrieved September 29, 2005.

students to resources and information, help them to frame the questions to ask, formulate the problems in clear language, explore alternatives, and make decisions. Students confront these problems in small groups, and pool their knowledge for successful solutions. These strategies give students the opportunity to use previous learning or evolving knowledge depending on the method used.

It was 4:36 a.m. She was in a cold sweat and having difficulty breathing. She felt as though she had run a marathon. Fear swept through her—something terrible was going to happen. Panic-stricken, she woke her husband, Jeremy.

"Denise, what is it? Is it a nightmare?" said Jeremy.

"No, it's like I'm having an asthma attack. I feel lightheaded and I can't catch my breath. My heart feels like it's beating a thousand times a minute."

Afraid to upset her husband further, Denise didn't tell him that an immense feeling of apprehension suddenly overcame her. She got up to drink some water and waited for the anxiety to subside. Her mind was racing. Jeremy was the one with the family history of heart disease. This couldn't be happening to her. It was his problem. A few months earlier, Jeremy was diagnosed with coronary artery disease. He was only 48 years old, the same age as Denise. The scare had encouraged him to gradually end years of chain smoking and adopt a healthier lifestyle. He was currently working on giving up the occasional cigarette for good.

"No," Denise thought to herself. *"There's no way this was a sign of heart troubles. I didn't have a pain in my chest, I'm physically fit, and I have no family history. There's just no way."*

After assuring herself of this, Denise was somehow able to fall back asleep.

Source: Adapted from: Rubin, L., & Herreid, C. F. (2002). Wake-up call. University at Buffalo, State University of New York. http://www.sciencecases.org/heart/heart1.asp. Retrieved September 29, 2005.

As in other group strategies, students should be allowed to work without instructor interference, and optimally within a group of three to eight participants. The instructor must be comfortable with ambiguity and with adopting the nontraditional roles of witness and resource, rather than authority. The instructor may provide the structure of a series of questions to guide group exploration and discussion. It is probably wise to reveal these questions slowly over time, rather than chance that students will rush to premature closure. Pay careful attention to the sequencing of the questions suggested in Box 10–8.

Box 10–8 Sample Questions to Facilitate Case Method/Problem-Based Learning

What evidence do you have?

How reliable is that evidence, and where do you need validation?

Are there any observations that are conflicting or serendipitous?

What additional information do you need?

Are any patterns observable in the scenario?

What are the assumptions in this situation, and should they be challenged?

Have there been errors in logic, reasoning, or the thought process? (Allow for different points of view.)

Have you had other experiences that could be extrapolated to this new situation?

Compare and contrast this situation with others you may have encountered that are similar.

How do your own biases affect this analysis?

What does research and expert opinion tell us? How credible are these sources?

Is there more than one solution/answer to this problem; and what is your opinion(s)?

Can we arrive at a decision as a group?

What are the consequences/implications of this decision(s)?

In case method, the materials may be an in-depth description, including present problems and background information. The case may demonstrate how concepts and theories learned in class are applied to clinical practice. Shorter cases, a few sentences to a paragraph, may only present essential information, and focus through questions on assessment, missing data, alternative decisions, and consequences. Case studies also may be developed to represent the unfolding of clinical situation over time. These are referred to as unfolding cases. After the student has answered questions about the current part, the scenario is modified. This can continue indefinitely (Oermann, 2004).

The format for cases or problem situations can take several forms. They can include the solution, allowing merely for analysis or suggested alternative solutions. Unfinished cases have the results withheld, either by design or reality. Situations may be fictional or real. In the situation where the teacher authors such material, care should be taken that the material is complex enough to challenge the student, yet not so obscure as to make solution impossible. The time involved in developing or securing these materials is a major obstacle to use of these techniques.

Grand rounds is another instructional method focusing on case material. The case material may either be real or fictitious, current or retrospective, one case or several. Presenting a case at grand rounds assumes some sophistication in presentation and knowledge. Faculty or senior students are often the presenters of case material and the facilitators of discussion. Criteria for grand rounds is presented in Box 10–9. Grand rounds may be conducted in the clinical area or the classroom. In some settings, they are videotaped for future review (Oermann, 2004). Grand rounds should include staff nurses, who are the appropriate role models for students.

Concept Mapping

A concept map is a visual (graphic) representation used to illustrate and facilitate understanding of relationships between one or more concepts, thus directly enhancing critical thinking. In addition, concept maps facilitate communication between students and faculty. Many nurse educa-

Box 10–9 Format for Nursing Grand Rounds

The oral presentation will include the following and last for 10–15 minutes:

- Presenting condition and relevant history
- Related pathophysiology and resulting symptomatology with a focus on multisystem involvement (include assessment here)
- Relevant diagnostic/laboratory data
- Impact of any intervention to date, including pharmacologic
- Top priority nursing diagnoses and plan of care
- Expected outcomes
- Teaching/counseling needs of client/family
- Transfer or discharge planning; referrals to community agencies
- Relevant research or research deficits associated with this patient's condition
- Ethical issues

For a satisfactory grand rounds presentation, the presenter should:

- Present materials in a professional manner
- Provide audience with supportive handouts
- Have audio-visual/multimedia materials to enhance the presentation
- Stimulate group participation

tors have in recent years adopted this teaching strategy, originating from the education discipline. Mapping has been well documented in the literature and given various labels, depending on the field and its intended use. It has been called cognitive mapping, idea mapping, patterned mapping, patterned note taking, and flow charting (Koehler, 2001).

There is no one right way to design a concept map. The learner should be oriented to mapping and to the logic behind the methodology, but then encouraged to be creative in the map design while still including all of the appropriate data. Ideally, the learner creates the map and the teacher can gain great insight into the nature and extent of the student's understanding of content by reviewing the maps. No two concept maps will ever be the same. Four main styles of concept maps are possible, yet there may be more. These are the spider map, hierarchical or chronological map, flow chart, and systems map. Refer to Figure 10–1 for samples.

Proposals have been made to use some form of concept mapping in lieu of traditional nursing care plans, but for our purpose we will be considering mapping as a strategy for learning. The benefits of concept mapping include the following: (Hanson, 2005)

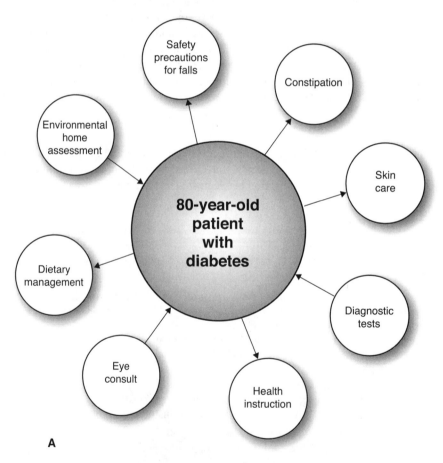

A

FIGURE 10–1 Designs for concept maps. (A) The spider map. (B) The hierarchical or chronological map. (C) The flow chart, linear progression. (D) The systems map. Adapted from: Hanson K. Concept mapping in health care management. South Dakota State University, College of Nursing, Continuing Nursing Education. http://learn.sdstate.edu/nursing/ConceptMap.html. Retrieved September 6, 2005.

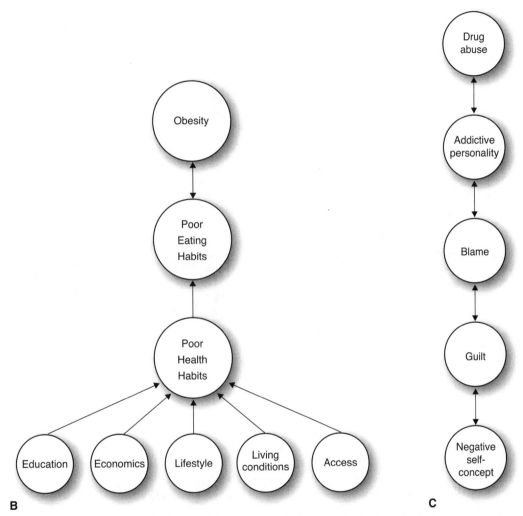

B   **C**

FIGURE 10-1 (B) The hierarchical or chonological map. (C) The flow chart, linear progression.

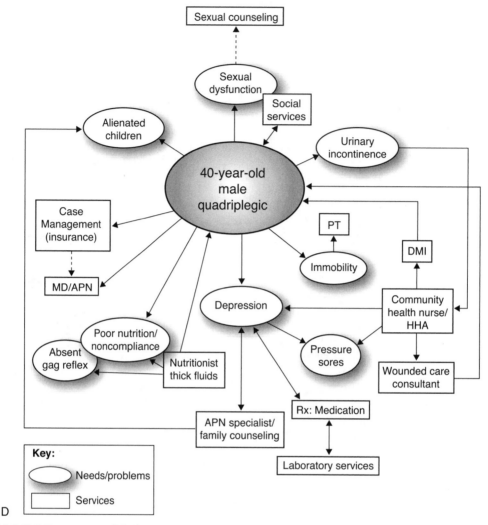

FIGURE 10–1 (D) The systems map.

- Improves the student's ability to organize a body of knowledge
- Allows the student to assimilate previously learned knowledge with newly acquired knowledge
- Demands critical thinking skills
- Provides a visual aid that may promote learning
- Allows the student to identify what they know about a topic and also what they must still learn

One person alone may construct concept maps or a group may collaborate in this work. In fact, the greater the number of students who participate in the map development, the more meaningful the discussion. These maps may be used in any content area, but the most common application is in the clinical setting. Mapping can be a successful tool in leading discussions during post-conference: the student(s) draws a map showing patient problems and how these problems are interrelated. The map illustrates relationships between one or more medical diagnoses, nursing assessment data, diagnostic test results, nursing diagnoses and collaborative problems, and interventions and treatments.

Students can be introduced to the idea of concept maps by the instructor's use of such tools. Use a blackboard, transparencies, or the computer to visualize lecture content in this format, without labeling it as such. Once students have been intrigued or found it useful to their understanding, invite them to participate in using this format.

Summary

The teaching strategies that have been presented here are just a start. These techniques will grow and multiply by combining them and making minor and major modifications. The secret is to trust your intuition and continuously assess your students and the pace at which they are growing in their learning.

Remember that as a teacher of students preparing for professional practice, your goal is to develop critical thinking skills adequate to support evidence-based practice. The student who thinks critically can ask appropriate questions, gather relevant information, efficiently and creatively sort through this information, reason logically from this information, and come to reliable and trustworthy conclusions about their practice.

Any of the strategies detailed here can facilitate the development of these skills. Lecture brings the perspective of an expert and models critical thinking. Group discussion, in all of its forms, when properly facilitated by the teacher, moves students to challenge one another, while sharpening their thinking skills. The jigsaw builds responsibility and independence through a group within group experience. Debates allow us to find new meaning and consider the opposing views of our arguments. Journaling provides the time to examine self and to process concepts. Role playing and simulation allow us to experience new situations without the inherent risk that reality would hold. Case studies offer an opportunity to apply concepts to novel situations, extrapolating from the familiar. Problem-based learning promotes a spirit of inquiry, confronting what we don't know as opposed to what we do know. The teacher's only restriction is her own creativity.

R e f e r e n c e s

Angelo, T. A., & Cross, K. P. *Classroom assessment techniques: A handbook for college teachers* (2nd ed.). Retrieved September 29, 2005 from
http://honolulu.hawaii.edu/intranet/committees/FacDevCom/guidebk/teachtip/assess-2.htm.
Arnold, E., & Boggs, K. (2003). *Interpersonal relationships* (4th ed.). Philadelphia: Saunders.
Aronson, E., Blaney, N., Stephan, C., Sikes, J., & Snapp, M. (1978). *The jigsaw classroom.* Sage Publications.
Bastable, S. B. (2003). *Nurse as educator* (2nd ed.). Boston: Jones & Bartlett.
Beeman, L. Appropriate Application of Human Simulation Technology Utilizing Benner's Model of Novice to Expert. *Clinical Simulation in Education.* Sigma Theta Tau International, 38th Biennial Convention— Clinical Sessions, November 12–13, 2005, Indianapolis, IN. Retrieved July 20, 2005 from
http://stti.confex.com/stti/bcclinical38/techprogram/meeting_bcclinical38.htm.
Bentley, G. (2002) Problem-based learning. In A. Lowenstein and M. Bradshaw, *Fuszard's innovative teaching strategies in nursing* (3rd ed., pp. 83–106). Gaithersburg, MD: Aspen.
Bloom, B. (1956). *Taxonomy of educational objectives.* New York: David McKay.
Bruce, S., Bridges, E. J., & Holcomb, J. B. (2003). Preparing to respond: Joint trauma training center and USAF nursing warskills simulation laboratory. *Critical Care Nursing Clinics of North America, 15*(2), 149–162.

Burch, K. (1997). A primer on problem-based learning: examples from international relations courses. University of Delaware, Newark, August 1997. Retrieved October 1, 2005 from **http://www.ntlf.com/html/lib/suppmat/82pblprimer.htm.**

De Cecco, J., & Crawford, W. (1974). *The psychology of learning and instruction* (2nd ed.). Englewood Cliffs, NJ: Prentice-Hall.

DeNeve, K. M., & Hepner, M. J. (1997). Role play simulations: The assessment of an active learning technique and comparisons with traditional lectures. *Innovative Higher Education, 21,* 231–246.

de Tornyay, R., & Thompson, M.A. (1982). *Strategies for teaching nursing* (2nd ed.). New York: John Wiley & Sons.

Dunn, R., & Dunn, K. (1978). *Teaching students through their individual learning styles: A practical approach.* Reston, VA: Reston.

Fitzgewrald, K. (2003). Instructional methods. In S. Bastable (Ed.), *Nurse as educator* (2nd ed.). Boston: Jones & Bartlett.

Farnsworth, S.T., Egan, T. D., Johnson, S. E, & Westenskow, D. (2000). Teaching sedation and analgesia with simulation. *Journal of Clinical Monitoring and Computing, 16*(4), 273–285.

Hancock, T., Mikhail, B. I., Santos, A., Nguyen, A., et al. (1999). A comparison of HIV/AIDS knowledge among high school freshmen and senior students. *Journal of Community Health Nursing, 16*(3); 151–163.

Hanson K. (2005). *Concept mapping in health care management.* South Dakota State University. Retrieved July 29, 2005 from **http://learn.sdstate.edu/nursing/ConceptMap.html.**

Herreid, C. F. (1994). Case studies in science: A novel method of science education. *The Journal of College Science Teaching,* Feb., 221–229. University at Buffalo, The State University of New York. Retrieved August 4, 2005 from **http://ublib.buffalo.edu/libraries/projects/cases/teaching/novel.html.**

Hodges, R., Kelley, L., & Wilkes, A. (1996). Benchmarking and networking through collaborative groups. *Journal for Healthcare Quality;18*(1); 26–31.

Koehler, C. (2001). Nursing process mapping replaces nursing care plans. In A. Lowenstein and M. Bradshaw. *Fuszard's innovative teaching strategies in nursing* (3rd ed., pp. 303–313). Gaithersburg, MD: Aspen.

Lowenstein A.J., & Bradshaw, M. J. (2001) *Fuszard's innovative teaching strategies in nursing.* Gaithersburg, MD: Aspen.

Moreno, J. L. (1957). *The first book on group psychotherapy.* Michigan University, self published.

Noveletsky-Rosenthal, H. (2001). Reflective practice. In A. Lowenstein and M. Bradshaw, *Fuszard's innovative teaching strategies in nursing* (3rd ed., pp. 107–112). Gaithersburg, MD: Aspen.

Oermann, M. H. (2004). Basic skills for teaching and the advanced practice nurse. In L. A. Joel (Ed.), *Advanced practice nursing: essentials for role development.* Philadelphia: FA Davis.

Ravert, P. (2002). An integrative review of computer-based simulation in the education process. *Computers, Informatics, Nursing, 20*(5), 203–208.

Rubin, L., & Herreid, C. F. (2002). Wake-up call. State University of New York at Buffalo. Retrieved September 29, 2005 from **http://www.sciencecases.org/heart/heart1.asp.**

Strohm, S. M., & Baukus, R. A. (1995). Strategies for fostering critical thinking skills. *Journalism and Mass Communication Educator 50*(1), 55–62.

Woodring, B. (1997). *Student evaluation of teaching effectiveness.* Unpublished manuscript.

Woodring, B. (2001). Lecture is not a four letter word! In A. Lowenstein and M. Bradshaw, *Fuszard's innovative teaching strategies in nursing* (3rd ed., pp. 65–82). Gaithersburg, MD: Aspen.

Yaeger, K. A., Halamek, L. P., Coyle, M., Murphy, A., Anderson, J., Boyle, K., et al. (2004). High-fidelity simulation-based training in neonatal nursing. *Advances in Neonatal Care, Dec;4*(6), 324.

REVIEW QUESTIONS

- What audio/visual materials could you use with a lecture on bonding during the post-partum period?
- Describe how you would handle a student who dominates during a discussion.
- In using journaling as an instructional method, what directions would you give the student?
- How would teaching patients about diabetic care differ from teaching beginning nursing students? Consider pacing, staging, content, and process.

CRITICAL THINKING EXERCISES

Develop the plan for a jigsaw focused on the nursing shortage. This would include the breakdown of the topic into parts manageable enough for study and complete enough to contribute to an understanding of the whole.

Construct a concept map of your choice to explain the process of education for self-care of a newly diagnosed diabetic.

Mrs. Jones has a terminal illness; she knows it, and wants her family's support. Her family knows the prognosis, but has never talked to her honestly and openly about her condition. Role play this situation with the patient and the family, both together and separate. The teacher's challenge will be to develop the objectives for the exercise, the story line, how the characters participate, and the role of the observers.

ANNOTATED RESEARCH SUMMARY

Alexander, J. G. (2002). Promoting, applying, and evaluating problem-based learning in the undergraduate nursing curriculum. *Nursing Education Perspectives, 23* (5), 248–253.

Since its development in the 1960s, problem-based learning (PBL) has become increasingly prominent in nursing education. In 1998, Stamford University received a grant from the PEW Charitable Trusts to promote, apply, and evaluate PBL in its undergraduate curriculum over 3 years. It has become integrated into the nursing curriculum in clinical and nonclinical courses. Descriptions of its implementation in specific courses are provided, and its usefulness in nursing education discussed. Evaluations and test scores indicate that PBL has had a positive effect on the students and exceeded the educational expectations.

Beers, G. W. (2005). The effect of teaching method on objective test scores: problem-based learning versus lecture. *Journal of Nursing Education, 44*(7), 305–309.

This study investigated the effect of teaching method on objective test scores of students in a school of nursing. The hypothesis stated there was a difference between objective test scores of students who were taught content on diabetes using problem-based learning (PBL) and students taught the same content using the traditional lecture method. A pre-test and post-test were administered to both groups of students. Both the pre-test and post-test scores of the two groups were compared using an independent test, and no statistically significant difference was found in the scores of the two groups. The results of this study show no difference in objective test scores based on teaching method.

Browne, M. N., Freeman, K. E., & Williamson, C. L. (2000). The importance of critical thinking for student use of the internet. *College Student Journal, 34*(4),

September 2000. http://static.highbeam.com/c/collegestudentjournal/septem-ber012000/

Students are increasingly so dependent on the Internet for their information that critical thinking programs that do not address the form and quality of persuasion on that medium are flirting with an anachronistic pedagogy. This paper documents the absorption of postsecondary students with the Internet as a source of "knowledge," spells out the attendant dangers, and suggests the essential first step in applying critical thinking to the Internet.

Burbach, M. E., Matkin, G. S., & Fritz, S. M. (2004). Teaching critical thinking in an introductory leadership course utilizing active learning strategies: A confirmatory study. *College Student Journal, 38*(3). http://static.highbeam.com/c/collegestudentjournal/september012004/

Critical thinking is often seen as a universal goal of higher education but is seldom confirmed as an outcome. This study was conducted to determine whether an introductory level college leadership course that encouraged active learning increased critical thinking skills. A pre- and post-assessment of critical thinking skills was conducted using the Watson-Glaser Critical Thinking Appraisal. Significant increases were found in the Deduction and Interpretation subtests, and total Critical Thinking. Student engagement in active learning techniques within the context of studying interpersonal skills for leadership appeared to increase critical thinking.

Cotton, K. (1988). Classroom Questioning Close-up No. 5. Portland, OR: Northwest Regional Educational Laboratory, May 1988.

This study synthesizes findings from 37 research reports on the relationship between teacher classroom questioning behavior and a variety of student outcomes. The study found that when teachers ask higher cognitive questions, conduct redirection/probing/reinforcement, and/or increase wait time, the cognitive sophistication of student responses increases.

Deeny, P., Johnson, A., Boore, J., Leyden, C., & McCaughan, E. (2001). Drama as an experiential technique in learning how to cope with dying patients and their families. *Teaching in Higher Education, 6*(1), 99–112.

Evaluated use of drama as a teaching method to familiarize nursing students with various scenarios of patient death. The combination of drama and group discussion was considered very effective by students, who requested more similar sessions.

Drummond, T. (2002). A brief summary of the best practices in teaching: Intended to challenge the professional development of all teachers. Seattle, WA: North Seattle Community College. http://northonline.sccd.ctc.edu/eceprog/bstprac.htm

A thorough summary of best practices in instructional methods.

Fry-Welch, D. K. (2004). Use of threaded discussion to enhance classroom teaching of critical evaluation of the professional literature. *Journal of Physical Therapy Education, 18*(2), 48–53.

Reflective thinking is important in developing critical-thinking skills necessary to critically evaluate the professional literature. Use of threaded discussion as an adjunct to in-class teaching engaged the students in reflective discussion prior to class sessions. This method of instruction allowed the professor to review the threaded discussion and assess student understanding of the discussion topic before class. Lecture then could be used to dispel areas of confusion and misinterpretation by the students. Web-based threaded discussion is a valuable pedagogical tool to use as an adjunct to on-campus courses.

Gough, D. (1991). Thinking about thinking. Alexandria, VA: National Association of Elementary School Principals.

This research summarizes five study reports concerning the nature of higher-order thinking skills and the most effective methods for teaching them. While focusing on different aspects of the topic, the authors of these reports are in agreement that thinking skills should be integrated across the curriculum rather than taught in isolation.

Hsu, I., & Hsieh, S. I. (2005). Concept maps as an assessment tool in a nursing course. *Journal of Professional Nursing, 21*(3), 141–149.

The results of this study indicated that the students developed their concept maps from a linear sequence of concepts at the beginning into a highly integrated web of concepts in the final draft. Students acquired problem-solving and critical-thinking skills by organizing complex patient data, analyzing concept relationships, and identifying interventions.

Isaacson, J. J. (2004). Nursing students in an expanded charge nurse role: A real clinical management nursing experience. *Nursing Education Perspectives, 25*(6), 292–296.

Ensuring that baccalaureate nursing students obtain a measure of management and leadership proficiency is a challenge for nurse educators. Having senior students manage juniors in a clinical course modeled in a peer hierarchical pattern that emulates advanced beginner practice is a creative approach that is both realistic and achievable.

Kennison, M. M. (2002). Evaluating reflective writing for appropriateness, fairness and consistency. *Nursing Education Perspectives, 23*(5), 238–242.

Nurse educators are divided about how to evaluate nursing students' reflective writings for evidence of critical thinking. This article reports on a study of consistency among faculty in grading writing in reflective journals. The results indicate a lack of consensus with regard to evaluation and differences among faculty with regard to how they view the purpose of such exercises.

Kirkpatrick, M., Brown, S., Atkins, A., & Vance, A. (2001). Using popular culture to teach nursing leadership. *Journal of Nursing Leadership, 40*(2), 90–92.

A nursing leadership course used analysis of films depicting cultural diversity, leadership and management styles, power, and teamwork. The experience promoted critical and reflective thinking and provided relevant and engaging examples of leadership.

Loving, G.L., & Siow, P. (2005). Use of an online case study template in nursing education. *Journal of Nursing Education, 44*(8), 387–388.

Combining the case study approach and the Internet.

Martin, C. (2002). The theory of critical thinking of nursing. *Nursing Education Perspectives, 23*(5), 243–247.

Case studies were applied in six courses to help students (1) understand complex and complicated issues and describe interrelated processes; (2) discuss policy- and decision-making ideologies that either are politically or socially charged; and (3) engage in informative and focused classroom discussion. Students' written comments and scaled responses suggest that the case method was an effective way to enhance student learning.

Nibert, A. T. (2005). Teaching clinical ethics using a case study family presence during cardiopulmonary resuscitation. *Critical Care Nurse, 25*(1), 38–43.

The presence of patients' family members during cardiopulmonary resuscitation (CPR) is an ethical issue debated among health-care professionals who routinely face life-threatening situations. Presentation of a case study involving a family's presence during CPR provides students in a critical care nursing course valuable experience in making ethical decisions that will prepare the students for the inevitable dilemmas faced by professional nurses.

Ogden, W. R. (2003). Reaching all the students: The feedback lecture. *The Journal of Instructional Psychology,* March 2003.
http://www.findarticles.com/p/articles/mi_m0FCG/is_1_30/ai_99983044

The feedback lecture was developed at Oregon State University at a time when questions regarding the changing nature of students seeking higher education came in conflict with existing staff and resources. The method, which involves pre-lecture activities, short lectures, discussion groups, and post-lecture activities, contributes directly to an instructional delivery system. The feedback lecture enables students to learn by their own strengths while providing ample opportunity for developing related strengths in other areas.

Russell, N. (2004). Student expressions: Journaling…. A nursing student's perspective. *SNRA Newsbulletin,* Feb/March.
http://www.srna.org/communications/newsbulletin.php

This Canadian student shares her frustrations and eventual conversion to journaling as a teaching method. She verifies that the purposes of journaling include one or more of the following: to develop critical thinking, to provide an opportunity for reflection, to give insight into the student's progression in nursing skills and clinical practice, and as a means of dialogue between faculty and student.

Schaefer, K. M. (2002). Analyzing the teaching style of nursing faculty: Does it promote a student-centered or a teacher-centered learning environment? *Nursing Education Perspectives, 24*(5), 238–245.

The purposes of this study were to (a) describe the predominant teaching style of a group of nursing faculty members, either as teacher centered or student centered, and (b) to compare teaching style to the instructional methods the faculty members used in the courses they taught and to their stated philosophies of teaching/learning. Findings indicate that the participants were more teacher centered than student centered; their written philosophies supported the teacher-centered approach. However, evidence that faculty used student-centered language, often in a teacher-centered context, indicates that participants in the study may recognize the need for a student-centered environment.

Shearer, R., & Davidhizar, R. (2003). Using role play to develop cultural competence. *Journal of Nursing Education, 42*(6), 273–276.

Role playing is a useful method for teaching cultural competence in nurse-patient situations. Successful implementation depends on identification of objectives and grading criteria, adequate time, guidelines for role specifications, monitoring of the process, delineation of the relationship to theory, and facilitation of constructive analysis.

Simpson, R. (2002). Virtual reality revolution: Technology changes nursing education. *Nursing Management, 33*(9), 14–15.

> Virtual technology can increase nursing students' clinical skills without risking harm to patients and can help prepare nurses for new practices, such as robotic surgery.

van Gelder, T. (2005). Teaching critical thinking: Some lessons from cognitive science. *College Teaching.* http://www.heldref.org/ct.php

> This article draws six key lessons from cognitive science for teachers of critical thinking. The lessons are: acquiring expertise in critical thinking is hard; practice in critical-thinking skills themselves enhances skills; the transfer of skills must be practiced; some theoretical knowledge is required; diagramming arguments (argument mapping) promotes skill; and students are prone to belief preservation.

Wikstrom, B. (2003). A picture of a work of art as an empathy teaching strategy in nurse education complementary to theoretical knowledge. *Journal of Professional Education, 19*(1), 49–54.

> Swedish nursing students conducted group dialogues about empathic understanding of the ill using Munch's painting "The Sick Girl" as a stimulus; a control group of 72 students discussed empathy without the visual prompt. The visual art group were more emotionally engaged in their learning.

Williams, B. (2001). The theoretical links between problem-based learning and self-directed learning for continued professional nursing education. *Teaching in Higher Education, 6*(1), 95–98.

> This study describes how the use of problem-based learning as an instructional methodology in undergraduate nursing curricula has been identified as one way to facilitate development of nursing students' abilities to become self-directed in learning. It discusses the theoretical links between problem-based learning and self-directed learning.

Yoder-Wise, P., & Kowalski, K. (2003). The power of story-telling. *Nursing Outlook, 51*(1), 37–42.

> This article presents the value of storytelling and offers guidelines for developing stories to use in teaching. It includes sections on presentation skills, overcoming pitfalls, and the power of telling stories.

Chapter Outline

ASSESSMENT AND EVALUATION STRATEGIES

11

Mary E. Partusch

Learning Outcomes

At the completion of this chapter, the reader should be able to:

- Identify a variety of assessment and evaluation strategies for program effectiveness.
- Design a course blueprint using outcome and evaluation methods for a course within the nursing program.
- Create test questions using the revised Bloom's Taxonomy.
- Develop an analytic or holistic rubric for a course assignment.
- Describe the three domains of learning.
- Evaluate test items using the Universally Designed Assessment Chart.

Key Terms

Affective domain
Analytical rubric
Cognitive domain
Holistic rubric
Program accreditation
Psychomotor domain
Question template
Rubrics
Test blueprint

The quality of a program, program outcomes, and course outcomes is fostered though ongoing assessment, feedback from those who have a stake in the program, and continuous use of data to foster improvements and promote quality. The strongest indicator of a successful nursing program is the NCLEX pass rate because it signals to all stakeholders that the graduate has met minimal educational standards to practice nursing. This is closely followed by graduate performance in the workplace, satisfaction of program graduates, and satisfaction of the graduates' employers. The assessment process of systematic evaluation that occurs at the program and course levels of a nursing program influences these indicators of positive outcomes. Assessment on the part of the faculty, students, graduates, and employers can provide ongoing feedback to promote program quality. The program faculty uses the internal course measurements—teacher-made tests, test bank, or a combination thereof, nontest classroom assessment methods, and clinical skills check-lists—to determine student course group achievement of knowledge. The external course measurements include standardized testing such as the Assesstest, and other commercially available tests. The ultimate external program measurement is NCLEX.

Program Assessment and Evaluation

The program level of assessment uses measures that will provide feedback on outcomes and processes. Feedback measures related to students receive the most attention because of the connection to a quality program product: the nurse graduate prepared for practice. Faculty focus groups or faculty surveys can provide internal feedback, based on faculty expertise and satisfaction. The measures of student exit interviews, exit surveys, pass rates on national qualifying examinations, graduate surveys, and employer surveys can provide patterns of information about the quality of the experiences and interactions, showing positive areas to enhance or negative areas to change for program improvement.

NCLEX-RN Pass Rates

The national qualifying examination (NCLEX-RN, or NCLEX-PN) pass rates provide quantitative data that can be benchmarked against quantitative data from other programs and the national average pass rate. Each program establishes a desired pass rate and works to achieve and maintain that pass rate. A program with a reputation for high-quality graduates may establish the standard of a desired national pass rate of 95% to 100%. A program that takes a larger number of higher-risk students with test anxiety or other challenges may establish the desired program pass rate to be at or above the national average pass rate. The respective state boards of nursing can provide pass rate data to the nursing program, and in some states, the low, average, and highest pass rates for all nursing programs are included in the report. Comparing the program pass rate to other nursing programs' pass rates and the national pass rate shows whether these program graduates are meeting state and national standards. When the desired group pass rate is achieved, programs continue to monitor assessment indicators, and incorporate additional measures when possible to promote program quality. Programs that do not achieve the desired group pass rate need to conduct a more detailed assessment to determine weak areas that need strengthening. A good place to start for a more detailed assessment of strong and weak areas is analysis of the NCLEX-RN group performance data for the respective school, which shows comparison to national standards.

Assessment of group performance on NCLEX content areas helps program faculty to determine strong curricular areas and areas in which the graduates as a group are not performing as well as national averages. There is NCLEX pass rate data provided to all programs, and the group curricular information related to a particular school is available for purchase. The curricular information may show a weakness across the group in a particular area, such as priority identification. Then for every course throughout the program, faculty needs to look at how priority identification is taught and student achievement is measured at progressively increasing levels. Closer inspection of what and how the respective content area is taught will reveal areas that can be strengthened. Assessment and testing measurement data may show this particular student group had more difficulty with priority identification on test items related to this topic. If standardized external testing has been used by the program, the faculty can compare standardized testing results to determine if the group scored lower on content related to the same areas as identified in the NCLEX results. Particular attention to strengthening priority identification skills of students in the last year of the program can result in the next year's NCLEX-RN takers achieving well in the area of priority identification. A word of caution here; strengthening one curricular area should not occur at the expense of another area. It is an ongoing challenge for nurse educators to strengthen and maintain all curricular areas to promote successful achievement of program outcomes and achieve a successful NCLEX pass rate.

Follow-up Surveys and Interviews

Assessment of graduates and employers provides qualitative and quantitative feedback about program quality. The assessment surveys need to have embedded program curricular outcomes to provide focus for the assessment, as well as measures related to satisfaction, employment, community service/involvement, and participation in professional organizations. Graduates are major consumers of the program. Interviews with and a survey of students graduating from the program provides immediate input related to program quality. Graduating students can provide feedback on challenging courses and faculty efforts to promote learning. Graduates can interpret if the challenge means it fostered achievement on their part, or hindered achievement, with suggestions for what worked well for them and what did not work. Group data from the graduate interviews and graduate surveys can show major program strengths, any areas that need strengthening, and overall satisfaction with the program. Follow-up surveys to graduates and their employers are conducted in 6 months to 1 year, and again in 2 to 3 years. The follow-up surveys provide data about areas for which the program strongly prepared the graduate, and any areas that need strengthening.

Many programs send out program-designed graduate and employer surveys. There also are commercial surveys available, such as those offered through the American Association of Colleges of Nursing (AACN). The commercial surveys can be administered online, analyzed, and followed by an evaluative report that is sent back to the school, and may contain an option to compare program results to those of nursing program results in other schools. A comparison of graduate exit, graduate follow-up, and employer survey data with NCLEX-RN pass rates and curricular data frequently shows areas of congruency.

Internal Feedback

Ongoing feedback for program assessment also comes from sources internal to the program, such as the current students and faculty. Individual input is important but can skew results from very happy or unhappy individuals and compromise privacy; therefore, all data are compiled together into group data. Current students can provide program input through surveys and group interviews. A focus group of representatives from the student body that is conducted on an annual or biannual basis gives group input on program strengths and improvements needed, primarily in areas to increase student satisfaction. The process can also reveal course weaknesses or clinical issues. Timely student group input can assist the program faculty in quickly addressing a difficulty before it becomes a major problem for the program.

Faculty surveys and faculty focus groups also provide input on ways to strengthen the program. The input could range from printer difficulties to team teaching or course difficulties, for example. Easier access to a printer may free up time for faculty to spend more time with students and in course preparation. If faculty group data show team teaching or course difficulties that may impinge on student achievement of outcomes, it may require more complex interventions. The yearly input from faculty and students is crucial for determining strengths and areas to be addressed in a timely manner to promote program quality.

Accreditation

Program accreditation by the Council of Collegiate Nursing Education (CCNE) or the National League for Nursing Accreditation Commission (NLNAC) provides a mark of quality against national standards met by other programs. Program accreditation is based on the faculty's assessment of systematic evaluation data from all sources, i.e., faculty, students, graduates, employers, consumers, and its use to maintain, strengthen, and revise the program when and if needed. Program chairpersons should have information about the CCNE and NLNAC accreditation standards, and additional information can be obtained from the respective Web sites. Accreditation of a nursing program signals to all stakeholders that the program is meeting nursing standards of higher education.

Course Assessment

Course assessment of student learning encompasses didactic (theoretical knowledge), college laboratory, and clinical assessment. The assessment measures must relate to student course outcomes and should progressively demonstrate student achievement of the course outcomes. Assessment measures tied to course outcomes and faculty modeling of desired behaviors can increase student modeling of desired professional behaviors and performing at higher levels on assessment measures (Ball & Garton, 2002). Development of a course blueprint that connects course outcomes to methods of evaluation can facilitate assessment. Regardless of the assessment measure used, it is important to have valid evaluative measures that reliably measure achievement of the same course content when used repeatedly. Evaluation methods and weighting of each method as a proportion of a course grade are stated in a course syllabus, providing clear expectations to promote learning and avoid misunderstandings between faculty and students. The course syllabus serves as a contract between faculty and student.

Outcome Blueprint

An outcome blueprint contains a pictorial blueprint of course outcomes and methods of evaluation. The use of a table format allows faculty to determine that all outcomes are being evaluated and shows the method used for the evaluation. The course outcomes stated in the course syllabus are listed down the side column, and methods of evaluation are listed across the top header row. Each course outcome should have one corresponding method of evaluation. After completing the blueprint, examine it to determine that there is at least one method of evaluation for each course outcome. If one course outcome is not being measured, determine if the course outcome is crucial, and if it is crucial, add a method of evaluation to measure student achievement of that outcome. If a method of evaluation is being used that does not correspond with any of the course outcomes, delete that method of evaluation or add a course outcome. The following table is an example of using a course blueprint to compare outcomes and methods of evaluation.

TABLE 11–1 Blueprint of Course Outcomes and Evaluation Methods **217**

Evaluation Method	Discussion	Research	Project	Exam
Course Outcomes				
1. Explore strategies used in patient education.	X	X	X	X
2. Design a teaching plan for patient teaching.			X	
3. Evaluate teaching strategies suitable for different learning needs.	X	X	X	X
4. Examine issues that can occur in teaching-learning situations.	X	X		X
5. Evaluate research on patient teaching.		X		X
6. Identify the components of learner assessment and evaluation.	X		X	X

Methods of Course Evaluation

Methods of evaluation can include written assessments, such as examinations, papers, literature critiques, and reflective journaling. Observations by student peers and faculty in the college laboratory and clinical setting are assessments that provide direct evaluation of student cognitive, affective, and psychomotor application of knowledge and skills. Assessment **rubrics** or rating scales for evaluating student achievement foster objectivity, alert the student to the level of course/faculty expectations, and focus on student learning.

Examinations, Test Development, Types of Questions, and Examples

Testing can include a range of multiple-choice, true-false, short answer, and essay items on a written examination; observation; self-evaluation; and peer evaluation. There are books and Internet resources dedicated to test development. The National Council of State Boards of Nursing (2006) provides e-learning resources, including assessment strategies and a test construction course available for faculty. Books and other Internet resources dedicated to test development are available.

Development of a **test blueprint** that is similar to a course outcome blueprint fosters measurement of all unit objectives. A test blueprint lists the unit or topical outline directly related to the course outcomes in the left column and the levels of Bloom's revised taxonomy across the header row. A complete description of Bloom's taxonomy occurs later in this chapter. For each component of the unit outline, determine the level of knowledge, such as comprehension or application, related professional values, and psychomotor skills that the student needs to function effectively at this level of nursing. If there are several units in a course, develop a blueprint for each unit that shows major content areas, number of test questions per content area, and the thinking level required, as reflected by the revised Bloom's taxonomy. Evaluation measurements, including test questions for courses at the end of the nursing program, require that students analyze information and evaluate possible solutions for the best alternative. Case situations in the test items can require varying levels of analysis and weighing of alternative solutions, which is reflective of a skill needed for nursing practice.

Multiple-Choice Testing

Testing with multiple-choice questions is the most common evaluation method for measuring student attainment of didactic knowledge. Many nursing textbooks now come with a test bank in the faculty resources accompanying the textbook. Because of differences in curriculum and courses across programs, the faculty reviews items in the test bank and select those most applicable to major content areas for the respective course. It is likely that not all test items in a test bank will be usable for a course, unless a course has been designed around a textbook.

Multiple-choice test questions can measure different levels of learning, including a range of how well students remember concepts and the ability to apply concepts, for example, concepts of nursing care with outcome criteria and evaluative measures. When developing a test question, ask about one idea in the stem of the question and avoid negative wording when possible. If words like "not" are used, underline them. If there are a series of multiple-choice questions that relate to the same situation, keep all of the questions in the series on the same page or screen as the situation; if this is not possible, repeat the situation on the new page. In a series of questions related to the same situation, the responses to one question should be independent of responses to other questions. In other words, the student should not need to go back to an earlier question, in order to respond to the current question.

There should be three to five possible responses to each multiple-choice question. Using three options for multiple-choice questions may decrease item difficulty as well as increase reliability and discrimination when detractors are removed. Placement of the correct response for each question should vary at random to avoid students guessing the correct answers based on a pattern. The incorrect answers should be plausible to avoid automatically eliminating a response and determining the correct answer by process of elimination. The response "all of the above" should be used cautiously, if at all; determining that at least two responses are correct would mean "all of the above" is correct, without requiring knowledge of the third response. It may be better to have only one correct response of three response options than to use "all of the above." Haladyna (1990) suggests development of a question structure that works well and then interchanging key information. For example, a format or **question template** of "*what intervention is used first when caring for the client with (fill in the blank)?*" can measure the student's ability to apply interventions and could be used with all topics in which application of interventions is tested (Haladyna, Downing, & Rodriquez, 2002).

True-False

True-false test questions can evaluate understanding of relationships between two concepts. For example, "The patient with cyanotic hands, lips, and toes has a lack of oxygen in the blood" can determine whether a student knows signs and symptoms of decreased blood oxygenation. Avoid reinforcing outdated information when writing questions that are false. The question, "Reddened areas over bony prominences should <u>not</u> be massaged with lotion" should be written in a manner to make the correct response "true," otherwise, it could reinforce an outdated and potentially harmful practice used in the clinical area, particularly by a weak student. True-false test questions are effective in measuring factual knowledge or relationships between concepts, but it is more difficult to write true-false questions that measure synthesis or evaluation.

Short-Answer and Essay Questions

Short-answer questions and essay questions can test beginning to higher-level thinking, and may be easier and less time consuming for instructors to create. They can take much longer to grade objectively, however. A short-answer or essay question can determine if students remember and are able to apply concepts. An example of an essay question is, "You are a community health nurse. Create a plan to address a community outbreak of influenza." This question requires the student to apply concepts of health promotion and disease prevention in the community setting, and requires creating the highest level of thinking in Bloom's revised taxonomy. Criteria for the correct response to the question should be written out and compared to the student responses when grading to increase effectiveness and objectivity.

Learning Level and Leveling Test Questions

The level of testing should correlate with the expected course outcomes and course placement in a nursing program. Concepts and outcomes introduced at the beginning of a program require student understanding to progress successfully through the program, and grasp concepts at the end of a program. In a beginning nursing course, testing on fundamental principles of nursing is important. A student may learn the concept of safety, for example, and test questions can determine student understanding of this concept on a basic or individual level. Testing the safety concept in a later course may include a higher level question that asks the student to create a plan to address community safety issues, such as how to prevent spread from an outbreak of influenza, mumps, or a highly contagious gastrointestinal illness.

Bloom's Taxonomy

The revised Bloom's taxonomy by Anderson and Krathwohl (2001) provides a framework for measuring cognitive (i.e., thought) processes, related to levels of thinking and action verbs that can be used in test questions. The original Bloom's taxonomy identified the **cognitive domain** with the following six knowledge levels: recall, comprehension, application, analysis, synthesis, and evaluation (Bloom, 1956). The revised taxonomy emphasizes the thinking levels: remembering, understanding, applying, analyzing, evaluating, and creating (Anderson & Krathwohl, 2001). Pohl (2000) provides examples of the original taxonomy compared to the revised taxonomy and sample questions that reflect levels of taxonomy. Assessment and testing throughout a nursing program should require increasing thinking ability levels as identified in the revised Bloom's taxonomy. There are also **affective** and **psychomotor domains** of learning. The affective domain relates to judgments and values. The psychomotor area relates to skill testing and demonstration; skill testing for an examination usually means the student demonstrates knowledge of sequenced activities or procedures in the college laboratory or clinical setting.

Following are two situations, the first of which requires understanding (revised taxonomy, second level) basic principles to prevent infection and applying (revised taxonomy, third level) this to a clinical situation. The second situation requires evaluating the situation (revised taxonomy, fifth level) and initiating action to determine cause and prevent further spread of the illness (revised taxonomy, sixth level of "creating").

Situation 1. There are five postoperative surgical patients in your work setting. What is the best way to prevent and avoid spread of possible infection?

1. Ask the nurse practitioner to order antibiotics.
2. Put patients with wound drainage on strict isolation.
3. Use good handwashing technique before and after caring for each patient.
4. Keep the patients as far from each other as possible.
5. Restrict visitors to those patients having no signs of infection.

Situation 2. A large number of students and teachers at a local school suddenly become ill with gastrointestinal symptoms of vomiting and diarrhea. They go home. As the school health nurse, what should you do next?

1. Contact the housekeeping department to clean the restrooms.
2. Check with the cooks about the food choices that day and suggest a lighter fare for the next day.
3. Contact the parents with information on follow-up care.
4. Immediately contact the public health department for follow-up on cause and infection control.

Written methods of evaluation primarily measure cognitive levels of thinking, rather than affective and psychomotor domains of learning. In the beginning nursing student, it is important for the student to understand handwashing and value the importance of handwashing to prevent the spread of infection. When the student actually takes the action of washing hands before working with clients, it shows that the student values the importance of handwashing. It also shows that the student has cognitive knowledge of the connection of handwashing to disease prevention, and whether or not the student has the psychomotor skill to demonstrate the correct handwashing procedure. In the clinical setting, the student would automatically initiate and use the correct handwashing technique before and after caring for a client, demonstrating the level of cognitive thinking, the affective value of applying the concept, and the ability to carry out the psychomotor procedure.

Universally Designed Assessment Methods

Thompson, Johnstone, Anderson, and Miller (2005) conducted a Delphi survey of test writers and developers to determine guidelines for assessment that is universally designed and accessible. Their research resulted in the table of considerations compiled in Table 11–2. Following these guidelines for test question development will make the test accessible to the broadest range of learners. These guidelines are also helpful when selecting test items from textbook-associated instructor test banks. There is a section in the table related to reading level of test items. The reading level of written tests, particularly in the year before taking national licensure examinations, should be consistent with the reading level of the national licensure examination. Many word processing programs allow the user to determine the reading level of a test. The use of medical terminology with multiple-syllable words can increase the reading level of a test and this should be taken into consideration when using reading level indexes.

Scoring and Determination of Item Difficulty and Discrimination

A good test question discriminates between the students who know the concepts and poor students who are guessing, and the more difficult a question, the more challenging it is for even good students. If weaker students get a question right and better students get a question wrong, the question does not discriminate correctly. Scoring programs for written tests can provide information on difficulty and discrimination of test items. If a scoring program is not available, a simple way to check for difficulty and discrimination of test items is to compare students with scores in the top third of the group to the students in the bottom third of the group for that examination. If a question is answered correctly by the top third of the class and the bottom third of the class answered incorrectly, it is likely that this question is more difficult and discriminates effectively. Checking difficulty and discrimination of test items is important, particularly if a large percentage of the class answered an item incorrectly. If a test question discriminates against a good student, the test item needs revision. Review of the test results with individual students can provide insight into student interpretation and misinterpretation of a question. After reviewing test results with several students and getting student input, faculty may determine ways to strengthen misleading items or response in the test, as well as determine topical or content areas that may need further clarification.

Does the item...

Measure what it intends to measure
- Reflect the intended content standards (reviewers have information about the content being measured)
- Minimize skills required beyond those being measured

Respect the diversity of the assessment population
- Accessible to test takers (consider gender, age, ethnicity, socioeconomic level)
- Avoid content that might unfairly advantage or disadvantage any student subgroup

Have clear format for text
- Standard typeface
- Twelve (12) point minimum for all print, including captions, footnotes, and graphs (type size appropriate for age group)
- Wide spacing between letters, words, and lines
- High contrast between color of text and background
- Sufficient blank space (leading) between lines of text
- Staggered right margins (no right justification)

Have clear pictures and graphics (when essential to item)
- Pictures are needed to respond to item
- Pictures with clearly defined features
- Dark lines (minimum use of gray scale and shading)
- Sufficient contrast between colors
- Color is not relied on to convey important information or distinctions
- Pictures and graphs are labeled

Have concise and readable text
- Commonly used words
- Vocabulary appropriate for grade level
- Minimum use of unnecessary words
- Idioms avoided unless idiomatic speech is being measured
- Technical terms and abbreviations avoided (or defined) if not related to the content being measured
- Sentence complexity is appropriate for grade level
- Question to be answered is clearly identifiable

Allow changes to its format without changing its meaning or difficulty (including visual or memory load)
- Allows for the use of braille or other tactile format
- Allows for signing to a student
- Allows for the use of oral presentation to a student
- Allows for the use of assistive technology
- Allows for translation into another language

Does the test...

Have an overall appearance that is clean and organized
- All images, pictures, and text provide information necessary to respond to the item
- Information is organized in a manner consistent with an academic English framework with a left-right, top-bottom flow

In addition to the other considerations, a computer-based test should have these considerations:

Layout and design
- Sufficient contrast between background and text and graphics for easy readability
- Color is not relied on to convey important information or distinctions

(table continued on page 222)

TABLE 11–2 Considerations for Universally Designed Assessment Items (continued)

- Font size and color scheme can be easily modified (through browser settings, style sheets, or on-screen options)
- Stimulus and response options are viewable on one screen when possible
- Page layout is consistent throughout the test
- Computer interfaces follow Section 508 guidelines

Navigation

- Navigation is clear and intuitive; it makes sense and is easy to figure out
- Navigation and response selection is possible by mouse click or keyboard
- Option to return to items and return to place in test after breaks

Screen reader considerations

- Item is intelligible when read by a text/screen reader
- Links make sense when read out of visual context ("go to the next question" rather than "click here")
- Nontext elements have a text equivalent or description
- Tables are only used to contain data, and make sense when read by screen reader

Test specific options

- Access to other functions is restricted (e.g., e-mail, Internet, instant messaging)
- Pop up translations and definitions of key words/phrases are available if appropriate to the test
- Students are able to record their responses and read them back (and have them read back using text-to-speech) as an alternative to a human scribe, but only if student has experience with this mode of expression and chooses it for the test

Computer capabilities

- Adjustable volume
- Speech recognition available (to convert user's speech to text)
- Test is compatible with current screen reader software
- Computer-based option to mask items or text (e.g., split screen)
- Computer software for test delivery is designed to be amenable to assistive technology

Source: Thompson, S. J., Johnstone, C. J., Anderson, M. E., & Miller, N. A. (2005). *Considerations for the development and review of universally designed assessments* (Technical Report 42). Minneapolis, MN: University of Minnesota, National Center on Educational Outcomes. Retrieved May 2, 2006 from http://education.umn.edu/NCEO/OnlinePubs/Technical42.htm.

Other Methods of Course Evaluation

Other methods of course evaluation can include papers; projects, both individual and group; presentations; observations; and concept mapping. These methods require a list of criteria on which the project will be graded. Use of assessment rubrics and grading scales increases objectivity in these methods of course evaluation.

Papers and Projects

Papers are used to determine higher levels of critical thinking, a student's ability to research, synthesize, and reflect on a topic, and to assess values associated with affective thinking. A student could write a paper about a case study situation from practice, researching the literature for current approaches to practice. Before clinical experiences, students can be assigned a nursing care plan or nursing concept map to show preparation and level of knowledge needed for the experience. A critical reflection paper could be required after a clinical experience to demonstrate analysis of a clinical situation. Another paper could require that a student explore an ethical dilemma encountered (or told about) in practice. The guidelines for the paper should include a list of items to be included and criteria for grading the paper. Components of the nursing process are frequently included in paper requirements for nursing problems. The paper structure and format should be specified including whether the paper can be hand-written or word-processed, and the number of references required. Specify the number of grading points assigned to the respective criteria. Length of the paper varies with the topic and purpose of the paper. A paper exploring an issue or policy may be seven to ten pages, requiring the student to synthesize and evaluate in a concise manner, whereas a research paper with extensive references may be longer. Papers take longer to grade than multiple-choice examinations and this should be factored in by faculty when determining paper requirements, keeping in mind that it can be more difficult to write a concise analytical paper; length does not automatically correlate with writing and thinking abilities. An assessment rubric, such as that in Figure 11–1 presented later in this chapter, can increase objectivity when grading papers. One way to increase grading reliability is to have two to three papers independently evaluated by a faculty peer. Papers can show that the student has effectively grasped the more complex concepts associated with course content and outcomes.

Projects done individually or in groups can require a psychomotor skill as well as cognitive and affective thinking. An individual project could entail designing and displaying a health-promotion poster in a community setting, or presenting projects to peers. The grading criteria should include a list of the project components with points and percentage of grade assigned to each component. Criteria related to content, references, layout, appearance, and reading level promote objectivity of evaluation and clue the learner into expectations for the desired product.

Group projects can promote collaboration and communication that reflect characteristics desired in professional practice. When group projects are assigned, specify expectations for group members that include criteria with points assigned. Group members could provide peer assessment using a rating scale of unsatisfactory to exemplary for criteria, such as quality of work, task accomplishment, timeliness, attitude, and contributions to group work, all of which reflect qualities of team work desired in nursing practice.

Classroom Presentations

Classroom presentations include components of both content and delivery skills. The evaluative criteria for the classroom presentation links to the course purpose of the classroom presentation. In some courses, students research topics not covered elsewhere and give an informal presentation to the class about the specific topic. Then the majority of the evaluative criteria are an outline of presenting content associated with the topic. If the purpose is to gain skills in professional nursing presentations and the nursing topic is secondary, more detailed criteria and grade points pertain to delivery of the presentation. Evaluative criteria for the presentation content includes an introduction, body, and concluding summary, similar to what is included in a written paper. If it is important that specific content be included in the presentation, include evaluative criteria pertaining to the specific content. For example, in a cardiovascular nursing course it may be important for the presentation to include pathophysiology and rehabilitation components specifically related to cardiovascular nursing. A general content outline embedded in the criteria conveys to the learner areas of importance and can avoid misunderstandings as well as missing content.

Criteria for the informal classroom presentation may include a clear introduction related to the topic, a presentation that can be heard, eye contact, and no detracting mannerisms (e.g., uhs, playing with hair, distracting hand/body movements). The delivery of informal classroom presentations can be secondary to the content associated with a topic. The informal classroom presentation may not require the student to dress other than in what is customary for the classroom; if more professional attire is expected, related evaluative criteria is stated.

Evaluative criteria for delivery of formal presentations should be consistent with expectations for professional presentations, level of formality, and the type of audience. The evaluative criteria include areas such as: a clearly articulated purpose or topic; gaining attention with an anecdote, startling statement, or unusual statistics; being knowledgeable and organized; maintaining listener (student peer) attention; varying pace and tone; time length, and a concluding summary that recaps key points and signals closure for the audience. McCullen (1997) offers criteria related to elocution and eye contact as part of a presentation rubric. Sample rubrics for assessing classroom presentations and oral expression have been developed by pre-college educators and are available online at TeAch-nolgy (1999–2006). These offer a good starting point for developing evaluative criteria for nursing classroom presentations. Evaluative criteria for classroom presentations embedded in a rubric convey to the student what is expected, can be used by peers, and add objectivity to the evaluation of classroom presentations (Allen, 2003).

Observations

An effective means of assessment is observation in the classroom and clinical laboratory. Observation requires assessment rating scales or rubrics to promote objectivity and clearly identify expectations for the student. A rating scale of "not demonstrated" or "demonstrated" can be included on a skills checklist. Facione and Facione (1994) developed a holistic critical thinking scoring rubric, which could be used to evaluate student critical thinking in an observation. Two faculty members (or two students) could independently assess a demonstration and then compare ratings; revise the tool as needed to increase reliability of measurement.

Concept Mapping

Concept maps can be used to evaluate whether a student can demonstrate relationships and connections between concepts. The concepts can be diagramed and clustered with arrows between concepts to show a visual representation of cause and effect. Such a diagram can demonstrate how a student connects—accurately or erroneously—patient assessment data, prioritizes information, and identifies nursing actions connected to the patient assessment data. Concept mapping is being used instead of the traditional nursing care plans (Koehler, 2004). Evaluation of a concept map requires criteria about content, size, and general guidelines. A sample concept map, included in the course syllabus, and a grading rubric provide student guidance and foster objectivity.

Rubrics for Grading and Assessment

An assessment rubric, such as the one in Figure 11–1, includes grading criteria for an assignment and signals to students the level of work expected on a grading scale of numerical or letter grades. Mertler (2001) describes **analytical** and **holistic rubrics.** The holistic rubric is designed to grade a process or product. A holistic rubric could be developed to score a class presentation, with characteristics of an excellent to poor presentation identified (Truemper, 2004). Moskal (2000) provides rationale for using rubrics and a linear example of a holistic rubric for grading a paper. The analytical rubric contains descriptive grading criteria for individual components of an assignment, as shown in Figure 11–1. A formal paper may have points assigned to the introduction, body, conclusion, format, and length. These components would be listed in the left hand column of a table, with rows across the table and a description of characteristics in each cell that correspond to a poor to excellent paper. The student learner then knows the level of work needed for the grade desired. The instructor using the grid increases objectivity when assigning grades. If a class is being team-taught, having faculty independently evaluate an assignment and then comparing evaluations can increase reliability of the tool, with modifications made as needed. Figure 11–1 provides a graphic example of a holistic rubric.

Grade Criteria	C	B	A
Introduction	**14 points** No introduction is given, the purpose of the paper is missing, or does not relate to course topics.	**16 points** The introduction is clear, states the purpose, and is related to course topics.	**20 points** The introduction is clear, has the purpose, is related to course topics, and presents the information in a creative way.
Body and content	**28 points** Content is unclear, outdated, not accurate, and/or information is not organized, does not fit, or is incomplete. No APA citations are given.	**32 points** The content is current, accurate, and organized around key points and clearly sequenced ideas. Four APA referenced citations are given.	**40 points** The content is current, accurate, and organized around key points and clearly sequenced ideas. Six APA referenced citations are given.
Conclusion	**14 points** No summary of topic, or it is unclear and/or contains no connection to purpose.	**16 points** Summarizes the topic clearly and concisely, with connection to purpose.	**20 points** Summarizes the topic in a clear, concise, and creative way, with connection to purpose.
Readability and technical aspects	**14 points** The text is not clearly written and/or is difficult to read, and/or lacks correct spacing. Text length is not 5-7 pages. Spelling, punctuation, and grammar errors distract or impair readability.	**16 points** The text is clearly written. In a few places the use of spacing detracts, or long paragraphs may interfere with readability. Headings are in APA format. Text length is 5-7 pages. There are some grammatical and spelling errors.	**20 points** The text is clearly written, and easy-to-read. Headings and subheadings foster readability and are in APA format. Text length is 5-7 pages. The document is free of grammatical and spelling errors.
Total Points Possible	**70 points or less**	**80 points**	**100 points**

FIGURE 11–1 Paper assessment criteria and grading rubric. Adapted from Ward, S. (2006). *Introduction to informatics.* Omaha: Nebraska Methodist College.

Summary

Ongoing assessment and evaluation of program components assists faculty to identify any problematic areas and strengthen program quality. Student and course evaluation contribute to overall program assessment. Course outcomes and methods of evaluation should demonstrate increasing levels of Bloom's revised taxonomy. Test items must be developed with increasing difficulty and discrimination throughout the program, and be designed around universal standards. Evaluative methods provide students with feedback on achievement of course content and outcomes. Grading rubrics for non-testing methods of evaluation illustrate expectations for levels of learning and foster grading objectivity. Faculty members compare internal and external standards in an ongoing assessment and systematic program evaluation to promote quality in and preparation of program graduates for the nursing profession.

Allen, M. (2003). Using scoring rubrics. Retrieved June 27, 2006 from **http://www.calstate.edu/acadaff/ sloa/links/using_rubrics.shtml.**

Anderson, L.W., & Krathwohl, D. R. (Eds.) (2001). *A taxonomy for learning, teaching and assessment: A revision of Bloom's taxonomy of educational objectives.* New York: Longman.

Ball, A. L., & Garton, B. L. (2002). Modeling higher order thinking in teacher preparation: Relationships between objectives, classroom discourse, and assessments. Retrieved April 20, 2006 from **http:// aaaeonline.ifas.ufl.edu/NAERC/2002/naercfiles/NAERC/Modeling%20HOT%20Ball-Garton2.pdf.**

Facione, P. A., & Facione, N. C. (1994). Holistic critical thinking rubric. Millbrae, CA: The California Academic Press.

Haladyna, T. (1990). Advances in item design. *Rasch Measurement Transactions, 4*(2), 103–104. Retrieved April 20, 2006 from **http://www.rasch.org/rmt/rmt42b.htm.**

Haladyna, T. M., Downing, S. M., & Rodriguez, M. C. (2002). A review of multiple-choice item-writing guidelines for classroom assessment. *Applied Measurement in Education, 15*(3), 309–334. Retrieved from **http://depts.washington.edu/currmang/Toolsforteaching/MCItemWritingGuidelinesJAME.pdf.**

Health Educational Systems Incorporated (HESI). (2002). HESIiNet Web delivery system. Retrieved April 20, 2006 from **http://www.hesitest.com/.**

Koehler, C. J. (2004). Nursing process mapping replaces nursing care plans. In A. J. Lowenstein & M. J. Bradshaw, *Fuszard's innovative teaching strategies in nursing* (3rd ed., p. 303). Boston: Jones and Bartlett Publishers.

McCullen, C. (1997). Presentation rubric. Evaluating student presentations. Developed by Information Technology Evaluation Services, NC Department of Public Instruction. Retrieved June 27, 2006 from **http://www.ncsu.edu/midlink/rub.pres.html**

Mertler, C. A. (2001). Designing scoring rubrics for your classroom. *Practical Assessment, Research & Evaluation, 7*(25). Retrieved May 5, 2006 from **http://PAREonline.net/getvn.asp?v=7&n=25.**

Moskal, B. M. (2000). Scoring rubrics: What, when and how? *Practical Assessment, Research & Evaluation, 7*(3). Retrieved May 31, 2006 from **http://PAREonline.net/getvn.asp?v=7&n=3.**

National Council of State Boards of Nursing (NCSBN). (2006). Advanced Assessment Strategies: Assessing Higher Level Thinking. Retrieved April 20, 2006 from **http://www.learningext.com/products/ assessmentstrategies/advancedcourse/advassess.asp.**

Pohl, M. (2000). Bloom's (1956) revised taxonomy. Retrieved April 20, 2006 from **http://eprentice.sdsu. edu/J03OJ/miles/Bloomtaxonomy(revised)1.htm.**

Thompson, S. J., Johnstone, C. J., Anderson, M. E., & Miller, N. A. (2005). Considerations for the development and review of universally designed assessments. (Technical report 42). Minneapolis, MN: University of Minnesota, National Center on Educational Outcomes. Retrieved May 2, 2006 from **http:// education.umn.edu/NCEO/OnlinePubs/TechReport42.pdf.**

Truemper, C. M. (2004). Using scoring rubrics to facilitate assessment and evaluation of graduate-level nursing students. *Journal of Nursing Education, 43*(12), 562–564.

Review Questions

- After reviewing the NCLEX pass rates for the graduating seniors, you note a significant decrease in the rates. What type of detailed assessment(s) should be performed to determine weak areas?
- You have been asked to evaluate the outcomes of your program using graduate and employer expectations. How would you proceed?
- Using a nursing management textbook of your choosing, develop learning objectives and evaluation criteria for an undergraduate course in nursing management.
- Review the course outcomes for a nursing course. Develop a blueprint of course outcomes and evaluation methods.
- Review a test from one of the nursing courses and determine the thinking levels for the questions as identified in the revised Bloom's taxonomy. Compare your results with the instructor test bank.

Critical Thinking Exercises

As a faculty member on the Curriculum Outcomes Committee, you have been asked to review the evaluation criteria for a course in nutrition for undergraduate students. You note that the syllabus has the following evaluation methods:

- Five quizzes, each worth 10%

- Concept paper on a specific diet, worth 20%

- Patient teaching brochure on a specific diet, worth 10%

- Final comprehensive examination, worth 20%

Discuss the assessment and evaluation components that should be addressed for each method. Create a rubric (analytic or holistic) for grading the patient teaching brochure.

Annotated Research Summary

Seldomridge, L. A. (2006). Evaluating student performance in undergraduate preceptorships. *Journal of Nursing Education, 45*(5), 169–176.

This article explores the challenges in evaluating student performance in preceptorships based on data collected during academic years 1999–2002, which revealed an usually large number of high grades and relatively few average grades. Multiple perspectives are explored, including preceptor issues of selection, orientation, recognition, role conflict, and experience with giving grades; faculty issues of role confusion and unclear expectations for student performance; and environmental issues of lack of control of the learning environment and differences in the values of education and workplace. Solutions are proposed, including an orientation for preceptors and faculty, ongoing faculty mentoring of preceptors, official preceptor recognition, clear articulation of expectations for student performance and faculty site visits, and creation of grading rubrics for various aspects of the course to be used by preceptors, faculty, and students.

Suits, J. P. (2004). Assessing investigative skill development in inquiry-based and traditional college science laboratory courses. *School Science and Mathematics, 104*(6), 248–257.

A laboratory practical examination was used to compare the investigative skills developed in two different types of general-chemistry laboratory courses. Science and engineering majors (SEM) in the control group used a traditional verification approach (SEM-Ctrl), whereas those in the treatment group learned from an innovative, inquiry-based approach (SEM-Trt). A scoring rubric was developed from their examination sheets to assess six component investigative skills. Results indicated that SEM students in the SEM-Trt group scored significantly higher than those in SEM-Ctrl for all six skills. Furthermore, nursing and applied science majors (NonSem) in the inquiry-based group (NonSEM-Trt) wrote significantly better discussions than did SEM students in SEM-Ctrol group. Overall, competency at the mid-range level of laboratory skills was attained by most SEM-Trt students (72.5%) but by only 30.5% of SEM-Ctrl and 28.6% of NonSem-Trt students.

Chapter Outline

Promoting Reflection in Groups of Diverse Nursing Students

12

Ruth A. Wittmann-Price

Learning Outcomes

On completion of this chapter, the reader will be able to:

- Describe the reasons for diverse groups of students in nursing education today.
- Understand the needs of traditional and nontraditional learners.
- Identify methodologies that enhance reflection through dialogue.
- Analyze the assets and deficits of each methodology.
- Discriminate between socialization techniques and learning interventions.
- Summarize the process of promoting caring in a diverse classroom.

Key Terms

Caring curriculum
Dialogue
Diversity
Emancipatory education
Reflection
Service learning
Value clarification

Nurse educators are faced with a multitude of challenges related to the changing demographics of students. In response to the publicized nursing shortage, school enrollments have increased and innovative programs have emerged all over the nation to attract large numbers of both traditional and nontraditional students (Holland, 2004). These innovative programs have changed the demographics of the nursing student population (see Table 12–1). In addition to attracting older, more mature students with diverse life experiences, minorities and men are increasingly entering schools of nursing. Accelerated programs, increased funding, availability of weekend and evening programs, and online theoretical components have done an outstanding job of bolstering nursing school enrollments (Heller, Oros, & Durney-Crowley, 2006; Karlowicz, Wiles, Bishop, & Lakin, 2003).

The welcome increase in student enrollment has created an educational challenge for current faculty. Because there is a substantial shortage of nurse educators, educational institutions are often unable to find qualified educators, and are finding creative ways to approach the dilemma produced by increased enrollments and lack of faculty. Schools are increasing class sizes, faculty

 TABLE 12–1 Frequency Distribution of Characteristics of Accelerated BSN Students

Demographic Variable	Percent %	
Previous baccalaureate degrees. (n = 29)	Psychology/social sciences	17.24
	Business/accounting	7.00
	Science	44.83
	Other	31.04
Length of time student has been out of school prior to coming into the accelerated BSN program. (n = 28)	1–5 years	62.10
	6–10 years	13.79
	11–15 years	17.24
	16 years or >	3.45
Current age of student. (n = 29)	18–25 years	34.48
	26–35 years	48.28
	36–45 years	13.79
	45 years old or >	3.45
Married.	Yes	34.48
	No	65.52
Have children.	Yes	20.69
	No	79.31
Currently employed.	Yes	44.83
	No	55.17
How many hours a week do you work? (n = 13)	5–15 hours	27.59
	16–25 hours	17.24
	26–30 hours	0
	31–40 hours	6.90
Do you think the accelerated BSN program is more demanding than your previous baccalaureate program?	Strongly agree—its more demanding	31.04
	Agree—it is more demanding	37.93
	Neither agree nor disagree	24.14
	Disagree—its not more demanding	3.45
	Strongly disagree that its not more demanding	3.45

Source: Godshall, M. (Dec, 2005). Survey of accelerated students. *Nursing Educational Experience,* unpublished results. Used with permission.

workload, and the number of adjunct faculty to assist with both clinical and classroom experiences. Schools are promoting dual appointments with hospital nursing personnel and, sadly, turning students away to compensate for the discrepancies in student to faculty ratios. The culminating effects of these sociological variables have caused classes today to look quite different from those of just 5 or 10 years ago. Today, a typical class is larger with diverse student populations of varying ages, educational backgrounds, life experiences, cultural histories, and different motivations for being enrolled in a nursing program.

The natural educational response to this scenario may be one of authoritarianism and control in order to keep the masses on the right track and preserve the current educational system. In effect, those pedagogical tactics fail within the context of large, diverse groups. Methodologies that promote humanistic education through interpretive pedagogies in the correct doses, along with traditional methodologies, are of utmost importance in these exciting educational times (Diekelmann, 2003). Methodologies must present the content along with critical thinking experiences to promote each student's individual learning experience. Various philosophies that promote humanism are emancipatory, caring, reflective educational experiences. **Emancipatory education** is humanistic because it values the worth of each individual by ensuring free speech, free choice, and freedom to use personal knowledge (Wittmann-Price, 2004). The methodologies to enact a humanistic philosophy will be explored in this chapter with suggestions for innovative "methodological mixing" of nontraditional methodologies with tried and true traditional methodologies. This combination will help promote a positive educational experience that enhances student-teacher relationships in order to foster a professional learning environment to promote growth for both student and teacher (Gillespie, 2002).

Philosophical Underpinnings

The current world view in nursing education rejects the punitive classroom of the past, which many educators are old enough to recall. Education today has turned toward a philosophical belief that in order to produce people who care at the bedside they must be cared for in the classroom and in clinical areas in which they learn. Caring is humanistic; it is treating each person as a unique, equal, and valuable individual. Caring begets caring. Caring can be role modeled by the educator and educators should never underestimate the influence they have on any student (Murray & Main, 2005). This section will describe the philosophical underpinnings of a humanistic education by describing the main components of two theories: emancipatory education and the **caring curriculum.**

Emancipatory Education

Paulo Freire (1970) viewed the educational systems of the world as more than just vehicles to gain knowledge. Freire proposed that schools were powerful enough to promote an emancipated society. He believed that educational institutions were actually microsystems of society and vehicles to change the entire socioeconomic stance of society. He recognized that society was oppressive to some groups and believed that oppression serves the purpose of dehumanization by producing a "culture of silence" that is exploited for political or economic gain. Because of this intellectual, emotional, and psychological enslavement, the oppressed develop a "fear of freedom" (Freire, 1970, p. 36) in exchange for perceived security.

Schools or educational institutions could actually combat oppression by developing an emancipatory culture within the classroom where both teacher and student are equal learners.

Freire (1998) challenges the teacher to be more than an information provider; he challenges the teacher to be a cultural worker by creating a microenvironment of equality and care. The mechanism by which this is done is the use of teaching methodologies that promote **dialogue, reflection,** communication, and responsiveness on a level that never tolerates punitive action, authoritarian lines, or dehumanization. The philosophy is not so much about what specific methodologies are but rather about how they are enacted. Even more traditional methodologies, such as conventional lecture learning (CLL) (Siu, Laschinger, & Vingilis, 2005) can be emancipatory if that lecturer or educator is open to discussion, questions, and reflections of personal experience.

Reflection

Reflection is a main component of Freire's emancipatory education model and is characterized by thinking critically about alternatives. Reflection can be in the form of dialogue or communication to produce an internal awareness, or it can be a thought process spurred by creative questioning or situational dilemma. Freire believed that traditional educational methods alone foster oppression because they do not encourage the reflection needed for critical thinking (Romyn, 2000). It is important to reflect on issues to recognize the inherent personal and social aspects. Reflection also encourages one to think critically about the information gained from personal and empirical knowledge in order to synthesize it into a decision for students, educators, and practitioners (Fahrenfort, 1987; O'Callaghan, 2005; Raymond & Profetto-McGrath, 2005). Dialogue, as characterized by true and honest communication, is one methodology that promotes reflection. Freire proposes the establishment of a collaborative climate in which dialogue is encouraged and students take responsibility for their learning. This is echoed in today's nursing education literature, which calls for an interpretive, caring curriculum (Diekelmann, 2003). Owen-Mills (1995) endorsed a wider vision of emancipation by stating, "The challenge for nurse educators . . . extends beyond the confines of an institution and into the homes, hospitals and communities where nursing is practiced. For a caring curriculum to be truly emancipating, its effects must become internalized as a way of being" (p. 1193). Methodologies that can promote emancipatory education include interactive learning experiences, such as gaming, small-group discussions, and reflective writing and dialoguing about professional experiences and what personal growth can be promoted from them. Every professional experience encountered by the student nurse in the classroom and in the clinical area can pose as a reflective learning experience for both student and teacher.

Caring Curriculum

The caring curriculum (Bevis & Watson, 2000) is a concept that draws from both critical social theory and feminist theory. Some of the main theory ideas are briefly described in Table 12–2.

The main idea is that nursing is a call to care for human beings, a service; and the educational setting needs to reflect that caring, value-based attitude. The paradigm has great implications for nursing education and is constructed under the following 11 assumptions:

- Education must liberate both students and faculty from the authoritarian restraints of behavioral objectives.
- It must acknowledge students' equal power in education.
- It must define curriculum as interaction between teaching and students with the intent that learning take place.
- Learning must be structured differently so the learners are actively engaged in learning pursuits.
- The curriculum cannot be purely content driven.
- It must be supported by an alliance between teachers, students, and clinical practitioners.

TABLE 12–2

235

Philosophical Underpinnings

Critical Social Theory	Feminist Theory
The main concept of critical social theory is that society applies unequal power that causes oppression. This is applicable to many human situations creating the need for emancipation (Hegel, 1960; Marx & Engels, 1976; Paley, 1998).	Societal power or domination can cause oppression and denial of equality, which can affect knowledge, education, and economy (Arslanian-Engoren, 2002; Perry, 1994).
Critical social theory identifies oppression by using immanent critique. Immanent critique is a method of examining a social system to uncover discrepancies between values and reality (Harden, 1996).	Liberal feminists stress equal opportunity for women in areas of individualism, privacy, equality, autonomy, and self-fulfillment (MacPherson, 1983).
In the 1960s, Habermas developed praxis for implementing equality to counteract the oppression described in critical social theory. He used a modality called, "communicative action" (Habermas, 1969). This methodology is said to reduce social injustice or oppression through true and meaningful human dialogue (Duchscher, 2000).	Radical feminists take into account women's ways of knowing as unique and different (not just separate) from men (Pohl & Boyd, 1993).
Communicative action can be operationalized as reflection, which can take the form of communication between two individuals or as an internal awareness process (self-dialoguing) (Mill, Allen, & Morrow, 2001).	Socialist feminist theory believes that society is driven by labor and proposes that there is inequality of assigned work roles between women and men and calls for planned social change (Jagger, 1988).
Through dialogue, relationships between phenomena and individuals can be explored (Habermas, 1969).	Feminist theory validates personal knowledge as true knowledge and has highlighted the fact that the majority of science has been built on a patriarchal tradition, which has established empirical knowledge as superior to other knowledge. Feminist theory recognizes that empirical knowledge is only one valid type of knowledge (Berragan, 1998).
Knowledge is recognized to include empirical analysis, hermeneutic interpretation, and critique of domination (Duchscher, 2000).	
Heidegger (1949) believed that person and reality are perceived and it is the interpretation of the lived experience that constitutes true knowledge. This implies that personal knowledge is a true and important knowledge because it comes from the experience of the individual.	
A person's experiences cannot be separated from the person and a person's interpretation of the experience is part of her personal knowledge (Polanyi, 1958).	

- It should be clinically focused.
- It should provide faculty with practical guidelines, not squelch creativity.
- It must acknowledge different ways of knowing.
- It should allow one entry into practice.
- It should offer a criticism model for assessing learning (Bevis & Watson, 2000, pp. 1–2).

Developing a caring curriculum based on the main assumptions that (1) education should be an equalized learning process for faculty and students; and (2) learning how to think may be more important than remembering content in nursing education, may not be without implementation difficulty (Miklancie & Davis, 2005). Conventional pedagogies and methodologies die hard and oppression in the educational environment is insidious.

Philosophically in a humanistic educational realm, to truly care one must provide the student with the freedom to develop as an individual. Control and authoritarianism negate true caring within the learning environment. Control is self-fulfilling whereas freedom to explore and learn is humanistic and caring. Developing methodologies that promote an emancipatory classroom in which the norm is communication and dialogue without intimidation should be today's educational goal. It is within this type of educational praxis that critical thinking can best be developed. In light of the incredible amount of knowledge acquisition that needs to take place in schools and colleges of nursing, methodologies to promote critical thinking are more important than ever. Educators are challenged to teach the learner how to learn and not just what to learn. "Deep learning" is learning that goes beyond the content to understanding and embracing the concepts of a subject. There are many metacognitive methodologies (August-Brady, 2005) that enhance critical thinking, but without a caring curriculum that fosters emancipatory learning these teaching-learning strategies may be difficult to implement. The classroom that contains diverse learners—be it **diversity** in age, educational background, or culture—is a challenge to any educational philosophy and calls for flexibility in methodology to reach all learning styles (see Chapter 6) and promote an emancipatory learning environment in which critical thinking is fostered and caring becomes the agreed upon culture.

Challenges of Diverse Learning

Many accelerated programs—averaging 11 to 18 months—have been developed to educate RNs in a short period of time. The applicants for these programs are both culturally and educationally diverse, including adult students, often with degrees in other disciplines. The motivation for returning to school to be a nurse differs greatly from person to person. For some adult learners, it is job security or an economically driven reason. Others return to school because they dislike or are burned out by their current or previous profession. Some students have verbalized the reason for returning as a calling to help people that developed somewhere along their life journey. Regardless of the reason for returning to school, every adult student brings with them a wealth of life experiences, which both enhance and complicate the learning environment.

One complicating factor in the learning environment is that the adult student or second degree student is often in the classroom with college-aged undergraduate students. The life experiences of the adult student may be intimidating to the younger student who has difficulty relating to them. The adult student often perceives the traditional students as naïve, inexperienced at life, and fortunate to have school as their only obligation. On the other hand, the adult students may be intimidated because they have been away from school for years and have no current experiences in education to draw upon. Adult students also are often intimidated by the current technology used in the educational settings of today. A divide in the classroom and clinical area with a diverse group can easily occur and must be guarded against by developing interactive methodologies and promoting dialogue of viewpoints. Adult students may readily share their opinions and experiences. The younger or reticent student may need encouragement to share their viewpoints or may need written outlets, such as reflection papers to feel included as a group member.

Adult students are said to view education more critically, goal-oriented, and with more objectivity (Bradshaw & Nugent, 1997). Adult students are not afraid to dialogue with instructors about their opinions and are sophisticated educational consumers (American Association of Colleges of Nursing, 2005). Adult students many times have self-sacrificed financially and socially to undertake a nursing program.

In contrast, the younger student may have a different educational perspective. The younger student is "in the swing of things" educationally, just emerging from high school, and is technologically savvy. The younger student views teachers as authority figures and course assignments as tasks rather than a means to an end. The younger student often lives on campus and has the educational institution's resources more readily available to them.

To deal with these differences, a classroom must encompass multiple methodologies that encourage group interaction, dialogue, and **value clarification** in an emancipatory, caring environment that has zero tolerance for oppression.

Developing a caring emancipatory curriculum seems like a monumental task for a nurse educator who may have 40 to 80 care plans to check, eight to 10 clinical groups to coordinate and 2 to 3 hours of lecture a week to "get all the content in." Nonetheless, educational methodologies that promote reflection, humanism, and cultural sensitivity can yield nursing students who understand the importance of collaborative caring as opposed to nursing students who are competing for attention, grades, and recognition. Interviews, electronic dialogues, and reflection papers are just a few of the many methodologies that can promote caring. A caring curriculum has the potential of creating caring students who will have learned to care for patients, regardless of student age. This approach also creates an environment in which individual differences are respected because they are acknowledged, explored, communicated, and understood. The following sections review some specific methodologies geared to increase understanding of diversity among students and promote an emancipatory, caring learning environment in the context of such diversity (Bankert & Kozel, 2005).

Methodologies Used to Promote Reflection Through Dialogue with Diverse Student Groups

Methodologies that promote reflection, when used in conjunction with traditional methods, have successfully (Oermann, 2003) enhanced the nursing curriculum in a course where accelerated adult students were mixed with traditional undergraduate students. These methodologies include value clarification exercises, interviews, **service learning**, and discussion and dialogue. Socialization is also discussed; although not exactly classified as a methodology, it creates a more cooperative learning environment and is important for students to identify with the culture of nursing.

Value Clarification

Value clarification means openly looking at what you hold true in your heart. Value clarification is a process that encompasses seven steps defined by Raths, Harmin, and Simon (1966):

1. Choosing freely
2. Choosing from alternatives
3. Choosing after consideration of the consequences
4. Prizing and cherishing the choice
5. Publicly affirming our belief

6. Acting on the valued choice

7. Acting consistently and regularly on this value

Value clarification assists nursing students to identify their feelings on nursing issues through awareness, validation, and social interaction (Uustal, 1977). It is an essential tool that "reflects sensitivity to human diversity" (O'Brien & Renner, 1998, p. 287). In education, it can assist to build an emancipatory, caring learning environment because it encourages students to share intimate thought processes and reflections with one another. It is a methodology in nursing education that was very popular in the 1970s but interest waned through the 80s, possibly as a result of increased discussion about technological and ethical issues. Value clarification may be applicable again as an advantageous teaching strategy within the large, diverse classroom. Value clarification exercises can safely explore feelings in the classroom and set the stage for the patients we care for. Uustal (1977) states:

> If you do not take time to examine and articulate your values you will not be fully effective with patients. The clearer you are about what you value, the more able you will be to choose and initiate a course of action that is consistent with what you say you believe in. The price paid for unexamined values and values conflicts often is confusion, indecision and inconsistency (p. 2058).

Value clarification as a methodology, can be used as a separate strategy up front or intertwined throughout the course with other classroom and clinical methodologies. Value clarification exercises can provide a good "jump start" for a large class of diverse learners. It opens dialogue, reflection, and awareness of differences in moral judgment and perspective. A value clarification exercise does not have to be overly time-consuming if used as an ongoing process. Different pieces can be used during different class times and one piece can build on another.

Value identification in nursing programs has been affirmed by accrediting bodies for quite some time (AACN, 1995) and the integration of values into the curriculum of nursing education is essential for developing a caring environment for patients (Bulfin, 2005; Weis, Schank, Eddy, & Elfrink, 1993). Value clarification exercises, modified from Uustal (1977) are illustrated in Figure 12–1. Coupling a traditional student with an adult learner for this exercise leads to insight for both students. These exercises also can be accomplished in small groups, as post-conference tools, and related to discussion about ethical dilemmas encountered in the clinical area.

Interview

Health interviews have long been used in nursing to elicit health histories and are a technique taught to nursing students to assess or gather information from patients. Besides learning about a person's health history, the interviewer often learns about the value the interviewee places on health. It uses techniques that facilitate information gathering: good communication skills, cultural tolerance, and caring. Students can use these techniques to interview each other to enhance collegial understanding. Everyone has a story to tell, but not everyone has a chance to tell it. It is a self-disclosing assignment so care needs to be taken to protect confidentiality. For those students who are uncomfortable with being interviewed by other students, an alternative interview can be arranged with a client. The interview should encompass more than just relaying information from mouth to pen about health status. The interview should be set up to ask specific questions about health promotion, cultural practices, family resources, complementary or alternative medicine use, and likes and dislikes.

The interview technique worked well in one class, for example, by encouraging traditional students and nontraditional students to interview each other. This class interview had specific guidelines and content related to the social, personal, and spiritual significance of a birth experience. The birth experience could be their own (many of the adult students are parents) or some-

Name Tag

1. Write your name in the middle of it.

2. In each of the four corners, write your responses to these four questions:

   a. What one thing would you like your colleagues to say about you?

   b. What single most important thing do you do to make your nurse-patient relationships positive ones?

   c. What do you do on a daily basis that indicates you value your health?

   d. Name one value you believe in strongly.

In the space around your name, write six adjectives that you feel best describe who you are.

What have you discovered about yourself?
Were any of the questions especially difficult to answer?
What values are reflected in the answers you gave?
What additional questions would you ask?

Note other value clarification exercises at the end of the chapter.

FIGURE 12–1 Value clarification exercise. Adapted from Uustal, D. (1978). *AJM*, 2058–2063.

one close to them (if a traditional student had no exposure to a birthing process they could look up a birth experience on the Internet and report on that as if they were the person). This assignment was used to enhance the content of a maternal-child health nursing course (Lee & Lamp, 2005) but other topics can be used as well, such as the student experience with an aging individual, an ill adolescent or child, or an adult who is nonadherent to a healthy lifestyle. This technique is useful in assisting students who normally may not interact with one another to dialogue with each other and create an understanding of where the other student "is coming from" in a semi-structured, safe environment. Just as interviewing is used in the clinical area, this technique may assist with behavior change, and help students to explore and resolve issues (Donnan, 2005).

Service Learning

Another methodology that encourages interaction, caring, and dialogue is service learning. A service-learning project can be integrated into the curriculum as an assignment. Service learning is getting the students out into the community in the form of a partnership. The students learn from the experience and they "give back" to humanity a needed service. Service learning is a philosophy of cultural awareness and does not count as clinical hours. Vanderhoff (2005) defines service learning as "giving students the opportunity to provide service to others while tying in learning objectives and a class project for professional development" (p. 36). It is more than volunteerism because students receive a percentage of their grade for it. It is more than just community service; it is course-based educational experience for credit (Bentley & Ellison, 2005). Service learning can take place in local community-based settings or even internationally (Perry & Mander, 2005). Service learning entails recognizing the needs of the community or a given patient population (Vanderhoff, 2005).

Service learning can be enacted in many ways and forms. One class, for example, developed a service-learning project in which students were randomly divided into groups for "Teddy Bear Clinics" on Sundays at different parishes in a local area. The Teddy Bear Clinics were advertised through the parish nurse and focused on teaching young children health promotion. Children came to the clinic with a stuffed animal and pretended to be a parent with a child. The children were escorted through stations by a nursing student. The stations each had a different theme, such as handwashing, teeth brushing, injury prevention, first aid, and safety. After the clinic, the students wrote a reflective paper on what they learned from the experience in relation to their experience and ability to communicate information to children and a diverse group of parents.

Another class took blood pressures at the mall and parishes and counseled people on healthy heart diets. This service project became more than just a blood pressure screening. Student journals indicated that it became a forum in which students learned to interact with the public in a professional role. This journal entry illustrates the effectiveness of service learning:

> I enjoyed this experience. I only took blood pressures on a few people, however, I thought there was more that we were doing. One elderly gentleman sat and talked with me for quite some time. I felt as though he really wanted to sit with someone and have them listen to him. It made me feel as though I had helped out much more than I had initially thought I would or could that day. It was very nice to be able to help those people out (Blackboard electronic journal from 1-22-06).

This project helped make students more culturally competent by breaking down barriers through reflection and discussion of real life experiences. It is very difficult for students working on a service-learning project together not to interact constructively. A cooperative purpose is always a powerful tool in education.

Service learning has increased in popularity in recent years and may be directly linked to the service-learning boom at the high school level (13 million high school students participate in service learning each year). Almost 30% of the 6.7 million students in public and private 4-year college settings participate in a course in which service-learning is integrated into the curriculum (National Service Learning Clearinghouse, 2004). Also, about 50% of the community colleges offer service learning courses throughout disciplines (National Service Learning Clearinghouse, 2004).

Bentley and Ellison (2005) called service learning a "powerful learning experience" (p. 287). It should have a two-fold purpose. It should meet both the students' needs and the community needs. Bentley and Ellison (2005) used service learning in a course in which 16 nursing students partnered with Head Start to assist teenagers to transition into parenthood. Qualitative data showed positive enrichment from the students. Quantitatively, it was evaluated against a control group on the Health Education Systems Incorporated (HESI) scores. The experimental or service-learning students scored higher on the comprehensive HESI, designed to test nursing knowledge, but not significantly (service-learning group, $\underline{M} = 92.01$; control, $\underline{M} = 90.22$). These results show a trend toward service learning as an educational enhancement in the understanding of nursing curriculum content.

The ingredients that have been identified for academic-community partnerships by Plowfield, Wheeler, and Raymond (2005) are applicable to service learning. The ingredients include time, tact, talent, and trust. Time must be invested by the teacher to establish the relationship with the agency or community service being utilized. Connections have to be established person to person and electronically to understand the needs of both groups and the resources available. Time is also a detriment to the process because establishing a service-learning curriculum is time-intensive on faculty who are already overextended. Tact is necessary to ensure a trusting relationship. Communication is a key element as is maintaining the vision of the project throughout the process of detail analysis. Tact calls for respect, which means prompt answers, attending to matters, answering questions, and anticipating problems. Talent is recognizing and celebrating different areas of expertise in situations. Plowfield, Wheeler, and Raymond (2005) state, "no one wants to invest time and resources when objectives are not clear or the path to achieving them is fraught with obstacles" (p. 219). Talent guards against this pitfall in service learning. Building trust is an ongoing process, forged through the other three values in a service-learning project. Trust is built through open dialogue and tact while working together on mutual goals (Plowfield, Wheeler, & Raymond, 2005).

Perry and Mander (2005) used an international service-learning model in which nursing students traveled abroad for a focused learning experience in maternal-child health. The experience started in well-developed countries where the students were acculturated into the health-care system, then it expanded to third world countries where the students provided service. Service was rendered through nursing care and bringing supplies and resources. The journaling comments from the students and faculty regarding the experience supported that these projects enhanced knowledge and cultural sensitivity in a way that could not be accomplished in a classroom. Consider one student's comment:

> It was unforgettable experience that I will treasure for the rest of my life. The trip has definitely empowered me as a future nurse and as a woman through the learning process of this great adventure (p. 151).

A long-standing, 8-year, service-learning project at Capstone College of Nursing of the University of Alabama, has students enrolled in a fundamental nursing class participate in a project that provides health screening and physical assessments on K through 12 school students. The outcomes of this project include enhancements in skill, clinical decision-making, and communication (Adams, 2004; Denner, Coyle, Robin, & Banspach, 2005).

Dialogue

Perry and Mander (2005) state, "Don't criticize or comment on differences, appreciate them" (p. 148). How does that appreciation develop? The first way would be to experience it—experience it through true dialogue. Someone cannot actually experience the history of another but can understand that history better through communication. Communication is the essential ingredient to promoting positive group dynamics, if the communication is open, honest, and done in a flexible environment (August-Brady, 2000).

Classroom discussion is a wonderful tool to create an environment of empathy and understanding. But due to curriculum demands, classroom time is limited. Other techniques, such as 10-minute diffusion time, and electronic discussion platforms, may be necessary to assist in facilitating communication to assist intercultural, intercollegial appreciation. These quick dialoguing techniques may help a group of diverse students "gel" and acquire a positive learning experience without undo time commitment.

10-Minute Diffusion Time

Setting 10 minutes aside at the end of class for storytelling enhances dialogue and understanding. Trying to pick a specific topic, such as "Who witnessed a birth this week?" or "Who felt more comfortable in clinical this week with a specific skill?" can start a story. This is different from post-conference because the entire group is together, not just the clinical group. Even though time allotted to this methodology is minimal, often the conversation spills over into the hall after class and students take time out to listen to each other and tell their own stories (Irvin, 1996).

Discuss Electronically

Opening the discussion board for threads about specific topics and nonspecific topics assists students to share and become aware of each other. One technique is to open an uncensored thread that is just for the students and promise not to enter the thread. Other discussion threads can be opened for specific student groups. Groups can be composed of students from the same clinical group or they can be random. Interest groups for a specific topic or dilemma have also been used. Discussion threads of random groups usually need a topic to begin the conversation. If the discussion is a class expectation, or takes the place of post-conference, it is easy to use a rubric that clarifies what the expectations of the discussion are (see Figures 12–2 and 12–3).

Socialization

Accelerated and weekend/evening programs place a very constraining schedule on the adult student. Although students are aware of the academic schedule when they enter the program, it is different once it is being "lived." Scheduled socialization breaks promote integration of the group, role modeling of the culture of nursing, and stress relief (Murray & Main, 2005). Understanding that the students in a classroom today have differences in culture, age, learning styles, and expectations can set up nurse educators for difficult teaching circumstances. Having "down" time in which students can mingle and dialogue on a different level than the classroom is a great way to

Points (Possible 16)	0	1	2
What was it like for you to have your children or choose not to have children?	Not answered	Partially answered	Well answered and described.
Can you remember what you were thinking or feeling when you had your children?	Not answered	Partially answered	Well answered and described.
What special things does your family do when people are pregnant or delivering?	Not answered	Partially answered	Well answered and described.
What was your nursing care like?	Not answered	Partially answered	Well answered and described.
What was the most positive thing that happened to you during that time?	Not answered	Partially answered	Well answered and described.
What was the most negative thing?	Not answered	Partially answered	Well answered and described.
If I decide to take care of moms and babies for the rest of my life, what advice would you give me?	Not answered	Partially answered	Well answered and described.

FIGURE 12-2 Interview rubric.

Discussions: Possible 6 points			
Objective	**0 points**	**1 point**	**2 points**
Participation in discussions	Posts infrequently.	Posts responses to most or all discussion board topics.	Posts thoughtful responses to all Discussion Board topics.
Content	Responses do not demonstrate an understanding of content, readings, or activities.	Responses demonstrate an understanding of module content, readings, and activities.	Responses demonstrate a thorough understanding of module content, readings, and activities.
Quality of feedback to others	Feedback is not given to class members.	Feedback to class members is general.	Feedback to class members is constructive, specific, and supportive.

FIGURE 12-3 Discussion rubric.

establish a trusting relationship that may not be fostered in the formal setting. Pizza parties, meet and greet sessions with light snacks, brown bag lunches, family nights, and movie nights are just a few examples of ways to enhance socialization. Nursing education is a rigorous curriculum that is stressful and affects the entire family. Downtime and socializing with faculty and other students in a different setting assists in relationship building and communication (Miklancie & Davis, 2005).

Summary

The nurse educator today is likely to face a classroom of students with much different demographics and numbers than in days past. Classes are larger and comprise more adult and returning students than ever before. Learning styles differ by individuality, culture, and age. Pedagogies that enhance interstudent understanding and caring can only promote understanding and caring in nursing practice. Using old standby pedagogies exclusively may not meet the expectations of today's learners. Methodologies that promote dialogue, value clarification, and caring are needed to help students socialize into a caring profession. Reflection and awareness of values, attitudes, bias, and appreciation for life experience must be integrated with content in a flexible educational environment. Our classrooms and clinical groups are microcosms of the patient-care area; caring for each other must be integrated to be realized in the professional role.

References

Adams, M. (2004). Faculty matters. *Nursing Educational Perspectives, 25*(5), 216–217.

American Association of Colleges of Nursing. (2005). Accelerated programs: The fast-track to careers in nursing. *AACN Issues Bulletin.* Retrieved 12-10-05 from **http://wwww.aacn.nche.edu/Publications/ issues/Aug02.htm.**

Arslanian-Engoren, C. (2002). Feminist poststructualism: A methodological paradigm for examining clinical decision making. *Journal of Advanced Nursing, 37*, 512–517.

August-Brady, M. (2000). Flexibility: A concept analysis. *Nursing Forum, 35*(1), 5–13.

August-Brady, M. (2005). The effect of a metacognitive intervention on approach to and self-regulation of learning in baccalaureate nursing students. *Journal of Nursing Education, 44*(7), 297–304..

Bankert, E., & Kozel, V. (2005). Transforming pedagogy in nursing education: A caring learning environment for adult students. *Nursing Education Perspectives, 26*(4), 227–229.

Bentley, R., & Ellison, K. (2005). Impact of a service-learning project on nursing students. *Nursing Education Perspectives, 26*(5), 287–290.

Berragan, L. (1998). Nursing practice draws upon several different ways of knowing. *Journal of Clinical Nursing, 7,* 209–217.

Bevis, E., & Watson, J. (2000). *Toward a caring curriculum: A new pedagogy for nursing.* New York: National League of Nursing.

Bradshaw, M. J., & Nugent, K. (1997). Clinical learning experiences of nontraditional age nursing students [News, Notes & Tips]. *Nurse Educator, 22*(6), 40–74.

Bulfin, S. (2005). Practice applications. Nursing as caring theory: Living caring in practice. *Nursing Science Quarterly, 18*(4), 313–319.

Denner, J., Coyle, K., Robin, L., & Banspach, S. (2005). Integrating service learning into a curriculum to reduce health risks at alternative schools. *Journal of School Health, 75*(5), 151–156.

Diekelmann, N. L., Editor. (2003). *Teaching the practitioners of care: New pedagogies for the health professions.* The University of Wisconsin Press.

Donnan, C. (2005). Mental health at work. *Occupational Health, 57*(11), 16.

Duchscher, J. E. (2000). Bending a habit: Critical social theory as a framework for humanistic nursing education. *Nurse Education Today, 20,* 453–462.

Fahrenfort, M. (1987). Patient emancipation by health education: An impossible goal? *Patient Education and Counseling, 10*(87), 25–37.

Freire, P. (1970). *Pedagogy of the oppressed.* New York: The Continuum International.

Freire, P., & Aravjo Freire. (1998). *The Paul Freire reader.* New York: The Continuum International.

Gillespie, M. (2002). Student-teacher connection in clinical nursing education. *Journal of Advanced Nursing, 37*(6), 566–576.

Godshall, M. (Dec, 2005). Survey of accelerated students. *Nursing Educational Experience,* unpublished results. Used with permission.

Habermas, J. (1969). *Toward a rational society: Student protest, science, and politics.* London: Heinemann.

Harden, J. (1996). Enlightenment, empowerment and emancipation: The case for critical pedagogy in nurse education. *Nurse Education Today, 16,* 32–37.

Hegel, G. (1960*). Hegel; highlights, an annotated selection by Wanda Orynski,* New York: Philosophical Library.

Heidegger, M. (1949). *Existence and being.* Chicago: Henry Regnery.

Heller, B. R., Oros, M. T., & Durney-Crowley, J. (2006). The future of nursing education: Ten trends to watch. NLN Publications. Retrieved June 29, 2006 from **http://www.nln.org/nlnjournal/infotrends. htm#top.**

Holland, S. (2004). Nursing Spectrum. Greater Philadelphia Area. August 23, 2004, 10–11.

Irvin, S. M. (1996). Creative teaching strategies. *Journal of Continuing Education in Nursing, 27*(3). 108–114.

Jagger, A. M. (1988). *Feminist politics and human nature.* Totawa, NJ: Rown & Littlefield.

Karlowicz, K. A., Wiles, L. L., Bishop, J. F., & Lakin, M. B. (2003). The promise and perils of a weekend nursing program. *Nurse Educator, 28*(2), 77–82.

Lee, C., & Lamp, J. K. (2005). The birth interview: Enhancing student appreciation of personal meaning of pregnancy and birth. *Nurse Educator, 30*(4), 155–158.

MacPherson, K. I. (1983). Feminist methods: A new paradigm for nursing research. *Advances in Nursing Science, 5*(2), 17–25.

Marx, K., & Engels, F. (1976). *The German ideology.* Moscow: Progress Publ.

Miklancie, M., & Davis, T. (2005). The second-degree acceleration program as an innovative educational strategy: New Century, new chapter, new challenge. *Nursing Education Perspectives, 26*(5), 291–293.

Mill, J., Allen, M., & Morrow, R. (2001). Critical theory: Critical methodology to disciplinary foundations in nursing. *Canadian Journal of Nursing Research, 33*, 109–127.

Murray, C., & Main, A. (2005). Role modeling as a teaching method for student mentors. *Nursing Times, 101*(26), 30–33.

National Service Learning Clearinghouse. (2004). Retrieved November 28, 2005 from **http://www.servicelearning.org/index.php.**

O'Brien, B., & Renner, A. (1998). Opening minds: Values clarification via electronic meetings. *Computers in Nursing, 16*(5), 266–271.

O'Callaghan, N. (2005). The use of expert practice to explore reflection. *Nursing Standard, 19*(39), 41–47.

Oermann, M. (2003). NLN Educational Summit, Breakout session. *Classroom teaching: Keep students active with these strategies.*

Owen-Mills, V. (1995). A synthesis of caring praxis and critical social theory in emancipatory curriculum. *Journal of Advanced Nursing, 21*, 1191–1195.

Paley, J. (1998). Misinterpretive phenomenology: Heidegger, ontology and nursing research. *Journal of Advanced Nursing, 27*, 817–824.

Perry, P. (1994). Feminist empiricism as a method for inquiry in nursing. *Western Journal of Nursing Research, 16*, 480–494.

Perry, S., & Mander, R. (2005). A global frame of reference: learning from everyone, everywhere. *Nursing Education Perspectives, 26*(3), 148–151.

Plowfield, L., Wheeler, E., & Raymond, J. (2005). Time, tact, talent and trust: Essential ingredients of effective academic-community partnership. *Nursing Educational Perspectives, 26*(4), 217–220.

Pohl, J. M., & Boyd, C. J. (1993). Ageism within feminism. *Image: Journal of Nursing Scholarship, 25*(3), 199–203.

Polanyi, M. (1958). *Personal knowledge: Towards a post-critical philosophy.* Chicago: The University of Chicago Press.

Raths, L. E., Harmin, M., & Simon, S. B. (1966). *Values and teaching.* Columbus, OH: Charles E. Merrill Books.

Raymond, C., & Profetto-McGrath, J. (2005). Nurse educators' critical thinking: Reflection and measurement. *Nurse Education in Practice, 5*(4), 209–217.

Romyn, D. M. (2000). Emancipatory pedagogy in nursing education: A dialectic analysis. *Canadian Journal of Nursing Research, 32*, 119–138.

Siu, H., Laschinger, H., & Vingilis, E. (2005). The effect of problem-based learning on nursing students' perceptions of empowerment. *Journal of Nursing Education, 44*(10), 459–469.

Uustal, D. (1977). The use of value clarification in nursing practice. *The Journal of Continuing Education in Nursing, 8*(3), 8–13.

Uustal, D. (1978). Values clarification in nursing application to practice. *American Journal of Nursing, 78*(12), 2058–2063.

Vanderhoff, M. (2005). Service learning: The world as the classroom. *PT Magazine,* May, 34–41.

Weis, D., Schank, M. J., Eddy, D., & Elfrink, V. (1993). Professional values in baccalaureate nursing education. *Journal of Professional Nursing, 9*(6), 336–342.

Wittmann-Price, R. (2004). Emancipation in decision-making in women's health care. *Journal of Advanced Nursing, 47*(4), 437–445.

REVIEW QUESTIONS

• What are the philosophical underpinnings that promote reflection?
• What are the socioeconomic reasons for the changing demographics of student nurses?
• What are the methodologies and how is each implemented to promote reflection?
• What other activities can be provided to enhance socialization of diverse groups of students?

CRITICAL THINKING EXERCISES

Reformulate the interview questions in Figure 12–2 to fit your course content.

Rework value-clarification exercises to fit an online format and place on a discussion board platform or in group folders and monitor student interactions.

Complete the value clarification exercises that follow.

Exercise 1: Patterns—Which words describe you?

Draw a circle around the seven words you feel best describe you as an individual.
Underline seven words you feel most accurately describe you as a professional person.
(Yes, you may circle and underline the same word!)

UNPREDICTABLE

AMBITIOUS   OPINIONATED

  SELF-DISCIPLINED   RESERVED

OUTGOING   INDEPENDENT

                          CONCERNED

EASILY HURT   ASSERTIVE

          GENEROUS   INDIFFERENT

     CAPABLE   ARGUMENTATIVE

SUSPICIOUS   THOUGHTFUL

                          FUN-LOVING   IMAGINATIVE

DYNAMIC   INTELLECTUAL

                          COMPROMISING   EASILY LED

RELIABLE   LIKABLE

          OBEDIENT   MOODY

HELPFUL   SLOW TO RELATE

Reflective Questions:

Are you happy with your patterns?
Do you like who you are?
Do you choose to change? Which ones? Why?
What values are reflected in your patterns?

Exercise 2: Forced-Rank Ordering

How would you prioritize the following alternatives?
Remember there is no correct set of priorities.
Probe your imagination and ask yourself why you feel the way you do.

1. With whom on a nursing unit would you become most upset with? The nurse who:
   A. Never completes assignments.
   B. Rarely helps others.
   C. Projects own feelings on patients.

2. Which would you rather have happen to you if you had a serious health problem?
   A. Not be told
   B. Be told directly
   C. Find out by accident

3. What makes you happiest at your work?
   A. Skills using your hands and caring for patients with complex needs.
   B. The ability to compile data and arrive at a nursing diagnosis.
   C. Being able to communicate easily and skillfully with patients.

4. What would be the most difficult for you to do?
   A. Listen and counsel a dying patient.
   B. Care for a person with serious burns.
   C. Work in CCU full time.

Reflection question:
What rank-ordering questions can you create?

Exercise 3: Value Continuum

Consider each of the following questions carefully and ask, "Where do I stand?" In each continuum, place an X on the line that best describes your feelings about the issue.

1. How do you feel about supporting a professional organization?

   _____

   I refuse to become a member of any   I belong to every professional group in existence.
   professional organization.

2. How do you feel about your decision-making skills?

   _____

   I am unable to make decisions without   Good decision maker and documents decisions.
   consulting others.

3. How do you feel about abortion?

   _____

   Not appropriate under any circumstance.   Abortion should be available on demand.

4. How do you feel about taking a re-licensure examination every 5 years?

   _____

   Absolutely not.   Definitely.

Exercise 4: Value Voting

This exercise demonstrates that there are many facets to every issue.
How do you determine your position?
What factors influence your thoughts and feelings?
Indicate your responses in the following manner.

5	4	3	2	1
Strongly Agree	Agree	Undecided	Disagree	Strongly Disagree

DO YOU BELIEVE

A. _____ Patients have the right to participate in all decisions related to their health.

B. _____ Continuing education should be mandatory.

C. _____ Patients should be told the truth.

D. _____ Badly deformed babies should be allowed to die.

E. _____ Abortion should be legal.

F. _____ There should be a law guaranteeing medical care for each person in this country.

Exercise 5: Unfinished Sentences

Complete the following sentences.

Use them to examine your attitudes, feelings, and values.

1. I feel most competent in my position in nursing when

_____ .

2. I wish nursing directors would

_____ .

3. A demanding leader makes me feel

_____ .

4. I get real pleasure in nursing from

_____ .

5. Patients are most anxious

_____ .

6. The primary purpose of nurse internship programs should be

_____ .

Exercise 6: A Planning Board for Healthy Relationships

Prioritize the alternatives below in the following manner:

1 = Choice you feel is MOST important in a nurse-patient

10 = Indicates the alternative you feel is LEAST important

_____ Empathetic listening

_____ Disclosing myself to a friend

_____ Being honest in answering questions

_____ Helping my friend in times of need

_____ Remaining objective about my friend's decisions

_____ Telling authorities if my friend is abusing alcohol

_____ Spending time with my friend

_____ Enjoying the same pastimes

_____ Reporting a potentially serious health problem my friend may be having

_____ "WILD CARD" add an alternative of your own_____

Adapted from: Uustal, D. (1978). *AJN*, 2058–2063.

ANNOTATED RESEARCH SUMMARY

Duke, M. (2001). On the fast track: Speeding nurses into the future: A two-year bachelor of nursing for graduates of other disciplines. *Collegian, 8*(1), 14–18.

Graduates of other disciplines entering nursing on a fast track program were studied in Australia. Academic scores of the accelerated group of students were higher than those of the traditional students 6 out of 7 years. Other findings noted that accelerated students were highly motivated and experienced increased stress while undertaking their nursing courses.

Kearns, L. E., Shoaf, J. R., & Summey, M. B. (2004). Performance and satisfaction of second-degree BSN students in Web-based and traditional course delivery environments. *Journal of Nursing Education, 43*(6), 280–284.

Two groups of accelerated students were studied and comparisons made on the data of course scores and composite examination scores. One group of accelerated students used Web-based courses and the other received traditional courses with Web enhancement. Students enrolled in the Web-based courses scored significantly higher on test measures while satisfaction scores of the students enrolled in the traditional course were higher.

Halkett, A., & McLafferty, E. (2006). Graduate entrants into nursing—are we meeting their needs? *Nurse Education Today, 26*(2), 162–168.

Qualitative investigation at the University of Dundee revealed themes identified as significant by accelerated nursing students. Three focus groups identified consistent themes of the accelerated BSN student. These included:

Usefulness of their first degree to their current program of study.
Course design and content.
Assessment strategies.
Placement issues.
Attitudes of others.

It has been suggested that these themes be taken into consideration when educators undertake program development.

Chapter Outline

MANAGEMENT STRATEGIES IN CLIENT CARE SETTINGS

13

Susan M.P. Scholtz

Learning Outcomes

On completion of this chapter, the reader will be able to:

- Describe perceived threats and stressors inherent within clinical education.
- Discuss the impact of perceived threats on learning outcomes within clinical education.
- List critical attributes of the concept of threat.
- Differentiate between the effects of challenge and threat on learning outcomes.
- Explain Pennebaker's expressive writing paradigm.
- Describe the correlation between prevention as intervention and expressive writing.
- Discuss the concept of reframing through cognitive restructuring.
- Explain Scholtz's theory of reframing threat apperception (STRTA).
- Describe an expressive writing exercise designed to decrease threat apperception prior to clinical education.

Key Words

Apperception
Challenge
Clinical education
Expressive writing
Threat
Threat apperception

Over the years, faculty strived to design a curriculum that will prepare the novice nurse to meet the health-care needs of society. Educators have been innovative in developing courses aimed to produce successful learning outcomes. Educational technology and active teaching/learning strategies have been incorporated into the classroom setting.

Although dramatic changes have occurred with the classroom setting, **clinical education** has remained somewhat stagnant. Clinical education is defined as "the integration of knowledge and skills associated with patient care" (Scholtz, 2000). Experienced nursing faculty members will agree that the basic model for clinical education has remained static for the past 25 years or longer.

For example, students (approximately 8 to 10) are assigned to a faculty member for a clinical rotation. Typically, the day before the experience, the instructor assigns each student to approximately two patients in the acute care setting. Students research the chart of each patient and document pertinent information. The student memorizes medications, reviews pathophysiology, and designs a nursing plan of care. The day of the experience, the instructor quizzes each student on the information. Basically, the student reiterates information from the chart or memorized knowledge. During pre-conference, as one student is being questioned, the remaining students are anticipating questions they may be asked by the instructor. The students proceed to deliver nursing care and regroup at the end of the day for post-conference. Again, the student basically remains focused on the individual assignment.

By consistently assigning a student to one or two patients per week, instructors put a limit on the number of situational experiences that may arise; thus, opportunities for clinical judgment are limited. In addition, the clinical experience remains prescriptive and static. The instructor's primary function becomes that of a supervisor of procedures as opposed to a facilitator of learning. The amount of critical thinking or clinical judgment that occurs during the course of the day is questionable. As the number of students in each clinical group increases, the amount of time available to engage in meaningful discussion and inquiry decreases proportionately.

Clinical Education for Today's Nursing Student

Although this model of clinical education may have sufficed in the past, clinical education must be revised for today's nursing student. Unpredictable client needs, early discharge, and limited available clinical sites require the student to integrate knowledge more efficiently.

Redesign Pre- and Post-Conferences

Because one learning outcome of pre-conference is to broaden the knowledge base and awareness of all students, weekly clinical rounds may be incorporated. This technique has been used in medicine for years and encourages students to assume an active role in decision-making. Instead of purging memorization of knowledge, the instructor can facilitate learning at the application level of learning. Students have the opportunity to know the patients' clinical picture in a particular zone as opposed to the one patient assigned to them. Their knowledge base is broadened and the experience offers additional dimensions.

At the risk of sounding blasphemous, daily post-conferences may be a thing of the past. In lieu of post-conference, the student may be given an alternative forum to process the events of the day in a group setting. Asynchronous dialogue allows the student to document his insights, feelings, or thoughts on a password-accessed Web site that is established specifically for the instructor and students. Students are encouraged to post responses to the logs of their peers.

Internet relay chat (IRC) can be used to set up synchronous chat rooms for the students. Students enter the room using a specific password at a designated time and can join ongoing dialogue. They can share their experiences with their clinical group or nursing students from other schools. The benefit of this strategy is that students can participate from the comfort of their rooms and actively engage in dialogue. A time can be set that is convenient for all and not necessarily at the end of an arduous clinical day.

Clinical Preceptors

The use of preceptors is not a new concept in nursing education, but the value of the strategy may have gained popularity. Instructors, who teach on a clinical unit but are not employed as nursing staff on the assigned unit, are basically "guests" on the unit. They are not as vested in the outcomes of the unit because they are generally instructing students for 1 or 2 days per week. With rising enrollment and high numbers of schools rotating through the same clinical sites, their engagement in the matters of the unit is limited.

Students, assigned instead to a preceptor who works as a professional nurse on the assigned unit, can learn from a permanent member of the unit. The preceptor can exercise independent decision-making that the nursing student can observe. Collaborating with a nurse preceptor in the care of four to six patients gives the student greater exposure to a variety of clinical scenarios.

Students could also have increased flexibility. For example, the senior nursing student may be assigned to schedule clinical hours with the preceptor on an evening shift or weekend. This schedule would allow the student to see the variations that occur within the unit and clinical practice on different shifts.

In order for preceptorships to be effective, the potential preceptors should be interviewed. The nurse should embrace the philosophy of the nursing program and not approach the experience with the perception, "This is how I was taught...so this is how I will teach!" Before the screening, a specific list of criteria should be designed to select a qualified preceptor. It is imperative that the nurse enjoy working with students and respect their learning needs. A letter of recommendation by the nurse manager or an instructor who has observed the nurse's interactions with students may be required. It is important to realize that many nurses are experts in clinical practice but novices in nursing education. Once an individual preceptor is selected, the instructor/faculty member should serve as a mentor to the newly assigned clinical instructor. Through the collaborative efforts of the expert instructor and preceptor, successful learning outcomes can be attained.

Student Perception of Clinical Education

Clinical education is a vital component in the pedagogy of nursing education and students anxiously await their first experience caring for a patient. The need to prepare nurses to provide holistic nursing care and to manage both complex problems and psychosocial issues is inherent within the scope of clinical education. Complicated procedures, nursing care plans, complexity of disease processes, and interrelationships with families and members of the health-care team are often stressful to the nursing student.

Individual differences and appraisal of the clinical learning environment may have an effect on whether students assess clinical experiences as either a **challenge** or a **threat** (Lazarus, 1999). Lazarus (1999) suggested that each person interacts differently with the environment; therefore, relational meanings of environmental stimuli are unique to the person. The nursing student who appraises the clinical experience as challenging has the potential for growth and mastery. Conversely, the student who appraises clinical education as a threat has the potential for stagnation and failure (Lazarus, 1999).

According to Scholtz (2000), critical attributes of threat include negative cognitive perception, future oriented, negative affective emotions, and the potential for harm. Threat triggers feelings of uncertainty, worry, and distress. The student who feels threatened may experience a threat to self-integrity, immobilized coping, and altered self-esteem (Scholtz, 2000). Challenge is the perception and anticipation of positive outcomes associated with a stimulus (Lazarus, 1991). A perception of challenge facilitates the student's desire and ability to perform and learn. Challenge is the opposite of threat. **Threat apperception** is the person's assessment of stimuli and the attribution of meanings and consequences to the threatening stimuli (Lazarus, 1999).

According to Neuman's systems model, repeated stressors, such as perceived threat, can cause instability within the person (Neuman, 1995). Tension-invoking stimuli have the potential to cause situational crises and may jeopardize the student's success within the educational program (Neuman, 1995). Learning within this context may be jeopardized in students who perceive clinical education as threatening (Kleehammer, Hart, & Keck, 1990). Because the quantity of time devoted to clinical education is limited, the quality of the experience must be maximized in order for the learner to have successful outcomes.

Recognizing that clinical education may be inherently stressful to students, nurse educators attempt to create an environment that enhances learning and promotes professional and personal development of the nursing student (Biggers, Zimmerman, & Alpert, 1988). Rather than intervening when the student is in crisis, perceived threat and performance anxiety could possibly be circumvented through prevention as intervention.

Characteristics of nursing students prone to stress related to clinical education have been studied with varying degrees of reported success (Beal, 1988; Godbey & Courage, 1994; Russler, 1991; Williams, 1993). The profile of a typical student prone to anxiety and stress is a conscientious and hard-working individual (Meisenhelder, 1987). The individual invests long hours in preparing for the clinical education experience and appears overly prepared. However, the student becomes intimidated when questioned by the instructor. Consequently, the true abilities of the student may be blocked by threat, which manifests as performance anxiety.

According to Williams (1993), the nursing major may be the most threatening of all academic majors in college due to its multidimensional nature. In an attempt to discover the threats inherent within nursing, Williams (1993) conducted a descriptive correlational study. Students identified fear of harming the patient and learning clinical procedures as concerns. These fears may be preconceived by the student; nonetheless, they are perceived as very real. Feelings of threat can be manifested during the initial clinical experience and persist throughout progression through the curriculum. One student may fear the "unknown" of the community experience; whereas, another student fears the high technology of the intensive care units.

Because the amount of time dedicated to clinical education is at a premium, nurse educators strive to use this time to maximize learning. Rather than take a reactive stance to students' needs and intervene after the stress has occurred, a more proactive approach may be to intervene in order to prevent the stress. A student who is threatened by the demands of clinical education may feel incapable of performing necessary skills. As a result, the context of the situation is the perception of a negative outcome and failure. Instead of working within the present framework of completing the task, concentration is focused on failure to succeed. One goal of nursing education is to promote a learning environment that is perceived by students as safe and nonthreatening. This goal may be accomplished through prevention as intervention. Neuman (1990) defines primary prevention through intervention as an action that occurs before a reaction to a stressor. Williams (1993) made a critical recommendation that the initiation of preventive measures that address the high levels of stress experienced by nursing students may enhance student learning and promote successful outcomes.

According to Pennebaker's expressive writing paradigm (1997), writing about an emotional experience decreases feelings of inhibition and promotes self-disclosure of thoughts and fears. The student who worries about an upcoming clinical experience can release and address these threats through **expressive writing.** Scholtz's theory of reframing threat **apperception** also addresses the use of expressive writing as a method to facilitate positive learning outcomes (Figure 13–1).

Expressive Journaling

The nursing student has a reciprocal interaction with the clinical environment. As the student prepares for the upcoming clinical experience (patient assignments, complex procedures, medication administration, etc.), the student appraises the potential for personal growth (challenge) or if the stimulus is incongruent with established goals (threat). For example, the student may be assigned to a client who receives multiple intravenous medications and treatments. Although the nursing instructor may perceive this assignment as a positive learning experience, the nursing student may feel threatened by the complexity of the assignment (threat apperception) and begin to experience feelings of anxiety or threat. The perception of the experience as incongruent to the successful attainment of positive outcomes can immobilize learning. Basically, the student fears that failure to perform successfully will result in a failing grade.

Expressive writing is an active process that enables the individual to express feelings of stress through affective discharge. It allows the student to "slow down" the velocity and intensity of the perceived threat. Moreover, expressive writing allows an individual to distance or short-circuit the emotional intensity of a threatening stimulus through reframing (Eckstein, 1997).

Written language is instrumental in reframing threat apperception. It can change the conceptual or emotional meaning of the context in which threat is experienced. Expressive writing enables the student to simply write about thoughts, feelings, and emotions before clinical education. It also prompts students to think about potential coping strategies and transcribe them into written language (Pennebaker, 1997).

Expressive writing is effective when used before a clinical education experience. Typically, nursing students are given client assignments the day before the experience. Once they have researched the client's chart, they begin to prepare for the upcoming experience. Based on the complexity of the case, students' anxiety may heighten. They may perceive the complex procedures as a threat. Instructors who use expressive writing ask the students to think about the upcoming experience. On the evening before clinical, the following prompt is given:

> Today, I want you to reflect on your deepest feelings and thoughts about going into the clinical setting tomorrow. In writing, you may want to explore your thoughts about what you may experience as you care for your client. Write freely about those feelings and do not censor your thoughts or emotions. Do not worry about spelling or grammar. Let your feelings come to life as you transform them into written language. Write for approximately 20 minutes.

Students may become anxious as they identify their anxieties. In order to prevent their anxieties from immobilizing learning, students are asked to approach the day proactively. In order to accomplish this task, they are asked to problem solve by identifying three things they may want to do that will help deal with any stresses, threats, or challenges that may occur during the clinical experience. See Box 13–1.

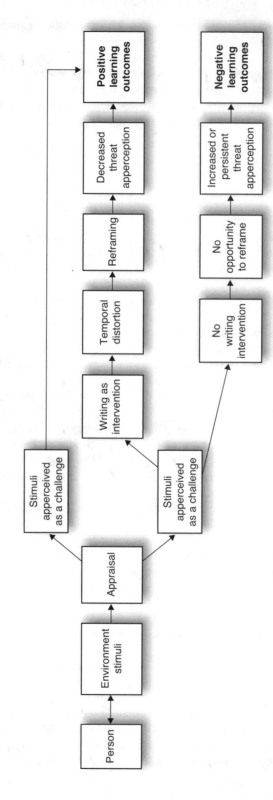

FIGURE 13–1 Scholtz's theory of reframing threat apperception. In this model, the student who perceives the environment as a "threat" can be led to a positive learning outcome by using writing as intervention. It helps to reframe the threat in a different perspective to decrease threat apperception. Without using writing as an intervention, the student who perceives the environment as a threat will have negative learning outcomes.

I just finished doing my research for tomorrow's patient assignment. I was surprised my instructor assigned me to take care of such a sick patient. My patient, Tavia, is only 5 years old. Her parents brought her to the hospital because they thought she had a malabsorption. I guess that when she began to limp because she had so much abdominal pain, the doctor ordered some more tests. According to the nurse who was taking care of her today, Tavia has cancer. When I read about it in my peds book, it sounds as though this is an aggressive type of cancer and that she probably won't live to see her next birthday. The doctor is going to meet with her family tomorrow and tell them.

In some ways, I wish they would tell the family when I am not there. Her mom and dad are my age. I saw them in her room and it looked as though they were both crying. I just hope I know what to do tomorrow when he tells them. Knowing me, I just hope I don't fall apart and don't start crying too. That is something no one needs! And what if Tavia asks me something I am unable to answer? Suppose she asks if she is going to die? Then what? She is a beautiful little girl and I know it will be a "good learning experience." But . . . I don't know if I am ready!

I think it may be helpful to talk with my instructor about how I feel before I go into Tavia's room. She probably can give me some ideas on how to handle Tavia. My instructor is open and I am pretty comfortable telling her I am nervous.

I guess the thing I fear most is of "losing it" when they tell the family. I will try and focus on Tavia and just let her know I am there for her. The instructors have said its okay to show some emotion, but if I do lose it . . . I will leave the room until I can get myself together. If she asks me, "Am I going to die?" I will answer her honestly . . . I don't know the answer to that. Her primary nurse did tell me that she would be Tavia's nurse again tomorrow . . . so I'll work closely with her too.

Students, who are able to reframe the experience, may perceive the once threatening experience as a challenge. The student may perceive the clinical education experience as a challenge in which mastery and success can occur.

Reflective Journaling

Journaling have long been used by educators as a way to process and assimilate personal experiences into knowledge. In the 1980s, instructors assigned process recordings, which were basically objective logs of the students' activities during the course of a clinical experience. Once written, students were asked to revisit the written logs and interpret the events in a prescriptive way. The directives for this assignment were often self-limiting; consequently, the student fell into the trap of writing for the instructor as opposed to writing for self-understanding.

In the early 1990s, Heinrich (1992) developed a model for a dialogue journal. The concept of this model was to encourage students to "write themselves into understanding" (p. 17). Students are often consumed with the activities within a clinical experience, such as completing procedures, delivering medications, and providing nursing care. Concurrently, the instructor is trying to meet the learning needs of the students and collaborate with the nursing staff. Meaningful dialogue between student and instructor can become almost nonexistent. Post-conferences, a 30 to 45 minute meeting with the nursing students following a clinical practicum, were once thought to be the arena whereby students could process the events of the day.

Ironically, instead of assimilating the experiences, students are often distracted and unable to focus. They can relate a log of their "hands on" experiences and tasks, but they may be unable or reluctant to share the meaningful experiences they have shared with a patient and the family. Possibly, the interaction may have been too personal, and the student hesitates to disclose the experience because of a sense of heightened vulnerability. Inner discomfort may be the result of an unsettling life experience yet, may result in deriving new meaning or knowledge. The right time to process and reflect may occur on the drive home from the experience or late in the night as the student tries to sleep.

Just as nursing students need to reflect, so too do instructors. The instructor may be working with a student and an assigned patient and notice connections between the patient and the student to which the student is oblivious. How many times has an instructor made a mental note to share an observation with a student only to forget about it? The "pearl of wisdom" is lost and the student does not benefit. Unfortunately, instructors may become caught up in praising or criticizing students' performance as they relate to tasks and fail to see the uniqueness of the student.

A reflective dialogue helps both student and instructor to not only process experiences of the day but also to create a unique connection. Both partners in the dialogue assume responsibility for sharing insights, thoughts, and ideas. Students no longer reflect on their day and submit their reflection to their instructor only to have the instructor make comments on the grammar and end the paper with a "Good job!" Instead, students are told to write with abandon and not censor their thoughts. Concurrently, the instructor must be open to the student's thoughts and remain nonjudgmental. Also, the objective is not to use this forum as an evaluative process but rather to facilitate learning.

Students are given some direction regarding completion of this assignment. Journaling is a therapeutic and educational process; therefore, students must complete the writing exercise within 24 hours of the experience. The rationale is that insights and emotions should be put onto paper as soon as possible to enable the student to relive the experience while it is still fresh in her mind. Inner dissonance often triggers meaningful reflection. Once the student begins to establish preconceptions, the risk for misconceptions increases.

Sometimes, the simple process of putting one's thoughts or anxieties onto paper can help the student distance herself from the emotion associated with the experience. Self-discovery occurs by "seeing ourselves and our reactions to life experiences as clearly as possible" (Selling, 1998, p. 13). Anxieties may be expressed and new inquiries may be formulated. Students may be encouraged to "journey back" and revisit the entries at a later date. They may notice that the experience has been reframed and look at the experience from a different perspective. New meaning can be found by looking at an event with a different lens.

Students are advised to find a comfortable, private place to write; write with abandon; not censor thoughts, spell check, or count words. This is probably the one scenario where imperfection in writing is allowed. It is imperative that students find the right time to write. For example, students report being unable to sleep after a meaningful clinical experience and purge themselves of their thoughts through reflective writing. Instructors can share their testimony of electronically receiving their most poignant journals from students during the wee hours of the morning. Electronic journaling may create an ambiance of anonymity. Students may share their innermost thoughts via writing as opposed to delving into their thoughts in a face to face dialogue.

Likewise, instructors are encouraged to respond to the journals in a sensitive and meaningful way. They should mentor the student through the process. For example, if the instructor views a situation differently from the student, it may be best to acknowledge the student's thoughts and then state his opinion. Instructors may initiate a therapeutic use of self approach and further guide the student to make meaning of the experience. There may be some situations where the instructor has made an observation about a connection between student and client and shared this in a dialogue. The fact that an instructor has not only made the observation but shared it with the student may have a significant impact on the student's learning and self-discovery. Criticisms and evaluative comments should be avoided in this dialogue.

One challenge inherent within journaling is that the instructor must wholeheartedly value the process as worthwhile. The instructor makes a commitment to read and respond to the journals in a thoughtful and insightful manner. Some instructors may assign more value to concrete exercises, such as medication profiles, concept maps, or other common clinical assignments. Although the educator will affirm the importance of gaining insight into emotions, and feelings, they may not subscribe to the fact that knowledge can be gleaned from this technique. The question arises: "If the journal is not graded, does it have value?" Students' perceptions may mimic those of the instructor: if there is no grade assigned, it probably is just a waste of time. Unless the instructor fully believes that writing can lead to self-discovery and learning, the exercise is merely a writing exercise without value. See Box 13–2.

Thematic Analysis

One method to use writing as a paradigm to learn is to use the reflective journals longitudinally as a qualitative learning process. Students may be required to write reflective journals over the course of a semester. For example, in one phenomenology of nursing course, students were assigned to observe professional nurses in the role of educator, clinician, counselor, advocate, and coordinator of care. The journals described the insights, experiences, and behaviors they encountered while interacting and collaborating with professional nurses. Upon completion of the fifth journal, the students were instructed to "journey back" through the entries and extrapolate themes or patterns that emerged. For example, the student may find that each nurse exemplified intuitive thinking; thus, intuition was a theme.

After each student reviewed the entries, they were assigned to collaborative groups of three. After discussion, the group members identified two emergent themes. These themes were further explored in the literature in a minimum of five peer reviewed nursing journals or books. Such themes as clinical judgment, critical thinking, the novice nurse, and conflict resolution were a few that emerged. The students prepared an oral presentation to discuss both themes and supporting research. Each group distributed the reference lists to all students electronically.

The presentation captured the student/nurse's lived experience in nursing care of the client/family. This assignment enabled the student to correlate information found in clinical practice with research. This assignment was a graded course requirement. Introspection, self-discovery, and dialogue among peers was established.

Overall, the effectiveness of the use of writing as a method to facilitate learning through self-discovery is well documented in the disciplines of psychology and education (Pennebaker, 1991). Writing techniques specifically linked to learning within the clinical setting have the potential to create connections, facilitate engagement, and create meaning among the nursing student.

Summary

Clinical education has remained relatively constant for many years. The paradigm of the past may no longer prove effective as a result of increasing nursing school enrollments and the skills needed to facilitate critical thinking in students to become reflective practitioners. Clinical education has always held a great potential to threaten students and some students are more prone to threat than others. Nurse educators can use different teaching strategies to create an environment that enhances learning and promotes professional and personal development of the nursing stu-

The following excerpt was written by a senior level nursing student following a clinical experience on pediatrics:

Today I was assigned to take care of a little girl named Tavia. She is no more than 5 years old. I remember looking over her chart last night when I did my research and thinking that there would not be much of a challenge in today's clinical assignment. From what I read, it seems as though she was admitted a few months ago and the doctors thought she had a lactose intolerance. I got to clinical a little early today and looked over her lab results that were not on the chart as of yesterday. Her results puzzled me. Her hemoglobin was really low, but I figured she did not have a diet that was rich in iron . . . so no big deal. As I cared for her throughout the day, I got this gut feeling that something was radically wrong with this picture. Her belly pain was so bad that she limped when she walked. I must say that I was really taken aback by her family. Her mom was not much older than my son and her grandmom is probably in her 40s, which is my age! After I gave her a bath, I decided to recheck her chart. Everyone is anxious, because the surgeon has the results of her biopsy that was taken.

The day got progressively worse! My primary nurse instructed me to "get a room ready" where the family would be told the results. From what she told me, a diagnosis of a fast growing type of cancer had been made and the family was soon to be told. Sue, I can't explain it . . . but I knew deep inside of me that something was radically wrong with her from the moment I started her care. I don't know if it was intuition because I am a mom . . . or maybe problem solving because I am a nurse . . . but I knew it! Maybe it's this thing you call clinical judgment or just plain intuition . . . You know, at first I was upset with myself that I had given into my emotions. Then I looked at you and my primary nurse and saw that you too had filled up with tears, and realized that this too is a part of nursing . . .

Instructor's Reflective Response:

You have offered many insights here, and yes, what you did show was clinical judgment or intuitions . . . both of which are critical as nurses. I too struggled with today's events. In fact, looking back, I saw myself more in the role of Tavia's nurse than in the role of the instructor. It's amazing, but I used to work in a pediatric oncology unit as a young nurse. Although the care of the patient has significantly changed over the years, what I have really noticed in myself are new insights. I always reached out to parents and their children before . . . but I wasn't a mother then. Now when a child is diagnosed with something deadly, I perceive things from a parent's point of view as well as a nurse . . . which can complicate things! The only thing that kept flashing through my mind was that every child I ever cared for with this diagnosis died. You did a great job today . . . your empathy and caring was instrumental in helping these parents cope. They will grieve the diagnosis but focus on their new challenges in their parenting role. I will keep you posted on her condition.

The dialogue between the instructor continued over the next few weeks. The discussions vacillated between concern and hope for Tavia's future. It was also an effective medium for support when the child succumbed to the disease.

dent. Some of those strategies include using technologically enhanced discussions, participating in grand rounds, and employing expert clinicians as preceptors on the clinical unit. A preventive paradigm shift is needed in clinical education rather than intervening when the student is in crisis. Perceived threat and performance anxiety can be circumvented through expressive writing that is tailored to increase connection and facilitate a positive learning experience for nursing students in any clinical area.

Beal, J. A. (1988). New directions for stress research with students. *Nurse Educator, 13*(2), 12–13.

Biggers, T., Zimmerman, R. S., & Alpert, G. (1988). Nursing, nursing education, and anxiety. *Journal of Nursing Education, 27,* 411–417.

Eckstein, D. (1997). Reframing as a specific interpretive counseling technique. *Individual Psychology, 53,* 418–428.

Godbey, K. L., & Courage, M. M. (1994). Stress management program: intervention in nursing student performance anxiety. *Archives of Psychiatric Nursing, 8,* 190–199.

Heinrich, K. T. (1992). Intimate dialogue: Journal writing by students. *Nurse Educator, 17*(6), 17–21.

Kleehammer, K., Hart, L., & Keck, J. F. (1990*).* Nursing students' perceptions of anxiety-producing situations in the clinical setting. *Journal of Nursing Education, 29*(4), 183–187.

Lazarus, R. S. (1991). *Emotion and adaptation.* New York: Oxford University Press.

Lazarus, R. S. (1999). *Stress and emotion: A new synthesis.* New York: Oxford University Press.

Meisenhelder, J. B. (1987). Anxiety: A block to clinical learning. *Nurse Educator, 12*(6), 27–31.

Neuman, B. (1990). Health as a continuum based on the Neuman systems model. *Nursing Science Quarterly, 3,* 129–135.

Neuman, B. (1995). *The Neuman systems model* (3rd ed.). East Norwalk, CT: Appleton & Lange.

Pennebaker, J. W. (1997). Writing about emotional experiences as a therapeutic process. *American Psychology Society, 8,* 162–166.

Russler, M. F. (1991). Multidimensional stress management in nursing education. *Journal of Nursing Education, 30,* 341–346.

Scholtz. S. (2000). Threat: Concept analysis. *Nursing Forum, 35,* 23–29.

Selling, B. (1998). *Writing from within: A guide to creativity and life story writing* (3rd ed.). Alameda, CA: Huner House.

Williams, R. P. (1993). The concerns of beginning nursing students. *Nursing and Health Care, 14,* 178–184.

REVIEW QUESTIONS

- What elements of clinical education are common threats to nursing students?
- What are the characteristics of a nursing student who may become intimidated by clinical education?
- How does Neuman's theory of prevention as intervention relate to minimizing stressors inherent within clinical education?
- How does expressive writing help to decrease apperception of threat in the nursing student before clinical education?
- Explain Scholtz's theory of reframing threat apperception and its relation to the student's ability to achieve positive learning outcomes related to clinical education.

CRITICAL THINKING EXERCISES

Interview a nursing student immediately before the initial experience in a clinical setting. Identify themes of challenges and threats identified by the student before the clinical experience.

Design an expressive writing exercise to be completed the day before an initial clinical education experience. Examine the proactive strategies the student identifies to minimize the threats.

Kuiper, R. (2005). Self-regulated learning during a clinical preceptorship: The reflections of senior baccalaureate nursing students. *Nursing Education Perspectives, Nov-Dec 26*(6); 1–6.

The researchers studied senior students who were being precepted in the clinical area. Reflection was done by speaking into audio tapes. The analysis of the tapes showed it a useful technique for self-regulating learning strategies and environmental structuring for metacognitive activities in the clinical area.

Plack, M. M., Driscoll, M., Blissett, S., McKenna, R., & Plack, T. P. (2005). A method for assessing reflective journal writing. *Journal of Allied Health, 34*(4), 199–208.

The researchers studied the extent reflection was evident in journal writing of students (N = 27). Forty-three journals were assessed and coded for nine elements of reflection. Interrater reliability was assessed using intraclass correlation coefficients. Analysis showed that 14.7% of the journals were assessed as showing no evidence of reflection, 43.4% as showing evidence of reflection, and 41.9% as showing evidence of critical reflection; the percent agreement between rater pairs for the overall assessment of the journals ranged from 67.4% to 85.7%. The tool or coding developed is promising for assessing written reflection.

Chapter Outline

ROLE TRANSITION: USING PARTNERSHIPS AND COGNITIVE APPRENTICESHIP TO BECOME A NURSE EDUCATOR

14

Judy Murphy

Learning Outcomes

On completion of this chapter, the reader will be able to:

• Describe methods to ease transition from nurse clinician to nurse educator.
• Distinguish literature and theory related to developing expertise.
• Identify how cognitive apprenticeship and partnerships can help facilitate role transition.
• Relate how clinical expertise can facilitate role transition.
• Analyze differences between preceptors, mentors, and partners.
• Discriminate between outcome-oriented, professional growth–oriented, and relationship-oriented partnerships.
• Summarize the process of developing competence as a nurse educator.

Key Terms

Cognitive apprenticeship
Competence
Mentor
Novice educator
Partnership
Preceptor
Reflection

This is an exciting, albeit challenging, time to become a nurse educator. It is challenging because health care is in crisis with the acute shortage of nurses. This shortage is compounded by the nurse faculty shortage that is projected to increase over the next decade (Rosseter, 2004). Many bright individuals who are interested in nursing as a career are being turned away because of an insufficient number of nursing faculty members. It is exciting because much is being discovered about brain physiology and its effect on learning; evidence-based teaching methods are the expectation, and the technology explosion has hit the classroom. Nurse educators today need expertise in pedagogy and nursing in order to effectively instruct the next generation of nurses.

The purpose of this chapter is to provide information and suggestions to ease the transition from nurse clinician to nurse educator, with a focus on developing expertise and achieving **competence.** The transition to nurse educator and leader in the profession can be facilitated by developing **partnerships** with colleagues, peers, and **mentors** in nursing education. "Partnerships are mutually beneficial, professional relationships between and among nurses" (Heinrich et al., 2005, p. 34). Developing expertise as an educator, transitioning from clinician to educator, and developing competence will be discussed using **cognitive apprenticeship.** Cognitive apprenticeship is a framework in which teaching is aimed at conveying the thinking process that experts use to handle complex tasks (Collins, Brown, & Newman, 1989). Learning to become a nurse educator involves being able to break down complex tasks into sequential steps to be explained or demonstrated to nursing students. The nurse educator also role models critical thinking and asks questions that promote critical thinking of nursing students. Cognitive apprenticeship, which refers to "the focus of learning through guided experience on cognitive and metacognitive processes" (Collins et al., 1989, p. 457), will help nurse educator students to master these teaching skills.

Although nursing education in the past focused on performing tasks and psychomotor skills development, nursing today requires critical thinking, reasoning, and judgment that must be developed as part of nurses' basic education. Teaching students how to learn, not just what to learn, is essential in this age of accelerated change and innovation (Murphy, 2005). Nurse educators must be experts at teaching and learning, as well as at nursing. Cognitive apprenticeship—which is found in literature on adult education, developing expertise, and teaching mathematical reasoning processes—can help. Linking cognitive apprenticeships and partnerships optimizes learning and professional socialization in that graduate students in nursing education will learn to share their gifts and talents with colleagues and foster a pass-it-on mentality. This offers a solution to the crisis of an insufficient supply of nurse educators. Using both the partnership perspective of fostering mutually beneficial relationships and the cognitive apprenticeship perspective of developing expertise will facilitate the transition from clinician to educator. Graduate education is a challenging but transformative experience, one that can be facilitated by supportive relationships. Caring for oneself is essential to being able to role model caring for others in the nurse educator role. Successful partnerships provide the care for self that is essential in nursing education.

Novice to Competent to Expert: A Progression

Novice nurses struggle when they first perform a physical assessment on a patient. Reading about the sequencing of skills and actually performing them is not the same. Although the novice nurse may have used the framework of head-to-toe assessment to guide performance, ease and fluidity are absent. According to the works of Benner (1984) and Dreyfus and Dreyfus (1986), the beginning nurse is a novice. For the novice, information is processed according to context-free rules and skills are performed according to a precise sequential process where modifications are unlikely. Benner, Dreyfus, and others (Ericsson & Smith, 1991; Itano, 1989) who have studied the novice-expert continuum in learning, report that skill acquisition is situational and dependent upon experience.

Like the novice nurse, the new nurse educator is a novice in this new role. Although the beginning nurse educator has content knowledge of nursing, her pedagogical knowledge and application is lacking. A novice nurse educator will need some help and support with setting priorities. By the end of a graduate education program, the former novice should be a competent nurse educator. Although proficiency and full expertise is generally not mastered until 10 years of job experience, competency takes 2 to 3 years to develop. Achieving competency results in the ability to analyze a situation and cope with problems abstractly. Expertise develops over time as the educator takes rule-based strategies and modifies or adapts them to fit in a variety of situations.

When considering the work on novice-expert progression, and developing expertise, experience is critical. Although many adult learning theorists believe that the learner's experience provides a rich resource for learning (Caffarella & Barnett, 1994; Dewey, 1938; Kolb, 1984; Mezirow, 1995), not all practical experience leads to learning (Brehmer, 1980). Unless the learner connects new experience to earlier knowledge, the learner misses an opportunity for learning (Dewey, 1938; Schon, 1991; Sheckley, 1997). It is generally understood that **reflection** on an experience—noting similarities that substantiate current understanding of the concept, and differences that enhance one's understanding—will provide a broad knowledge base. From a learning perspective, more experiences will lead to the development of a prototype in which the most common elements seen in practice form the basis for an expectation of the usual course associated with that practice. Over time, however, the expert comes to recognize that the unusual may occur. The unusual events (considered outliers in a normal curve) broaden one's understanding of a concept (Medin & Ross, 1989; Sternberg & Horvath, 1995). For example, even though most students respond well to constructive feedback, sometimes a student will respond defensively. Predicting which students will become defensive and intervening before the situation escalates is a skill that the expert nurse educator will possess.

Graduate education shows us that although gaining competence takes time and experience; experiences upon which students do not reflect may not lead to learning. So how does one smoothly move down the path from novice nurse educator to expert educator? Partnerships and cognitive apprenticeship can help move novices along their career path. Box 14–1 shows the expectations of the preceptee functioning in the role of learner.

Achieving Competence

According to Kelly (2002), "Competence is the possession of knowledge, attitudes and skills necessary to meet a certain standard of practice" (p. 27). Benner (1984) identified "competent" as one of the stages in her novice-expert model of developing expertise. In stage three, the competent nurse begins to see "his or her own actions in terms of long-range goals or plans of which he or she is consciously aware" (Benner 1984, pp. 25–26). For the competent nurse, a plan establishes a perspective or prioritization of importance of aspects of a situation. The plan is based on considerable conscious, abstract, analytic contemplation of the problem. A competent nurse educator will most likely be able to: (1) plan clinical or classroom experiences based on identified objectives; (2) anticipate student problems or concerns; and (3) be prepared to circumvent or resolve issues as they arise. For example, matching patient assignments to students' readiness and skill can be challenging even for the expert educator but supporting students by anticipating anxieties and providing resources helps to optimize the experience for both student and patient. The

The preceptee is expected to perform in the role of learner, participant observer, student-educator, and budding scholar.
Responsibilities include:

- Determining learning goals for the experience.
- Collaboratively planing assignments, activities, timelines, and projects with preceptor to meet learning objectives.
- Seeking supervision and guidance from preceptor on an ongoing basis.
- Regularly scheduling evaluative meeting with preceptor to analyze learning activities and objectives.
- Maintaining a journal of practicum experience articulating reflections on experience and connecting reflections to required readings.
- Prioritizing specific learning to meet individual needs.
- Informing the preceptor and faculty advisor *immediately* of any problems/concerns arising during placement.
- Notifying agency and preceptor in a professional and timely manner if unable to meet commitments.
- Performing within the administrative guidelines of the affiliating agency.
- Completing a self-evaluation of performance according to learning objectives and preceptor expectations within academic program guidelines.

competent educator is able to anticipate problems and seize the teachable moment to make the most of the experience.

Developing Competence in Students

Developing competence in students is analogous to developing competence as a nurse educator. Nourish students' efforts and practice, and expect success. Research (Wlodkowski & Ginsberg, 1995) has shown that expectation leads to the reality in practice and apprenticeships. Development of competence will be enhanced if students and their **preceptors,** teachers, and partners expect them to succeed. Developing competence can be achieved best through guided practice. In essence, the need for feedback and guided practice early in the program in nursing education depicts the role modeling, coaching, and scaffolding of cognitive apprenticeship. In the beginning, reliance on others for coaching may be necessary, but as students become more proficient, they increase their self-efficacy and self-regulation of learning (Glaser, 1996; Wlodkowski & Ginsberg, 1995). Balance independence in learning with a commitment to being helped and helping others.

Developing Competence in Nurse Educators

Competence as a nurse educator cannot be achieved without practical experience. Literature on developing competence and, ultimately, expertise (Chi, Glaser, & Farr, 1988; Ericsson, 1996; Ericsson, Krampe, & Tesch-Romer, 1993) indicates that reflective practice and a variety of experiences promote the development of expertise. A variety of experiences means working with more than one preceptor, in more than one setting to broaden one's perspective on nursing education. Settings include clinical, laboratory, and class. Students in graduate programs should participate in opportunities in which they work with several preceptors over the course of the program of study. Student educators can maximize their learning opportunities by being open to the lessons offered by each individual helping to shape their future practice. Expectation of success and multiple experiences are two key concepts that will enhance the development of competence as a nurse educator.

Transition from Clinician to Educator

How does one transition from being a good nurse clinician to being a competent nurse educator? Qualities that draw one into nursing are also essential to nursing education. The term nursing, which comes from the Latin term *nutricus*, means to nourish. Just as nurses nourish, support, and care for their patients, nurse educators nourish, support, and care for their students. Educators serve as role models of caring in our interactions with both students and patients. Caring can be role modeled and shared by setting up partnerships for the purpose of promoting nursing education. Partnering with peers and faculty on this journey transitioning from clinician to educator can lay the foundation for success. Other qualities that are similar to both educators and clinicians are listed in Box 14–2.

What Clinicians Bring to the Educator's Table

Considering the knowledge that a clinician has within the three domains of learning will help **novice educators** appreciate the skills clinicians bring to the profession. According to Bloom, Hastings, and Madeus (1971), the three domains of learning include: cognitive-knowledge, affective-feelings or attitude, and psychomotor-physical skills. Learning in the cognitive domain occurs when there is a change in knowledge and intellectual skill development. The intellectual skill development encompasses Bloom's taxonomy of increasing levels of intellectual skill including: knowledge, comprehension, application, analysis, synthesis, and evaluation. Learning in the affective domain occurs when there is a change in attitude or feelings; the recipient receives the phenomena, responds to the phenomena, values, organizes, and internalizes values, thus changing attitude. Learning in the psychomotor domain includes stages from perception of sensory cues of activity to be learned, through origination, in which the learner is able to create new patterns in response to different situations for the activity.

Previous learning related to nursing practice in these three domains will facilitate the transition from practitioner to educator in the following ways. Clinicians have a solid knowledge base

Box 14–2 Qualities Similar to Both Educators and Clinicians

- Quality assurance
- Accountability
- Dedication
- Good interpersonal skills
- Professional affinity
- Accountability for practice
- Bound by professional regulations
- Adherence to safety
- Quality care
- Good interpersonal skills
- People professions
- Desire to help others should be core principle

and a variety of experiences that give them a broader picture of a concept than that described in a nursing text. The novice educator brings this clinical knowledge to the educational setting. Telling narrative accounts of experiences is a particularly helpful teaching strategy (Lovin, 1992; Mattingly, 1991; Sparks-Langer & Colton, 1991). Narratives provide a forum for learning in both the cognitive and affective domains as the narrator describes an experience, dilemma, feelings, values, and attitudes. The description of the patient, assessment findings, and pathophysiology provide the cognitive learning whereas articulation of feelings and/or attitudes experienced by the nurse provides for learning in the affective domain. Equally important, educators can use their narratives to develop case studies or problem-based learning assignments to promote active learning for their students.

Moreover, clinicians' experience performing actual nursing skills is essential for teaching the foundations of nursing practice. Most nurses have learned a few helpful strategies not found in the nursing literature. It is only through hands-on practice that one truly learns the psychomotor skills necessary in nursing. Simple tricks like stretching a transparent occlusive dressing to break the adhesive fibers to ease removal of the dressing can only be learned by doing. In other words, reading the performance steps in a procedure manual or text involves the ability to perceive the information, but the actual mechanism of the action and complex overt response, also known as skillful performance, does not occur until one has carried out the procedure enough times for the skill to be achieved.

Although clinical experience will help facilitate the transition from clinician to educator, experience alone does not ensure learning (Brehmer, 1980; Sheckley & Keeton, 1997). A critical analysis of one's experience is essential before passing one's tips along to students. Critical analysis includes reflecting on one's experience and noting where and when the lived experience matches the theoretical, research findings. Nurse educators must be aware of the need to teach evidence-based practice. Learn to ask questions such as, Why does this work? Is this more effective than what's currently in print? If so, why is it more effective?

Recognizing and using clinical talents in the educational setting is accomplished best in a supportive environment. Setting up partnerships, whether they are peer partners, preceptor-student partners, or teacher-student partnerships, can facilitate role transition from clinician to nurse educator.

Cognitive Apprenticeship and Partnerships Ease Transition from Novice to Expert, Clinician to Educator

In academia, we have been socialized under a hierarchical structure using the work of cognitive developmental theorists like Perry (1981) and King and Kitchener (1994) who describe a linear or categorical model of development as individuals progress from one level of thinking to the next. The concept of connected relationships is linked to Riane Eisler's (1987) work on partnerships, in which she first described the "partnership way." In her work, she envisioned a society where mutual respect and trust, a low degree of fear and social violence, and an equal valuing of men and women are the norm. "The partnership way" offers a power-with rather than a power-over relationship between teachers and students, among peers and colleagues. Kathleen Heinrich and others (Heinrich et al., 2005) described how nursing education can be transformed through partnerships. A "How can I help you? How can you help me?" way of thinking can benefit both partners while promoting scholarship for both students and faculty. Rather than going it alone, graduate nursing students should develop partnerships with peers and teachers as they seek to advance in their nursing career. Sharing one's gifts and talents with others provides an opportunity for both individuals to grow. Several nurse educators (Heinrich & Scherr, 1994; Jacobi, 1991; Krawczyk, 1978; Paterson, 1998) have recognized the power of partnerships and peer-mentoring activities not just as a strategy for learning but also as a way to invigorate the profession and "promote reciprocal learning" (Eisen, 2001, p. 30) between professionals.

Setting Up a Partnership/Apprenticeship

So how does one go about setting up a partnership and a cognitive apprenticeship? Critical aspects of setting up a successful partnership/apprenticeship include trust and mutual respect. Learners must trust that their role model (preceptor) is proficient in skill and in ability to impart knowledge. Expert educators/preceptors must trust that their apprentice is willing to work with them and learn from them while providing a safe environment. A safe environment will be provided by the preceptor who does not expect the student educator to supervise or evaluate nursing students in an unfamiliar setting or situation. For example, a student educator should not be expected to be solely responsible for providing feedback to nursing students who have been known to be defensive when given constructive criticism. Mutual respect is essential in that both the partnership preceptor/role model and student educator should respect that each has gifts and talents that they bring to the partnership. Learning is not a one way street. Instructors can always learn from students whether they be nursing students or student educators.

Setting up a contract in advance where preceptor roles and student roles are well defined will help to ensure that both parties are cognizant of the expectations and will foster a climate of trust (see Box 14–3). A mechanism should be in place for renegotiating terms of the contract as changes in learner needs and preceptor abilities arise.

Box 14–3 Contract for Preceptor

The preceptor is expected to perform in the role of coach, facilitator, teacher, resource person, and evaluator. Responsibilities include:

Meeting with the preceptee before the preceptorship to review objectives and planned activities and reevaluate as needed.

Serving as role model, supervisor, and clinical expert of the preceptee.

Collaboratively planning assignments, activities, timelines, and projects with preceptee to meet learning objectives.

Providing scaffolded support by promoting increased independence and self-direction on the part of the preceptee in relation to meeting learning objectives.

Sharing stories of personal experience and knowledge with preceptee.

Providing a variety of opportunities for the preceptee to experience the real-life lived experience of a nursing educator.

Providing constructive feedback to the preceptee about their progress and performance.

Informing the faculty advisor *immediately* of any problems/concerns arising during placement.

Evaluating preceptee performance and progress toward meeting learning objectives.

Participating in joint conferences between preceptee and faculty advisor as scheduled.

It is essential that both apprentice and expert have mutual goals for the experience and a willingness to work together to achieve those goals. Setting the stage with a "How can I help you? How can you help me?" expectation will provide an opportunity for both preceptor and apprentice to gain from the experience. For example, one graduate student worked with a diabetic nurse clinician who was responsible for educating and evaluating pregnant women with diabetes. This student designed her learning experience in such a way that she not only learned from her preceptor but also shared her knowledge with the preceptor, and gave something back to the affiliating facility. The student, experienced in literacy and patient education, redesigned a patient diabetic education pamphlet to be more visually appealing and linguistically easier for all patients to read. In this way, both preceptor and student benefited from the experience.

If at all possible, apprentices should select their mentor/preceptor. If a student educator is assigned to a preceptor that she does not know, there exists the potential for a lack of congruence on goals/expectations or interaction style.

Preceptors, Mentors, and Partners

Preceptors, mentors, and partners all differ but each serves a positive role in easing the transition from clinician to educator. A preceptor is a specialized tutor who gives practical training to the student. Use of preceptors to coach, role model, and evaluate in nursing education is becoming increasingly common. Preceptors are used on both the graduate and the undergraduate levels. In addition, they have become popular in the practice setting where hospital nursing education departments have been pared down because of a lack of resources. The roles that a preceptor might be expected to assume include teacher, coach, facilitator, resource person, and evaluator. Preceptors ease the transition from clinician to educator by providing one-on-one instruction. In this environment, the learner is able to ask questions of his preceptor without the distraction of other student educators. Preceptors provide the real-life experience of what it is like to be a nurse educator and how to deal with a variety of issues or problems that may arise. For example, in one preceptor-student educator dyad, the student educator described how much she learned from this one-on-one experience. She not only learned by watching the preceptor teach in a variety of environments; she also gained confidence through the positive comments, coaching, and opportunities for experience offered by her preceptor.

A mentor differs from a preceptor in that a mentor relationship may be more informal than a preceptorship and usually is in place for a longer period of time. Vance (1982) defines a mentor as "someone who serves as a career role model and who actively advises, guides, and promotes another's career and training." Partnerships differ from mentor relationships in that partnerships are mutually beneficial to both partners. Although preceptoring and mentoring are usually confined to career development, partnerships can be beneficial in both professional and personal domains. Partnerships can be short-term, outcome-oriented, or long-term, such as professional growth–oriented and relationship-oriented partnerships (Heinrich et al., 2005). Outcome-oriented partnerships are those that focus on a specific, predetermined outcome; they have a finite ending or goal that defines and limits the terms of the partnership. One example of an outcome-oriented partnership is working with a colleague to develop a presentation. Partnerships can be more open-ended, such as those formed in professional growth–oriented partnerships and in relationship-oriented partnerships. Professional growth–oriented partnerships are evolving and ongoing in nature and include activities that foster personal professional growth. These partnerships might include activities such as designing innovative clinical education strategies, expanding the role of academic advisor, enhancing skills and knowledge surrounding learning styles, and working effectively with students with diverse abilities. Relationship-oriented partnerships develop and exist for the sole purpose of building camaraderie. These types of partnership activities might include interdisciplinary partnerships with other faculty, networking with clinical/community partners, and building friendships and support systems. Partnerships ease the transition from clinician to educator mainly by providing support and expertise to the novice educator.

Finding a Preceptor

Often, the student's advisor or professor may make suggestions based on connections with affiliating agencies. Choosing a preceptor solely based on proximity or ease of formulating a contract with the individual is not the best strategy. Graduate students should be advised to get to know leaders in their area of interest and make connections before the start of their practicum experience. As much as it is important that the preceptor have the expertise and agree to precept the student, equally important are relational qualities and personal affiliation. Preceptors and graduate students should be able to work collaboratively in the experience. Communication should be facile and collegial. Defining roles and responsibilities in advance can help to set forth and maintain boundaries and expectations and thus alleviate stress.

Getting the Most From a Preceptorship

Students should enter the experience with an open mind and a willingness to learn from the expert. Be prepared with questions concerning boundaries and expectations for working with the preceptor's patient population or student group. Develop a good rapport with the preceptor so any problems, questions, or issues can be addressed as they arise. Respect limits delineated by preceptors, such as the amount or type of feedback you will be allowed to give the nursing students. For example, does the preceptor want the student educator to evaluate a nursing student's performance? If so, under what circumstances would you use which evaluative tool or model? In what situations should the student educator avoid giving feedback? The preceptor-student educator relationship is complex in that the preceptor is serving in a dual role: that of teaching both nursing students and a student educator simultaneously. The student educator is in a dual role: that of both teacher and student. Recognizing the complexity of the situation will help the student educator to respect role boundaries. In addition, student educators and preceptors need to build planning and evaluation time into the practicum. Planning will include activities such as developing objectives for the experience, timelines, and a workable schedule. Evaluation should be ongoing throughout the practicum and should include both preceptor evaluation of the student educator performance and both parties' evaluation of their relationship. Offering to help the preceptor can set the stage for a more fulfilling preceptorship for both parties. What started out as a preceptor-graduate student relationship may evolve into a partnership in which both parties learn and receive satisfaction.

From Preceptor to Mentor

A preceptor-graduate student relationship usually is intended for a predetermined length of time, with set objectives for the relationship and with expected roles for the relationship. Although a preceptor model may be one used in academia to provide one-on-one learning opportunities for the novice, it does not necessarily foster long-term relationships. On the other hand, Vance and Olson (1998) have done extensive research on mentor relationships in nursing and found that mentored nurses are more likely to become leaders in their profession. Furthermore, 83% of influential nurses reported having one or more mentors. With the "graying" of nursing faculty, the future of nursing is at stake. We need to recognize that the way to entice more nurses to become educators is by nurturing, supporting, and encouraging their pursuit of graduate education. What better way to do this than by participating in a mentoring relationship? Specific help provided by mentors included career advice, guidance, promotion, professional role modeling, intellectual and scholarly stimulation, inspiration, idealism, teaching, advising, tutoring, and emotional support.

Graduate nursing students should be on the lookout for a good mentor to support further career development. The prospective mentor may be a preceptor, an educator, or a peer.

Mentors to Partners

In today's literature, we find that a mentoring relationship can be more of a partnership in which participants help and are helped by one another (Heinrich, Cote et al., 2003; Vance & Olson, 1998). This type of relationship has long-term benefits both for the individuals involved and the profession as a whole. You may ask, "Can every preceptor be a mentor/partner?" The answer is maybe, maybe not; much depends on the shared commitment and affinity that both partners have for a mutually beneficial relationship.

When mutual benefits are present in a mentorship (Vance & Olson, 1998), "[m]entoring assumes caring; a connecting with one another. Connections of caring are sources of power and influence for both mentor/leader and protégé/rising star" (pp. 30–31). One can see that both partners benefit from sharing one another's perspective and expertise. It is time that nurse-educators stop trying to go it alone in nursing and reach out to others, to share gifts, talents, and insights. A partnership relationship in which both participants reap the rewards from working with one another can help nurses individually and collectively be more satisfied in their professional and personal life (Eisen, 2001; Heinrich et al., 2005; Heinrich, Cote et al., 2003; Heinrich & Scherr, 1994). Mentoring partnerships created for the purpose of professional growth can help not only to ease the transition from clinician to educator, but also to achieve competence for the new nurse educator.

Cognitive Apprenticeship Specifically

Learning from an expert can best be accomplished by working closely, apprenticing, with the expert. Future nurse educators are not just apprenticing in the skill of teaching, they are also learning the thinking, reasoning, and critical thinking necessary. Cognitive apprenticeship provides a framework from which to plan teaching-learning experiences. Cognitive apprenticeship is a framework (Box 14–4) in which learning is depicted as a social process occurring within communities of practice (Lave & Wenger, 1991). Participation begins in the periphery of the occupation being learned, and through novice-expert relations, the learner becomes increasingly more involved in complex, higher-order issues. "Cognitive apprenticeship derives its power from knowledgeable, proficient people showing learners how to do something and stating aloud what they are thinking while doing the activity" (Brandt, Farmer, & Buckmaster, 1993, p. 75). In the cognitive apprenticeship process, learners work with a master (expert) who teaches by the methodologies listed in Box 14–5.

Preceptors and Cognitive Apprenticeship

The cognitive apprenticeship framework described earlier can be used by preceptors, mentors and, in some cases, partners. Cognitive apprenticeship has been shown to facilitate learning from expe-

Box 14–4 Cognitive Apprenticeship Strategies

Preceptor/expert strategies	Learner/novice activities
Role modeling	Reflection
Coaching	Articulation (journal writing, discussion)
Scaffolding support	Experience/practice

Box 14–5

275

Setting Up a Partnership/Apprenticeship

An expert is a teacher who exemplifies the following methodologies (with examples).

- Role models the behavior/skill: when a preceptor demonstrates how to coach and support a student nurse through giving his first injection.
- Coaches apprentices (novice educators) as they practice: when the preceptor coaches the nurse educator in correcting and providing feedback on student nurse concept maps or care plans.
- Provides scaffolded support: when initially the preceptor gives the student educator much feedback and encouragement on running a post-conference, but over time reduces the amount of feedback given.
- Encourages reflection: when the preceptor tells the student educator to think back on her practice session and analyze positive and negative events from the session.
- Encourages articulation: when the preceptor tells the student educator to discuss her analyses of her practice either in written form or in a dialogue.
- Provides opportunities for experimentation: when the preceptor gives the student educator a chance to teach in clinical, class, and laboratory settings.

rience. A preceptor or mentor can use cognitive apprenticeship strategies. Strategies, such as modeling, coaching, scaffolding support, promoting reflection, promoting articulation, and providing a variety of experiences, can help teach future nurse educators. Consider how cognitive apprenticeship can be used in graduate education within the preceptorship experience.

Preceptors, those specialized tutors who give practical training to student educators, are an integral part of graduate education. Both the preceptor and learner have a role in the apprenticeship process. The preceptor serves as a *role model* for the student educator in that he has expertise in the field. Preceptors model their expertise when they help the student educator develop a teaching-learning plan that includes learning objectives, time frames, and learning activities. During the course of the preceptor-student relationship, the preceptor will share stories from her practice that exemplify practical knowledge, as well as values and attitudes essential in nursing education. Preceptors will *coach* their student educators as they take on more responsibility for teaching. In the coaching role, the preceptor provides encouragement and support as the student tests the waters of being a nurse educator. The preceptor encourages the student to be as self-directed as possible in taking on the role of nurse educator. Learning is an active process that involves individual construction of knowledge based on one's earlier experience. Coaching and providing *scaffolded support* are key strategies where the amount and intensity of support is gradually diminished as the student takes on more responsibility and accountability. Although the preceptor's presence is felt, reliance on the preceptor's knowledge and experience decreases over time. The preceptor should be available to answer questions as needed, but must recognize the value in self-directed learning and push the student to become more independent in her learning over time. Student educators should be encouraged to seek new ways of looking at experiences, ever questioning, reflecting on experience, and refining knowledge construction. Coaching and scaffolding provide the challenge and support necessary for students to consider their practice and evaluate their performance continuously as they transition from practitioner to educator.

Reflection, articulation, and experience are strategies that the graduate student should use in the teaching-learning process. The graduate student should analyze and determine goals for the preceptored experience. Students should be encouraged to *reflect* on their *experience* in order to optimize learning. Reflection-in-action entails thinking during practice, and reflection-on-action (Schon, 1991) involves thinking back on the practice session and analyzing decisions/events that occurred. Both enhance learning and aid in the process of evaluation. While graduate students are being precepted, they should write a journal for each day of their experience; they should write about the experience and connect what they have seen or done during their practicum with literature that they are reading for the course.

Students are encouraged to question any problems/concerns they encounter during their precepted experience. They can *articulate* this reflection either in writing or through discourse. Much research supports the importance of thinking about one's thinking and responses in a situation to maximize learning from experience (Mattingly, 1991; Schon, 1991; Sheckley, 1997). Reflection on experience and articulation of an experience promote critical analysis and expand learning opportunities. For example, when a student educator reflects on a nursing student performing an injection for the first time and describes the performance in her journal, she realizes that only one domain of learning should be focused on at a time in order to optimize skill development. The student educator who does not reflect and articulate theory to practice connections, in this instance, domains of learning, would not make this connection. Consequences of a lack of reflection and critical analysis are that the future educator may ask cognitive questions while a nursing student is performing a psychomotor skill, thus interfering with skill development. Graduate student responsibilities therefore include elaborating and prioritizing specific learning to meet needs, meeting with the preceptor to develop a tentative schedule of activities to meet learning objectives, and seeking feedback from the preceptor on an ongoing basis. Discussing and evaluating the boundaries and expectations of the preceptor relationship uses both reflection and articulation to enhance learning from experience.

Summary

Like learning, role transition from nurse to nurse educator can at times be a painful process. This chapter has offered some suggestions to facilitate the transition by developing partnerships and using cognitive apprenticeship as a framework to ease the transition. The cognitive apprenticeship model has been used in studies of developing expertise and learning from experience. It is particularly applicable to professional development as it incorporates reflective strategies that are essential for competent practice. Reflective practice can be enhanced by bouncing ideas off of a partner. A reciprocal learning relationship helps both partners to grow, as ideas, thoughts, and problems are analyzed from multiple perspectives. Going it alone is an antiquated belief that has perpetuated the current faculty shortage. It is time that nurse educators develop a pass-it-on mentality and work together to invite colleagues to join them in educating the next generation of nurses. Working together, learning from one another, and developing power with relationships rather than power over student-teacher relationships will not only ease the transition to nurse educator but will invite others to join the league of nurse educators.

Belenky, M. F., Clinchy, B. M., Goldberger, N. R., & Tarule, J. M. (1986). *Women's ways of knowing.* Cambridge: Basic Books.

Benner, P. (1984). *From novice to expert: Excellence and power in clinical nursing practice.* Menlo Park: Addison Wesley.

Bloom, B. S., Hastings, T. J., & Madeus, G. F. (1971). *Handbook on formative and summative evaluation of student learning.* New York: McGraw-Hill.

Brandt, B. L., Farmer, J. A., & Buckmaster, A. (1993). Cognitive apprenticeship approach to helping adults learn. In D. D. Flannery (Ed.), *Applying cognitive learning theory to adult learning* (pp. 69–78). San Francisco: Jossey-Bass.

Brehmer, B. (1980). In one word: Not from experience. *Acta Psychologica 45,* 223–241.

Caffarella, R. S., & B. G. Barnett. (1994). Characteristics of adult learners and foundations of experiential learning. In L. Jackson & R. S. Caffarella (Eds.), *Experiential learning: A new approach.* San Francisco: Jossey Bass.

Chi, M. T. H., Glaser, R., & Farr, M. J. (1988). *The nature of expertise.* Hillsdale, NJ: Lawrence Erlbaum Associates.

Collins, A., Brown, J. S., & Newman, S. E. (1989). Cognitive apprenticeship: Teaching the crafts of reading, writing, and mathematics. In L. B. Resnick (Ed.), *Knowing, learning, and instruction.* Hillsdale, NJ: Lawrence Erlbaum Associates.

Dewey, J. (1938). *Experience and education.* New York, Collier Books.

Dreyfus, S., & Dreyfus, H. L. (1986). *Mind over machine.* New York: The Free Press.

Eisen, M. J. (2001). Peer-based professional development viewed through the lens of transformative learning. *Holistic Nursing Practice, 16*(1), 30–42.

Eisler, R. (1987). *The chalice and the blade: Our history, our future.* San Francisco: Harper and Row.

Ericsson, K. A. (1996). The acquisition of expert performance: An introduction to some of the issues. In K. A. Ericsson (Ed.), *The road to excellence.* Mahwah, NJ: Lawrence Erlbaum Associates.

Ericsson, K. A., Krampe, R. T., & Tesch-Romer, C. (1993). The role of deliberate practice in the acquisition of expert performance. *Psychological Review, 100*(3), 363–406.

Ericsson, K. A., & Smith, J. (1991). Prospects and limits of the empirical study of expertise: An introduction. In K. A. Ericsson & J. Smith (Eds.), *Toward a general theory of expertise.* New York: Cambridge University Press.

Glaser, R. (1996). Changing the agency for learning: Acquiring expert performance (pp. 303–311). In K. A. Ericsson (Ed.), *The road to excellence.* Mahwah, NJ: Lawrence Erlbaum Associates.

Heinrich, K. T., Cote, J., Solernou, S. B., Roth, K. A., Chiffer, D. K., Bona, G. A., et al. (2003). From partners to passionate scholars: Preparing nurse educators for the new millennium. In K. T. Heinrich & M. H. Oermann (Eds.), *Annual review of nursing education.* New York: Springer.

Heinrich, K. T., Pardue, K. T., Davison-Price, M., Murphy, J. I., Neese, R., Walker, P. & White, K. B. (2005). How can I help you? How can you help me? Transforming nursing education through partnerships. *Nursing Education Perspectives, 26*(1), 34–41.

Heinrich, K. T., & Scherr, M. W. (1994). Peer mentoring for reflective teaching. *Nurse Educator, 19*(4), 36–41.

Itano, J. K. (1989). A comparison of the clinical judgment process in experienced registered nurses and student nurses. *Journal of Nursing Education. 28*(3), 120–125.

Jacobi, M. (1991). Mentoring and undergraduate success: A literature review. *Review of Educational Research, 61*(4), 505–532.

Kelly, C. M. (2002). Investing in the future of nursing education: A cry for action. *Nursing Education Perspectives, 23*(1), 24–28.

King, R., & Kitchner, K. (1994). *Developing reflective judgment.* San Francisco: Jossey Bass.

Kolb, D. A. (1984). *Experiential learning.* Englewood Cliffs, NJ: Prentice Hall.

Krawczyk, R. M. (1978). Peer participatory conferences: A dynamic method of nursing instruction. *Journal of Nursing Education, 17*(8), 5–8.

Lave, J., & Wenger, E. (1991). *Situated learning legitimate peripheral participation.* Cambridge, MA: Cambridge University Press.

Lovin, B. K. (1992). Professional learning through workplace partnerships. *New Directions for Adult and Continuing Education, 55*(Fall), 61–69.

Mattingly, C. (1991). Narrative reflections on practical actions: Two learning experiments in reflective story-telling. In D. A. Schon (Ed.), *The reflective turn case studies in and on educational practice.* New York: Teachers College Press.

Medin, D. L., & Ross, B. H. (1989). The specific character of abstract thought: Categorization, problem solving and induction. In R.J. Sternberg (Ed.), *Advances in the psychology of human intelligence.* Hillsdale, NJ: Lawrence Erlbaum Associates.

Mezirow, J. (1995). Transformation theory of adult learning. In M. R. Welton (Ed.), *In defense of the life-world.* Albany, NY: State University of New York Press.

Murphy, J. I. (2005). How to learn, not what to learn: Three strategies that foster lifelong learning in clinical settings. In K. T. Heinrich & M. H. Oermann. *Annual review of nursing education* (Vol. 3, pp. 37–55). New York: Springer Publishing.

Paterson, B. (1998). Partnership in nursing education: A vision or a fantasy? *Nursing Outlook, 46,* 284–289.

Perry, W. (1981). Cognitive and ethical growth: The making of meaning. In A. Chickering (Ed.), *The modern American college* (pp. 76–116). San Francisco: Jossey-Bass.

Rosseter, R. (2004). Nursing faculty shortage fact sheet. Retrieved August 30, 2005 from American Association of Colleges of Nursing website: **http://www.aacn.nche.edu/Media/Backgrounders/facultyshortage.htm.**

Schon, D. (1991). *The reflective practitioner.* San Francisco: Jossey-Bass.

Sheckley, B. G. (1997). Reflection promotes complex thought. *Community Youth Roles, 4*(1), 4–5.

Sheckley, B. G., & Keeton, M. T. (1997). *Perspectives on key principles of adult learning.* Chicago: The Council for Adult & Experiential Learning.

Sparks-Langer, G. M., & Colton, A. B. (1991). Synthesis of research on teacher's reflective thinking. *Educational Leadership*, (March), 37–44.

Sternberg, R. J., & Horvath, J. A. (1995). A prototype view of expert teaching. *Educational Researcher, 24*(6), 9–17.

Vance, C., & Olson, R. K. (Eds.). (1998). *The mentor connection in nursing.* New York: Springer Publishing.

Vance, C. N. (1982). The mentor connection. *The Journal of Nursing Administration, 12*(4), 7–13.

Wlodkowski, R. J., & M. B. Ginsberg (1995). A framework for culturally responsive teaching. *Educational Leadership,* September, 17–21.

REVIEW QUESTIONS

- Describe the concept of "partnership" and how it is mutually beneficial to novice and expert educators.
- A student argues that the mark given on a care plan is not justified. The student followed the rubric but did not go into depth in the psychosocial area of the client. Describe how a novice educator might be apt to handle the situation and how an expert educator would also handle the situation.
- Integrate some creative teaching methodologies that would help a novice educator gain competence.
- Reflect on some important issues you would address in a contract with the novice educator you are about to begin mentoring.

CRITICAL THINKING EXERCISES

Mary Jane is a new nurse educator. She has just finished teaching medical and surgical asepsis as part of a fundamentals of nursing course. She is expected to submit 15 multiple-choice questions for the unit exam. Although Mary Jane took a course in test construction in graduate school, she is uncertain about having sole responsibility for developing these questions.

Select either cognitive apprenticeship or partnerships and describe how either strategy could be used to help Mary Jane accomplish this task.

Donna has worked in staff development in an acute care setting for a number of years. She has just taken on a new position as a clinical faculty member in a baccalaureate program. Donna is having difficulty with one of her students who has been consistently unprepared for clinical. Although Donna has had a number of conversations with the student, the student does not seem to recognize the gravity of the situation. Donna is used to working with professionals who respond well to constructive criticism by seeking to improve their performance.

Select either cognitive apprenticeship or partnerships and describe how either strategy could be used to help Donna develop and initiate a plan to improve this student's understanding of the situation.

ANNOTATED RESEARCH SUMMARY

Duncan, S. L. S. (1996). Cognitive apprenticeship in classroom instruction: Implications for industrial and technical teacher education. *Journal of Industrial Teacher Education, 33*(3), 66–86.

This study examined the effects of incorporating the instructional methods of cognitive apprenticeship into community college writing classrooms. A nonequivalent control group design was used in which nine volunteer instructors and 159 students participated in this study; both qualitative and quantitative data were collected. Student results on the dependent variable, a standardized writing assessment, were significantly greater for the students who had received role modeling, articulation, or scaffolded support strategies—all cognitive apprenticeship methods.

Cope, P., Cuthbertson, P., & Stoddart, B. (2001). Situated learning in the practice setting. *Journal of Advanced Nursing, 31*(4), 850–856.

This phenomenological study was constructed as an analysis of the experiences of nursing students under two different curriculums. A random sample of 10% of each cohort answered questions in semistructured interviews to compare the lived experiences of these two cohorts of nursing students. This paper reported on the section of the interview that dealt with the practice placement and difficulties with theory and practice. Data were examined for emerging categories. To ensure inter-researcher reliability, each transcript was examined by two people and the emerging categories were confirmed by comparison of findings. One of the main conclusions of this paper is that knowledge via the expert's contribution can be passed on by situating knowledge in authentic contexts and by utilization of cognitive apprenticeship techniques.

Glaser, R. (1996). Changing the agency for learning: Acquiring expert performance. In K. A. Ericsson (Ed.), *The road to excellence* **(pp. 303–311). Mahwah, NJ: Lawrence Erlbaum Associates.**

This chapter found in this book on excellence promotes understanding about how the agency for learning shifts as competence develops. Learners become much more self-regulated in their learning as they progress along the path from novice to expert. In the beginning, they need a great deal of support and guided practice. For the development of expertise, knowledge must be acquired in such a way that it is highly connected and articulated. The learner who apprentices in a complex environment where there are opportunities for problem solving, analogy making, and interpretation of events will acquire the structured knowledge necessary for developing competence.

Ironside, P. M. (2005). Working together, creating excellence: The experiences of nursing teachers, students, and clinicians. *Nursing Education Perspectives, 26*(2), 78–85.

In this exploratory study using hermeneutic methodology, participants were asked to describe excellence in nursing. One of the themes identified from the study data involved working together, creating partnerships among teachers and students. Developing partnerships and working together were paths to excellence that promoted innovation and reform.

Chapter Outline

ACHIEVING EXCELLENCE IN NURSING EDUCATION: THE NATIONAL LEAGUE FOR NURSING PERSPECTIVE

15

Theresa M. Valiga and Mary Anne Rizzolo

Learning Outcomes

On completion of this chapter, the reader will be able to:

- Explore the interrelation among faculty preparation, ongoing faculty development, and innovation, as well as the relevance of these concepts to achieving excellence in nursing education.
- Discuss the concept of excellence as it relates to nursing education.
- Describe how innovation, evidence-based teaching practices, and a science of nursing education can transform nursing education.
- Discuss the Core Competencies of Nurse Educators© as a framework of essential knowledge, skills, and attitudes relevant to the educator role.
- Describe the growing role of technology in the nursing education environment.

Key Terms

Certification
Evidence-based teaching practices
Excellence
Innovation
Science of nursing education

Throughout its more than 100-year history, the National League for Nursing (NLN) has worked to advance **excellence** in nursing education. For many years, the NLN was the only nursing organization that attended to education-related issues, and its initiatives have improved the quality of education designed to prepare tomorrow's nursing workforce and the future leaders of the nursing profession. This work continues into the 21st century, as the National League for Nursing strengthens its position as a leader in nursing education. This chapter will explore the current state of nursing education, along with its continued development and growth in the future.

The Current State of Affairs in Nursing Education

For the past few decades, the broad higher education community has placed great emphasis on research productivity and on securing grants to fund such endeavors. In nursing, our desire to document the uniqueness of nursing and the outcomes of nursing interventions have led to an increased emphasis on developing the science of nursing practice and carving out roles for nurse practitioners, nurse midwives, and nurse anesthetists. As a result of these converging circumstances, concerns about the preparation and ongoing development of faculty have been minimized, reward systems typically have not valued expertise in teaching, and the academy has failed to replace the many faculty members who are retiring.

In addition to these broad issues, faculty members in nursing typically do not encourage undergraduate students to become nurse educators, nor do they help students consider a career path in education. As a result, the profession now faces a significant faculty shortage, one that most recently led to approximately 125,000 qualified applications unable to be accepted for admission to various types of RN programs (NLN, 2004). Moreover, fewer and fewer individuals now fulfilling faculty roles and teaching in nursing programs actually have been prepared for the teaching role. These individuals typically have not studied the research on how students learn. For the most part, they have not been educated regarding curriculum design, curriculum integrity, or program evaluation. And far too many have a limited repertoire regarding innovative teaching/learning strategies and evaluation methods.

Without enough adequately prepared faculty members, the potential for decline in the quality of educational programs is real. And this is happening precisely at a time when the changing student population, the increased use of educational technology, and dramatic changes in the practice of nursing demand new approaches to and the transformation of nursing education.

One of the reasons why today's faculty members need to be prepared for their role relates to the fact that today's students are more diverse and experience very different life circumstances than those we have known in the past. Many students are working while they attend school; many do not have the educational foundations needed to succeed in college; and many have overwhelming family responsibilities that compete with study time. In addition, an increasing number of students are from countries outside of the United States and present faculty with values and cultural practices that are quite different from their own. Faculty, therefore, needs to know how to meet individual learning needs, be more skilled in the ability to advise and counsel students, and design curricula that are more flexible and accommodating.

In addition to the increased diversity in the student population with which faculty interact, today's students have grown up with technology as a natural part of their lives, and technology is becoming an increasingly integral aspect of the educational enterprise—from asynchronous approaches to teaching and learning to collaborative learning strategies; from high-tech simulators to PDAs. All expectations are that technology will become increasingly integral to the learning process, and nursing education must change to accommodate and, indeed, benefit from this.

The health-care arenas in which graduates of today's nursing programs will practice also are very different from those of the past, and the role of the nurse continues to evolve. Practice environments are characterized by uncertainty, ambiguity, chaos, conflicting information, constant change, and challenging ethical dilemmas. Health-care professionals collaborate through interdisciplinary teams to plan and implement care for patients, families, and communities. And increasingly sophisticated technology abounds. Graduates of nursing programs, therefore, need to be prepared to think critically, manage uncertainty and ambiguity, be technologically proficient, work effectively on multidisciplinary teams, be comfortable with complexity and conflict, and be leaders who advocate for change that will benefit the recipients of care. This amounts to a tall task for those educating them to fulfill this demand.

Finally, students, legislators, parents, and communities are demanding greater accountability on the part of institutions of higher education. There is an expectation that outcomes of the educational enterprise will be documented and that schools will be able to demonstrate that the experience has made a difference in how students think, their openness to new perspectives, their abilities to communicate effectively, their self-understanding, their ability to synthesize enormous amounts of potentially conflicting information, and their ability to provide true leadership that leads to change.

All of these differences require that current faculty members *unlearn* how they were taught so they can *re-learn* strategies and approaches that are more relevant for today's learners and today's issues. It means that our old ways of educating nurses are no longer appropriate, and we must give up many of the "sacred cows" that have become entrenched in nursing education.

We must become more innovative, rather than continue the way we have always done it. We must strive to achieve excellence, rather than settle for mediocrity. We must help faculty prepare for and stay current in their role as educators. We must begin to expect that the practice of teaching will be evidence-based.

While this presents an enormous challenge to the nursing education community, it is not an insurmountable one. And there are many initiatives currently underway to facilitate this transformation, to encourage more nurses to go into nursing education, and to help faculty develop in this role.

Transforming Nursing Education

There are a number of initiatives at work to transform nursing education. Underlying all of these initiatives are the themes of promoting excellence and **innovation,** as well as integrating evidence-based nursing education. Using technology to its best advantage is another necessity in transforming nursing education.

Promoting Excellence

The literature suggests that "excellence means striving to be the very best we can be in everything we do—not because some . . . 'authority' figure pushes us to do that, but because we cannot imagine functioning in any other way" (Valiga, 2003, p. 275). It means setting high standards and holding ourselves to those standards despite challenges encountered when striving to reach that level of performance or pressures placed upon us to accept less than the very best. Those who strive for excellence are unwilling to accept the status quo; they ask why things are done the way they are; they examine the assumptions that underlie existing practices; and they are willing to invest enormous amounts of time and energy to design, implement, and evaluate the effectiveness of new approaches.

The National League for Nursing has developed an *Excellence in Nursing Education Model*© (NLN, 2005b) (Fig. 15–1) that depicts the many elements that must be in place if we are to achieve excellence. As noted, excellence in nursing education will be attained if we have clear program standards and hallmarks that raise expectations, well-qualified faculty, administrators who create healthful work environments for faculty, interactive learning, and innovative curricula, among other things. For example, if the standards that guide program development are static and seek only acceptable levels of attainment, it is unlikely that we will achieve excellence. If faculty complements do not include expert teachers and educational "architects" as well as researchers and clinicians, academic programs may become irrelevant and fail to prepare graduates for the health-care arena in which they will practice.

In addition to developing a visual model that depicts the elements needed to achieve excellence in nursing education, the National League for Nursing has formulated *Hallmarks of Excellence in Nursing Education* (NLN, 2005c) that describe targets toward which faculty should strive in order to attain excellence in their programs (see Fig. 15–2). For example, excellence is characterized by students who are excited about learning, exhibit a spirit of inquiry and a sense of wonderment, and commit to lifelong learning. It also is reflected in:

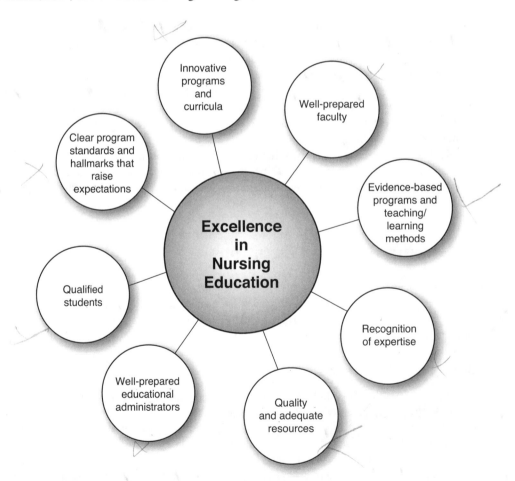

FIGURE 15–1 Excellence in Nursing Education Model.© Copyright, National League for Nursing, 2005. Reproduced with permission of the National League for Nursing.

HALLMARKS OF EXCELLENCE IN NURSING EDUCATION®

STUDENTS
- Students are excited about learning, exhibit a spirit of inquiry and a sense of wonderment, and commit to lifelong learning
- Students are committed to innovation, continuous quality/performance improvement, and excellence
- Students are committed to a career in nursing

FACULTY
- The faculty complement includes a cadre of individuals who have expertise as educators, clinicians, and, as is relevant to the institution's mission, researchers
- The unique contributions of each faculty member in helping the program achieve its goals are valued, rewarded, and recognized
- Faculty members are accountable for promoting excellence and providing leadership in their area(s) of expertise
- Faculty model a commitent to lifelong learning, involvement in professional nursing associations, and nursing as a career
- All faculty have structured preparation for the faculty role, as well as competence in their area(s) of teaching responsibility

CONTINUOUS QUALITY IMPROVEMENT
- The program engages in a variety of activities that promote excellence, including accreditation from national nursing accreditation bodies
- The program design, implementation and evaluation are continuously reviewed and revised to achieve and maintain excellence

CURRICULUM
- The curriculum is flexible and reflects current societal and health care trends and issues, research findings and innovative practices, as well as local and global perspectives
- The curriculum provides experiential cultural learning activities that enhance students' abilities to think critically, reflect thoughtfully, and provide culturally-sensitive, evidence-based nursing care to diverse populations
- The curriculum emphasizes students' values development, socialization to the new role, commitent to lifelong learning, and creativity
- The curriculum provides learning experiences that prepare graduates to assume roles that are essential to quality nursing practice, including but not limited to roles of caregiver, patient advocate, teacher, communicator, knowledge worker, change agent, coordinator, user of information technology, collaborator, and decision maker
- The curriculum provides learning experiences that support evidence-based practice, multidisciplinary approaches to care, student achievement of clinical competence, and, as appropriate, expertise in a specialty role
- The curriculum is evidence-based

TEACHING/LEARNING/EVALUATION STRATEGIES
- Teaching/learning/evaluation strategies are innovative and varied to facilitate and enhance learning by a diverse student population
- Teaching/learning/evaluation strategies promote collegial dialogue and interaction between and among faculty, students, and colleagues in nursing and other professions
- Teaching/learning/evaluation strategies used by faculty are evidence-based

FIGURE 15–2 Hallmarks of Excellence In Nursing Education.® Copyright, National League for Nursing. (2005). Hallmarks of Excellence in Nursing Education. New York: Author. Reproduced with permission of the National League for Nursing. *(continued)*

RESOURCES
- Partnerships in which the program is engaged promote excellence in nursing education, enhance the profession, benefit the community, and expand service/learning opportunities
- Technology is used effectively to support teaching/learning/evaluation processes
- Student support services are culturally-sensitive, innovative, and empower students during the recruitent, retention, progression, graduation, and career planning processes
- Financial resources of the program are used to support curriculum innovation, visionary long-range planning, faculty development, an empowering learning environment, creative initiatives, continuous quality improvement of the program, and evidence-based teaching/ learning/evaluation practices

INNOVATION
- The design and implementation of the program is innovative and seeks to build on traditional approaches to nursing education
- The innovativeness of the program helps to create a preferred future for nursing

EDUCATIONAL RESEARCH
- Faculty and students contribute to the development of the science of nursing education through the critique, utilization, dissemination or conduct of research
- Faculty and students explore the impact of student learning experiences on the health of the communities they serve

ENVIRONMENT
- The educational environment empowers students and faculty and promotes collegial dialogue, innovation, change, creativity, values development, and ethical behavior

LEADERSHIP
- Faculty, students, and alumni are respected as leaders in the parent organization, as well as in local, state, regional, national, or international communities
- Faculty, students, and alumni are prepared for and assume leadership roles that advance quality nursing care; promote positive change, innovation, and excellence; and enhance the power and influence of the nursing profession

---

**National League for Nursing. (2005). *Hallmarks of Excellence in Nursing Education*. New York: Author.

Reproduced with permission of the National League for Nursing.

FIGURE 15 – 2 (continued)

- Curricula that are flexible and dynamic, rather than static and rigid.
- Curricula that emphasize students' values development, as well as gains in their cognitive learning and ability to perform psychomotor skills.
- Environments that empower students and faculty and promote collegial dialogue, innovation, and creativity.

   Nurse educators who strive for excellence are passionate and "inflamed" by their work (Diers & Evans, 1980). They are guided by the *Excellence in Nursing Education Model* and the *Hallmarks of Excellence in Nursing Education* as they design curricula, design appropriate teaching/learning strategies and evaluation methods, engage in **evidence-based teaching practices,** and implement the full scope of the faculty role. In addition, they are open to new ideas and are innovative.

"Innovation [in nursing education] must call into question the nature of schooling, learning, and teaching and how curricular designs promote or inhibit learning, as well as excitement about the profession of nursing, and the spirit of inquiry necessary for the advancement of the discipline" (Diekelmann, 2001). "New pedagogies are required that are research-based, responsive to the rapidly-changing health care system, and reflective of new partnerships between and among students, teachers and clinicians. Our students and recipients of nursing care deserve no less" (NLN, 2003a, p. 1). If nurse educators are to meet this challenge, they must be creative in their approaches to teaching/learning, evaluation of learning, and program design. This is no small challenge for many of today's faculty members, however.

Most of today's faculty members have experienced curricula that are content-laden and highly structured. Their orientation has been on *what* to teach, rather than on *how* to teach, and they focus on covering content more than on the process of learning. Such a model is no longer appropriate to prepare graduates for the chaotic, ambiguous, uncertain world that characterizes 21st century nursing practice, nor is it adequate to prepare graduates who can serve as leaders in helping the profession create its preferred future.

Instead, what is needed are new interactive, student-centered pedagogies, such as narrative pedagogy and collaborative learning, that call upon nurse educators, students, consumers, and nursing service representatives to "form partnerships that will dramatically reform [nursing education] and the relationships between and among students, teachers, researchers and clinicians" (NLN, 2003a). Conversations about innovation must not focus on the content or subject matter to be covered in, added to, or updated in nursing curricula. Rather, nurse educators must reconceptualize our overall approach to and design of nursing education to ensure that it focuses on learning, is student-centered, allows for multiple ways to achieve intended outcomes, and acknowledges the importance of unintended outcomes.

Evidence-Based Nursing Education and the Science of Nursing Education

Nurses are becoming more knowledgeable about the concept of evidence-based clinical practice, and the Institute of Medicine (2003) has asserted that this is one of the concepts that must be integral to all health professions education. The National League for Nursing asserts that nurse educators must become more knowledgeable about the concept of evidence-based teaching and base their teaching practices and curriculum designs on research (NLN, 2002, 2005e). See Box 15–1, Suggestions for Future Research.

Many research questions need to be addressed if nursing education is to continue to prepare graduates who can function effectively in a practice role, advance the science of nursing and nursing education, and provide leadership to our profession. Faculty must be equipped to tackle the problems we face today, so that we can create a better tomorrow.

Guided by the *Priorities for Research in Nursing Education* (NLN, 2003b), nurse educators must be supported in their efforts to ask important questions about teaching practices, study the most effective and efficient ways to prepare graduates for 21st century nursing practice, and disseminate such pedagogical research. Efforts such as these are essential to building the **science of nursing education,** a science that will be built through the concerted efforts of faculty, graduate students preparing for a teaching role, and educator/scholars in all types of programs. Indeed, the development of one's ability to engage in the scholarship of teaching (Boyer, 1990) must become part of the preparation and continued development of nursing faculty.

In order to base our teaching on evidence, we need more basic research on how individuals learn, along with applied research that will help us understand better what it means to learn the practice of nursing. We need faculty who possess all the core competencies previously outlined, who engage in the scholarship of teaching and evidence-based teaching practices, and who actively contribute to the ongoing development of the science of nursing education. Such educator/scholars will help provide answers to questions such as the following:

- Is teaching theory and practice concurrently the best approach?
- What specialty areas provide students with clinical experiences that best facilitate their thinking, communication skills, team/collaborative skills, and patient care abilities?
- Should we continue to teach specialty areas such as pediatrics, obstetrics, psychiatry/mental health in our basic programs, or are these areas of specialty or advanced practice?
- What teaching/learning strategies can develop students' critical thinking and problem solving abilities, reflective thinking and practice, ability to engage in teamwork and collaboration, and delegation and supervision skills?
- What teaching/learning experiences will prepare graduates to function in a society where bioterrorism, genetic engineering, and cloning are real?
- What content areas can students learn best through technology (distance learning approaches, computer-based programs, etc.), and which require close student/teacher interaction?
- What is the right "mix" of faculty expertise for a given program, including individual expertise in areas such as assessment, curriculum design, and so on?
- How can we use clinical faculty and preceptors most effectively in the learning process?

distance learning v. online
(past) *(present)*

Technology in Nursing Education

The rapid technological advances of the past 25 years have been truly remarkable, as evidenced by how the Internet and the World Wide Web have changed the health-care arena and the educational environment. The pace of technological change will continue to advance at an ever-increasing rate, and the kind of technology that becomes integral to our educational worlds will change dramatically. It is impossible to discuss changes in nursing education without including and integrating concomitant changes in technology. *Mosby modules*

Many of our computer-based educational products are currently tied to screens and keyboards, but advances in virtual reality are already allowing users to interact with objects and feel as though they are "virtually there." Imagine learning anatomy and physiology by getting inside a virtual human body and exploring its structure and complex physiological interactions. Imagine placing students on a virtual hospital unit, complete with patients, staff, and equipment. *simulation lab*

We now have patient simulators that can speak and display physiological parameters appropriate for specific conditions, and at an affordable cost. It is now possible to move a learner through a simulation, with the degree of complexity and fidelity increasing as the learner's knowledge and skills increase. Students can begin by managing a fairly simple patient, with a limited number of variables present and, as they progress, be assigned to manage a patient whose condition changes unexpectedly and presents them with additional data, some relevant and some irrelevant. Once students have achieved proficiency with one dynamic, evolving patient simulation, they can be challenged to manage the care of two patients, and then an entire group of patients, for whom they must prioritize, delegate responsibility to others on the team, and assess progress.

In order to create more complex and dynamic patient simulations, however, faculty must be able to set up and manage those patient scenarios. Findings from educational research studies could provide faculty with the information they need to direct commercial companies to preprogram hundreds of patients. Faculty could then select a nursing care problem from that list, and the humanoid (i.e., simulator) would exhibit signs and symptoms of the problem, requiring students to make appropriate decisions to manage it or manage the complications that arise if the initial problem is not addressed appropriately or efficiently. To carry this future even one step farther, the computer would analyze the patient care interventions of an individual student and those of the group as a whole, select the next simulated experience that advances all learners to a more challenging problem, or present a new situation that is tailored to the learning style and meets the individual learning needs of each student.

All of this is most exciting. But while technology has the potential to assist faculty and students in the teaching/leaning process, it is not the answer to all of our educational problems. Students need to be exposed to a wide range of ideas and concepts that will help them develop the knowledge, skills, and values needed to engage in nursing practice, help them manage an increasingly complex and chaotic world, spark their personal interests, cultivate their individual talents, and sow the love of learning and leadership that help our profession to grow.

Preparation for and Continued Development in the Faculty Role

The NLN began its work on exploring the preparation of nurse educators for today and the future by convening a think tank on graduate preparation for the nurse educator role to define clearly the knowledge and skills that nurse educators need.

Think Tank

Members of the think tank included faculty and administrators from all types of nursing education programs, as well as representatives from staff development and the general higher education community. One outcome of this meeting was NLN's *Position Statement on the Preparation of Nurse Educators* (NLN, 2002), which states, in part, that:

> In light of the looming crisis in the supply of faculty to teach in schools of nursing, the time has come for the nursing profession to outline a preferred future for the preparation of nurse educators. This crisis must be used as an opportunity to recruit qualified individuals to the educator role, to ensure that these individuals are appropriately prepared for the responsibilities they will assume as faculty and staff development educators, and to implement strategies that will serve to retain a qualified nurse educator workforce.

The position statement concluded with a set of recommendations for faculty, administrators, and program development. They proposed actions such as early identification of talented neophytes; mentoring novice faculty; reinstating the educator track in master's programs, including learning experiences related to teaching and learning in all doctoral programs; finding innovative ways to use retired faculty; supporting faculty development; and rewarding expert educators.

A second outcome of the think tank was a preliminary list of core competencies for nurse educators.

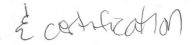

The list of core competencies developed by think tank participants was given to a Task Group on Nurse Educator Competencies, which operated under the guidance of NLN's Nursing Education Workforce Development Advisory Council. This group of nurse educators conducted an extensive search of the literature to determine if the eight competencies identified by the think tank participants were documented in evidence-based literature, or if there was a need to modify them. They worked for 2 years on this task and disseminated their work to the broad nurse educator community for comment. Based on this feedback, the task group refined the competencies and produced a manuscript, currently in press, that documents core competencies from the literature, identifies gaps in the literature, and proposes research questions that need to be addressed.

The Core Competencies of Nurse Educators© (NLN, 2005a) (see Fig. 15–3) have been incorporated into the *Scope of Practice for Academic Nurse Educators* (NLN, 2005d), and already are being used to provide direction for the development of graduate programs that prepare nurse educators. They provide a framework of essential knowledge, skills, and attitudes relevant to the educator role. In addition, they formed the basis for the development of the first and only **certification** program for academic nurse educators by providing the foundation for the items that were included in the practice analysis, an essential first step in the creation of a certification examination.

Development of the Academic Nurse Educator Certification Program

Certification in any field is a mark of professionalism. For academic nurse educators, it establishes nursing education as a specialty area of practice and an advanced practice role within professional nursing. It recognizes the academic nurse educator's specialized knowledge, skills, and abilities, and creates a means for faculty members to demonstrate their expertise in this role. Finally, it communicates to students, peers, and the higher education community that the highest standards of excellence are being met.

To begin the process of developing a certification program, members of the Certification Test Development Committee created task statements for each competency (see Fig. 15–3) in order to create a practice analysis survey. A random sample of nurse educators was invited to complete this survey, and statistical analyses of the results determined the blueprint for the certification examination. Another group of nurse educators created and approved all test items, and a governance committee established the policies and procedures pertinent to certification. Two hundred and six nurse educators took the pilot examination in September of 2005; 174 of them were the first to append the letters CNE^CM as their credential and mark of distinction.

Summary

Nursing education has been mired in old paradigms of teaching and learning for too many years, and the time is right to move out of that morass. We need to ask serious questions about the kinds of educational experiences we design for our students and whether those experiences prepare them to practice in the health-care systems of today and tomorrow. Only a research-based approach designed to create and continually refine a science of nursing education will challenge existing practices, such as the following:

• Lock-step curricula that allow for few student choices or exploration of areas of interest.
• Content-driven curricula that emphasize content coverage more than student learning.
• Teacher-centered as opposed to learner-centered approaches to nursing education.
• Specific days, hours, and locations for clinical experiences that provide little opportunity for students to experience the continuum of care.
• Evaluation and assessment practices that focus primarily on cognitive gains, objective measures, and passing the licensing exam.

CORE COMPETENCIES OF NURSE EDUCATORS©
AND TASK STATEMENTS

COMPETENCY 1 – FACILITATE LEARNING

Nurse educators are responsible for creating an environment in classroom, laboratory, and clinical settings that facilitates student learning and the achievement of desired cognitive, affective, and psychomotor outcomes. To facilitate learning effectively, the nurse educator:

- Implements a variety of teaching strategies appropriate to learner needs, desired learner outcomes, content, and context
- Grounds teaching strategies in educational theory and evidence-based teaching practices
- Recognizes multicultural, gender, and experiential influences on teaching and learning
- Engages in self-reflection and continued learning to improve teaching practices that facilitate learning
- Uses information technologies skillfully to support the teaching-learning process
- Practices skilled oral, written, and electronic communication that reflects an awareness of self and others, along with an ability to convey ideas in a variety of contexts
- Models critical and reflective thinking
- Creates opportunities for learners to develop their critical thinking and critical reasoning skills
- Shows enthusiasm for teaching, learning, and nursing that inspires and motivates students
- Demonstrates interest in and respect for learners
- Uses personal attributes (e.g., caring, confidence, patience, integrity and flexibility) that facilitate learning
- Develops collegial working relationships with students, faculty colleagues, and clinical agency personnel to promote positive learning environments
- Maintains the professional practice knowledge base needed to help learners prepare for contemporary nursing practice
- Serves as a role model of professional nursing

COMPETENCY 2 – FACILITATE LEARNER DEVELOPMENT AND SOCIALIZATION

Nurse educators recognize their responsibility for helping students develop as nurses and integrate the values and behaviors expected of those who fulfill that role. To facilitate learner development and socialization effectively, the nurse educator:

- Identifies individual learning styles and unique learning needs of international, adult, multicultural, educationally disadvantaged, physically challenged, at-risk, and second degree learners
- Provides resources to diverse learners that help meet their individual learning needs
- Engages in effective advisement and counseling strategies that help learners meet their professional goals
- Creates learning environments that are focused on socialization to the role of the nurse and facilitate learners' self-reflection and personal goal setting
- Fosters the cognitive, psychomotor, and affective development of learners
- Recognizes the influence of teaching styles and interpersonal interactions on learner outcomes
- Assists learners to develop the ability to engage in thoughtful and constructive self and peer evaluation
- Models professional behaviors for learners including, but not limited to, involvement in professional organizations, engagement in lifelong learning activities, dissemination of information through publications and presentations, and advocacy

COMPETENCY 3 – USE ASSESSMENT AND EVALUATION STRATEGIES

Nurse educators use a variety of strategies to assess and evaluate student learning in classroom,

FIGURE 15–3 Core Competencies of Nurse Educators © and task statements. National League for Nursing. (2005). *Core Competencies of Nurse Educators*. New York: Author. Reproduced with permission of the National League for Nursing. *(continued)*

laboratory and clinical settings, as well as in all domains of learning. To use assessment and evaluation strategies effectively, the nurse educator:

- Uses extant literature to develop evidence-based assessment and evaluation practices
- Uses a variety of strategies to assess and evaluate learning in the cognitive, psychomotor, and affective domains
- Implements evidence-based assessment and evaluation strategies that are appropriate to the learner and to learning goals
- Uses assessment and evaluation data to enhance the teaching-learning process
- Provides timely, constructive, and thoughtful feedback to learners
- Demonstrates skill in the design and use of tools for assessing clinical practice

COMPETENCY 4 – PARTICIPATE IN CURRICULUM DESIGN AND EVALUATION OF PROGRAM OUTCOMES

Nurse educators are responsible for formulating program outcomes and designing curricula that reflect contemporary health care trends and prepare graduates to function effectively in the health care environment. To participate effectively in curriculum design and evaluation of program outcomes, the nurse educator:

- Ensures that the curriculum reflects institutional philosophy and mission, current nursing and health care trends, and community and societal needs so as to prepare graduates for practice in a complex, dynamic, multicultural health care environment
- Demonstrates knowledge of curriculum development including identifying program outcomes, developing competency statements, writing learning objectives, and selecting appropriate learning activities and evaluation strategies
- Bases curriculum design and implementation decisions on sound educational principles, theory, and research
- Revises the curriculum based on assessment of program outcomes, learner needs, and societal and health care trends
- Implements curricular revisions using appropriate change theories and strategies
- Creates and maintains community and clinical partnerships that support educational goals
- Collaborates with external constituencies throughout the process of curriculum revision
- Designs and implements program assessment models that promote continuous quality improvement of all aspects of the program

COMPETENCY 5 – FUNCTION AS A CHANGE AGENT AND LEADER

Nurse educators function as change agents and leaders to create a preferred future for nursing education and nursing practice. To function effectively as a change agent and leader, the nurse educator:

- Models cultural sensitivity when advocating for change
- Integrates a long-term, innovative, and creative perspective into the nurse educator role
- Participates in interdisciplinary efforts to address health care and educational needs locally, regionally, nationally, or internationally
- Evaluates organizational effectiveness in nursing education
- Implements strategies for organizational change
- Provides leadership in the parent institution as well as in the nursing program to enhance the visibility of nursing and its contributions to the academic community
- Promotes innovative practices in educational environments
- Develops leadership skills to shape and implement change

COMPETENCY 6 – PURSUE CONTINUOUS QUALITY IMPROVEMENT IN THE NURSE EDUCATOR ROLE

Nurse educators recognize that their role is multidimensional and that an ongoing commitment to

FIGURE 15-3 (continued)

develop and maintain competence in the role is essential. To pursue continuous quality improvement in the nurse educator role, the individual:

- Demonstrates a commi(c)ent to life-long learning
- Recognizes that career enhancement needs and activities change as experience is gained in the role
- Participates in professional development opportunities that increase one's effectiveness in the role
- Balances the teaching, scholarship, and service demands inherent in the role of educator and member of an academic institution
- Uses feedback gained from self, peer, student, and administrative evaluation to improve role effectiveness
- Engages in activities that promote one's socialization to the role
- Uses knowledge of legal and ethical issues relevant to higher education and nursing education as a basis for influencing, designing, and implementing policies and procedures related to students, faculty, and the educational environment
- Mentors and supports faculty colleagues

COMPETENCY 7 – ENGAGE IN SCHOLARSHIP

Nurse educators acknowledge that scholarship is an integral component of the faculty role, and that teaching itself is a scholarly activity. To engage effectively in scholarship, the nurse educator:

- Draws on extant literature to design evidence-based teaching and evaluation practices
- Exhibits a spirit of inquiry about teaching and learning, student development, evaluation methods, and other aspects of the role
- Designs and implements scholarly activities in an established area of expertise
- Disseminates nursing and teaching knowledge to a variety of audiences through various means
- Demonstrates skill in proposal writing for initiatives that include, but are not limited to, research, resource acquisition, program development, and policy development
- Demonstrates qualities of a scholar: integrity, courage, perseverance, vitality, and creativity

COMPETENCY 8 – FUNCTION WITHIN
THE EDUCATIONAL ENVIRONMENT

Nurse educators are knowledgeable about the educational environment within which they practice and recognize how political, institutional, social and economic forces impact their role. To function as a good "citizen of the academy," the nurse educator:

- Uses knowledge of history and current trends and issues in higher education as a basis for making recommendations and decisions on educational issues
- Identifies how social, economic, political, and institutional forces influence higher education in general and nursing education in particular
- Develops networks, collaborations, and partnerships to enhance nursing's influence within the academic community
- Determines own professional goals within the context of academic nursing and the mission of the parent institution and nursing program
- Integrates the values of respect, collegiality, professionalism, and caring to build an organizational climate that fosters the development of students and teachers
- Incorporates the goals of the nursing program and the mission of the parent institution when proposing change or managing issues
- Assumes a leadership role in various levels of institutional governance
- Advocates for nursing and nursing education in the political arena

---

** National League for Nursing. (2005). *Core Competencies of Nurse Educators*. New York: Author.

Reproduced with permission of the National League for Nursing.

FIGURE 15–3 (continued)

We need nurse educators with the background in teaching/learning, curriculum development, program assessment, academic citizenry, and other skills to design new approaches to education. We need educator/scholars to examine the effectiveness of those approaches. We then need dedicated faculty to implement and continually test "proven" approaches with students. Until our nursing education environments are characterized in these ways, it will be difficult to meet the learning needs of diverse student groups, use technology to its fullest, and transform the way we prepare students for nursing practice roles.

References

Boyer, E. L. (1990). *Scholarship reconsidered: Priorities of the professoriate.* Princeton, NJ: The Carnegie Foundation for the Advancement of Teaching.

Diekelmann, N. (2001). Narrative pedagogy: Heideggerian hermeneutical analyses of lived experiences of students, teachers, and clinicians. *Advances in Nursing Science, 23*(3), 53–71.

Diers, D., & Evans, D. L. (1980). Excellence in nursing (Editorial). *Image, 12,* 27–30.

Institute of Medicine. (2003). *Health professions education: A bridge to quality.* Washington, DC: National Academies Press.

National League for Nursing. (2002). *The preparation of nurse educators* (Position Statement). New York: Author.

National League for Nursing. (2003a). *Innovation in nursing education: A call to reform* (Position Statement). New York: Author.

National League for Nursing. (2003b). *Priorities for research in nursing education.* New York: Author.

National League for Nursing. (2004). *Startling data from the NLN's comprehensive survey of all nursing programs evokes wake-up call.* New York: Author.

National League for Nursing. (2005a). *Core competencies of nurse educators.* New York: Author.

National League for Nursing. (2005b). *Excellence in nursing education model.* New York: Author.

National League for Nursing. (2005c). *Hallmarks of excellence in nursing education.* New York: Author.

National League for Nursing. (2005d). *The scope of practice of academic nurse educators.* New York: Author.

National League for Nursing. (2005e). *Transforming nursing education* (Position Statement). New York: Author.

Valiga, T. M. (2003). The pursuit of excellence in nursing education (Headlines from the NLN). *Nursing Education Perspectives, 24*(5), 275–277.

REVIEW QUESTIONS

- What is excellence and how can it be achieved in nursing education?
- How can innovation, evidence-based teaching practices, and a science of nursing education be employed to transform nursing education?
- Give an example of how your current practice as a nurse educator reflects each of the eight core competencies. If you are a graduate student preparing for the nurse educator role, give an example of how you intend to use each of these competencies as you develop in your new role.
- Select one new technology. Discuss its impact on nursing education today, and speculate about how it will impact nursing education in the future.

CRITICAL THINKING EXERCISES

Select three of the major elements in the Excellence in Nursing Education Model and show how they relate to one or more of the *Hallmarks of Excellence in Nursing Education.*

Outline the steps you would take to help your faculty colleagues focus less on covering content and more on the processes of learning. What challenges do you anticipate in helping them make this transition? Where do you expect you would find support for this endeavor?

Select one task statement associated with any of the *Core Competencies of Nurse Educators* and generate three research questions related to that task. Discuss how findings from your proposed research would advance the science of nursing education.

Select one new technology and generate examples of how it can be used to facilitate the development of critical thinking in students. Outline a brief research proposal to test your hypothesis.

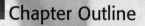

Chapter Outline

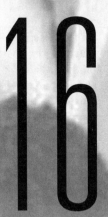

AACN Shaping a Future Vision for Nursing Education

16

Joan M. Stanley

Learning Outcomes

On completion of this chapter, the reader will be able to:

- Explain the changes, internal and external, to the health-care system that are having a significant impact on nursing education.
- Describe the forces that are creating a mandate for change in nursing education.
- Discuss the vision for future nursing education being proposed by the American Association of Colleges of Nursing.

Key Terms

Advanced practice registered nursing (APRN)
Associate degree nurse (ADN)
Baccalaureate degree in nursing (BSN)
Baccalaureate education
Clinical nurse leader (CNL)
Clinical nurse specialist (CNS)
Competencies
Doctoral education
Doctor of nursing practice (DNP)
Generalist
Master's degree in nursing (MSN)
Nurse practitioner (NP)

The American Association of Colleges of Nursing (AACN) has entertained an ongoing dialogue over the past decade and taken a leadership role in moving toward a preferred future of nursing education. The dialogue began in response to changing global demographics, a health-care system plagued with reports of large numbers of medical errors and system breakdowns, and drastic shortages of nurses and other health-care professionals. The dialogue, including a broad representation of stakeholders internal and external to nursing, has focused on the knowledge, skills, and **competencies** needed by professional nurses to address the demands of an evolving global society and health-care system. New models of nursing education have emerged from this dialogue. This vision for nursing education does not necessarily represent the vision of the association as a whole. Rather, this chapter represents the vision of one individual who has been actively engaged in this ongoing dialogue within and outside nursing. Where conversations are ongoing and future education models are being explored, this is noted. Where the association has taken a formal position, this is noted as well. Due to political, market, and societal forces, there is no way to predict exactly what form future nursing education will take. Regardless of its form, nursing education must respond to external forces and evolve if nursing is to remain a viable and important component of the health-care workforce able to make a significant impact on unmet health-care needs. To be successful, this evolution will require a true partnership between nursing education and practice.

Call for Change in Nursing Education

Although not the first indicator of the need to transform the health-care system, the report that first grabbed the public's attention was issued in 1999 by the Institute of Medicine (IOM). *To Err is Human: Building a Safer Health System*, which extrapolated data from two previous studies, estimated that somewhere between 44,000 and 98,000 Americans die each year as a result of medical errors (IOM, 1999, p. 1). More recent estimates say that these numbers may be much higher (Leape & Berwick, 2005, p. 2385). Even at the lower levels, these unnecessary deaths exceed the number of people who die from motor vehicle accidents, breast cancer, or AIDS. Total national costs of preventable adverse events (medical errors resulting in injury) were estimated to be between $17 billion and $29 billion of which health-care costs represented more than half (Johnson et al., 1992). In addition, medication-related and other errors that do not result in actual harm not only are extremely costly but have a significant impact on the quality of care and health-care outcomes. The IOM report focused on the fragmented nature of the health-care delivery system as being a major contributor to the high and inexcusable error rate. This fragmentation leads to a lack of continuity and multiple patient handoffs.

In addition to the growing concern over health-care outcomes, the United States is in the midst of a nursing shortage that is expected to intensify as baby boomers age and the need for health care grows. Dr. Peter Buerhaus and colleagues (2000) reported in the *Journal of the American Medical Association* that the United States will experience a 20 percent shortage in the number of nurses needed in our nation's health-care system by the year 2020. This translates into a shortage of more than 400,000 registered nurses nationwide. The fall 2004 survey of nursing programs conducted by AACN revealed that enrollment in entry-level baccalaureate nursing programs increased by 14.1 percent nationwide since fall 2003 (Berlin, Wilsey, & Bednash, 2005). Still, this increase is not sufficient to meet the projected demand for nurses. According to Peter Buerhaus and colleagues (2003), enrollment in nursing programs would have to increase at least 40 percent annually to replace the nurses expected to leave the workforce through retirement.

Other recent landmark reports focus on the nursing shortage, the crisis in the health-care system and proposed strategies for addressing these critical issues. The IOM in two follow-up reports in 2001 and 2003 stressed that the health-care system as currently structured does not, as a whole, make the best use of its resources and called on all health-care organizations and professional groups to promote health care that is safe, effective, client-centered, timely, efficient, and equitable (IOM, 2001, p. 6). The IOM Committee on the Health Professions Education Summit urged that all health professionals be educated to deliver patient-centered care as members of an interdisciplinary team, emphasizing evidence-based practice, quality improvement approaches, and informatics (IOM, 2003). The Joint Commission on Accreditation of Healthcare Organizations (JCAHO, 2002) has called for transforming the workplace, aligning nursing education and clinical experience. The Robert Wood Johnson Foundation (Kimball & O'Neill, 2002) has taken a broad look at the underlying factors driving the nursing shortage and urges the reinvention of nursing education and work environments to address and appeal to the needs and values of a new generation of nurses.

> It is evident . . . that leadership in nursing . . . is of supreme importance at this time. Nursing has faced many critical situations in its long history, but probably none more critical than the situation it is now in, and none in which the possibilities, both of serious loss and of substantial advance, are greater. What the outcome will be depends in large measure on the kind of leadership the nursing profession can give in planning for the future and in solving stubborn and perplexing problems . . . if past experience is any criterion, little constructive action will be taken without intelligent and courageous leadership (Stewart, 1953, p. 326).

Isabel Maitland Stewart wrote those words more than 50 years ago in her petition for education reform in nursing. Perhaps the most staggering revelation is that despite all of progress nursing has made in recent decades as a profession, nursing remains at the same "critical" juncture that it was at the end of World War II. Despite the promise of university-based education for professional nursing, the health-care system is in yet another nursing shortage with yet another call for "intelligent and creative leadership" requiring insight and innovation. Nursing as a profession must look beyond what currently exists and think beyond personal experience to what could be.

The *good* news is that nursing can provide many of the answers to the predominant health-care dilemmas of the future, including:

• The problems associated with normal human development, particularly aging
• Chronic illness management in all ages
• Health disparities associated with socioeconomic dislocations such as global migration, classism, and sexism
• Strategies for health promotion and disease prevention

Each of these prevailing health problems is suited to the nursing paradigm. Their amelioration is what nursing students are educated to do. The advancement of medical science and technology has changed the landscape of health and illness. Not only are people living much longer, they are living with chronic illnesses that would have been fatal 20 years ago. This is true in adults and children, resulting in the need for providers who can manage the ongoing health needs of persons of all ages. The necessity for practitioners who focus on the promotion of health and wellness and the prevention of disease has emerged. Such a focus addresses escalating medical costs and improves the health of the nation and global community (AACN, 2003).

Although there is ample evidence for the need to produce many more nurses to meet the pressing health-care needs of society, this is not just a matter of increasing the volume of the nursing workforce. Nurses, particularly those working in hospitals, are dissatisfied with their work (41 percent), and an inordinate number, particularly young nurses, plan on leaving their job (30 percent) (Aiken et al., 2001). Further, research by Linda Aiken and others also has shown that hospitals with a higher percentage of nurses with baccalaureate and higher degrees demonstrate lower mortality rates and lower failure to rescue rates (Aiken et al., 2003).

One of the natural responses to the changes in health care, new technologies, and calls for a better educated workforce has been to expand current educational requirements. Course requirements, clinical hours, and credit hours required for graduation from **associate degree (ADN),** **baccalaureate (BSN),** and **master's degree in nursing (MSN)** programs have grown exponentially. The result has been an increase in expectations for each of these degrees far beyond expectations and requirements for equivalent degrees in many other disciplines. Despite the growth in these requirements, graduates and employers still identify additional content and experiences needed to practice in today's health-care environment, including business principles of health care, evidence-based practice, and emerging areas of science such as genomics and environmental health.

The Institute of Medicine, American Hospital Association, the Robert Wood Johnson Foundation, and other groups external to nursing have called on all the health professions to change the way future health professionals are educated. New ways of educating health professionals, including inter-professional education and practice, and new practice models must be developed.

AACN Actions Shaping the Future of Nursing Education

In response to the calls for change within nursing education, AACN, over the past several years, has taken a leadership role in shaping the future of nursing education.

Recent AACN Actions Affecting Baccalaureate Nursing Education

In 2004, the AACN Board of Directors reaffirmed its position that **baccalaureate education** is the minimum education required for entry into professional nursing practice in today's complex health-care environment. Despite articulation mechanisms between associate degree programs and baccalaureate or master's degree programs in almost every state, only 16% of nurses educated in ADN or diploma programs continue their education beyond their entry-level degree (Spratley, Johnson, Sochalski, Fritz, & Spencer, 2001). Therefore, the AACN Board also reaffirmed the need for strong articulation mechanisms between ADN and BSN and MSN programs. The board urged the nursing community to create opportunities and incentives for nurses to pursue higher degrees in nursing, citing the Department of Veterans Affairs (1998) as one outstanding example of an organization that has provided such incentives and opportunities.

Recent AACN Actions Affecting Master's Nursing Education

In 2004, the AACN Board voted to accept the recommendations of a task force and to pilot a new professional nursing role at the master's degree level (AACN, 2004a). This new role, the **Clinical Nurse Leader**[sm] **(CNL),** grew out of several years' work by two task forces charged with examining the future needs of the health-care delivery system and potential education models. See section on the CNL for additional detail.

Recent AACN Actions Affecting Doctoral Education in Nursing

The AACN task force charged with revising the position statement on the *Quality Indicators for Research-Focused Doctoral Programs in Nursing* recommended further examination of the history of, need for, and criteria for practice doctorate programs in nursing. In October 2004, the AACN membership passed the *Position Statement on the Practice Doctorate in Nursing* (AACN, 2004b). This position statement sets the **doctorate of nursing practice (DNP)** as the highest level of preparation for clinical nursing practice. Nursing practice is broadly defined as "any nursing intervention that influences health care outcomes for individuals or populations, including the direct care of individual patients, management of care for individuals and populations, administration of nursing and health care organizations" (p. 3).

AACN member institutions also voted to move the current level of preparation necessary for advanced nursing practice roles from the master's degree to the doctorate level by the year 2015. See the section on the DNP for additional detail.

To facilitate the transition within nursing education to the practice doctorate by the target date of 2015, the AACN board created two task forces with representation from diverse nursing specialties and institutions. The first task force was charged with creating an "Essentials" document for practice doctorates, which outlines the basic competencies that must be built into these educational programs. This document is similar in nature to the other Essentials documents originated by AACN for baccalaureate and master's degree education.[1] The second task force, the roadmap task force, is focused on implementation of the new position statement and issues related to this transition, including moving existing **Advanced Practice Nurse (APN)** programs to the doctoral level and providing efficient bridge programs for master's prepared nurses interested in pursuing a DNP degree.

The Clinical Nurse Leader and Future Master's Nursing Education

In this possible new vision for nursing education explicated here, master's education programs would prepare advanced **generalists** in nursing, either as entry into the profession or in post-baccalaureate nursing education programs. The Clinical Nurse Leader (CNL), launched as a demonstration project, is being developed in collaboration with multiple stakeholders from practice and education. Currently, 90 schools, in partnership with more than 185 health-care facilities, are piloting a master's CNL curriculum and working to develop a new health-care delivery model. Other possible master's degree tracks may include preparation for middle management and informatics roles.

The CNL is an advanced generalist prepared at the master's degree level. Some of the key characteristics of the CNL role include (AACN, 2003):

- Implementation of evidence-based practice in all health-care settings for diverse and complex patients
- Risk anticipation, evaluating, and anticipating risks to client safety with the aim of quality improvement and preventing medical errors
- Lateral integration of care for a specified cohort of patients
- Accountability for evaluation and improvement of point of care outcomes
- Mass customization of care
- Client and community advocacy
- Client education for individuals, families, groups, and other health-care providers

---

[1] As the national voice for baccalaureate and higher degree nursing programs, AACN has established the educational standards and curricular guidelines through a series of *Essentials* documents that delineate the essential components and outcomes of baccalaureate and graduate nursing programs.

- Information management—using information systems and technology at the point of care to improve health-care outcomes
- Delegation and oversight of care delivery and outcomes
- Design and provision of health promotion and risk reduction services for diverse populations
- Team leadership and collaboration with other health professional team members
- Development and leveraging of human, environmental, and material resources

As a generalist, the CNL is not an **Advanced Practice Registered Nursing (APRN).** APRNs are prepared in an advanced specialty area of practice. The CNL collaborates with and complements APRN roles, including the **Clinical Nurse Specialist (CNS)** and the **Nurse Practitioner (NP),** to improve patient care outcomes.

The graduate level education of the CNL builds on professional nursing baccalaureate degree competencies and practice (AACN, 1998). The graduate of a CNL master's program is prepared as a generalist to provide care at the point of care and specific clinical leadership throughout the health-care delivery system.

The nursing profession must produce quality graduates who:

- Are prepared for clinical leadership in all health-care settings.
- Are prepared to implement outcomes-based practice and quality improvement strategies.
- Will remain in and contribute to the profession, practicing at their full scope of education and ability.
- Will create and manage microsystems of care that will be responsive to the health-care needs of individuals and families (Batalden, Nelson, Edwards, Godfrey, & Mohr, 2003; Mohr et al., 2003).

Unless nursing is able to create a professional role that will attract the highest quality men and women into the profession, nursing will not be able to fulfill its covenant with the public.

Specialty Nursing Practice and the Doctor of Nursing Practice

The Position Statement on the Practice Doctorate in Nursing, approved in Fall 2004 by the AACN membership, recommends moving all specialty nursing education to the doctoral level by the year 2015. With this recommendation, all current APRN education, which includes certified registered nurse anesthetist, certified nurse midwife, clinical nurse specialist, and nurse practitioner roles, would evolve to the doctoral level by 2015. The recommendation does NOT intend that all currently practicing APRNs will be required to obtain this new degree. It is intended that currently practicing and credentialed APRNs will maintain authority to practice just as occurred when, in the 1970s, NP education evolved from certificate to master's education.

The Essentials of Doctoral Education for Advanced Nursing Practice (AACN, 2006) addresses those areas of competency necessary for all **doctor of nursing practice** graduates and includes:

- Scientific underpinnings for practice
- Organizational and systems leadership for quality improvement in systems thinking
- Clinical scholarship and analytical methods for evidence-based practice
- Information systems and technology for the improvement and transformation of patient-centered health care
- Health-care policy for advocacy in health care

- Interprofessional collaboration for improving patient and population health outcomes
- Clinical prevention and population health for improving the nation's health
- Advanced nursing practice for specialty roles

The Essentials document has a format similar to that of the AACN *Essentials of Master's Education for Advanced Practice Nursing* (AACN, 1996) and includes the core competencies for all DNP graduates. The specialty role competencies, an essential component of the DNP curriculum, will be identified by the specialty nursing organizations. A diagram of the DNP curriculum, as currently envisioned, in shown in Figure 16–1.

An individual may enter a DNP program following a baccalaureate nursing education program, a master's advanced generalist program such as a CNL program, or one of the current master's APRN programs. Therefore, the DNP Essentials or end-of-program competencies include all of the post-baccalaureate nursing competencies necessary upon graduation from a practice doctorate in nursing program. Following the transition to this new model of specialty nursing education, it is possible that the current *Essentials of Master's Education* may be retired, having been replaced by the new *Essentials of the Doctor of Nursing Practice* and possibly a new set of guidelines for advanced generalist education at the master's level.

A New Model for Nursing Education

With the proposed future changes in nursing education, a number of differing models are possible. One such model for future nursing education and the entry points and pathways that could be taken throughout the model are presented here.

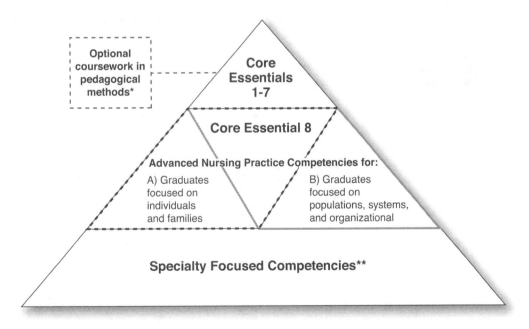

* For those students who may choose a career in health-care education or academia, additional pedagogical courses should be provided.

**Competencies, content, and practica are delineated by specialty nursing organizations.

FIGURE 16–1 Proposed DNP curriculum model.

Educational Pathways

For the health of the profession, nursing must maintain a robust pipeline of entry-level clinicians and provide seamless pathways to higher levels of educational achievement. Mechanisms must be strengthened to allow articulation or transition from one nursing degree program to another. These pathways should ensure that individuals receive appropriate academic credit for previous education and clinical experiences, that appropriate course and credit requirements are assigned to appropriate degrees, and that program requirements are not redundant. Ensuring these transition mechanisms also should standardize nursing education program expectations, including length of programs and ranges of credit and clinical requirements, and should improve access to the continuum of nursing education programs.

Completion of each degree should be based on documentation of end-of-program competencies delineated in the Essentials for each degree (baccalaureate, master's, and doctoral). This requires nursing, just as the rest of higher education is doing, to examine and develop new mechanisms for assessing outcome competencies, such as virtual testing, simulations, and portfolio development (AACU, 2004).

Individuals will enter the profession through a number of entry points. One point of entry is the BSN program offered through an articulation agreement between a community college and upper degree granting institution or solely by the upper degree granting institution. Graduates of a BSN program are prepared to sit for the nursing licensure exam (NCLEX).

A second point of entry into the profession is at the master's degree level. Individuals entering a master's in nursing program must have completed a baccalaureate degree in another field or a pre-nursing baccalaureate degree. This model parallels other health professions' education, including medical education. A pre-nursing degree would include a broad base of physical and social sciences and other general education courses. If entering the nursing profession at the mas-

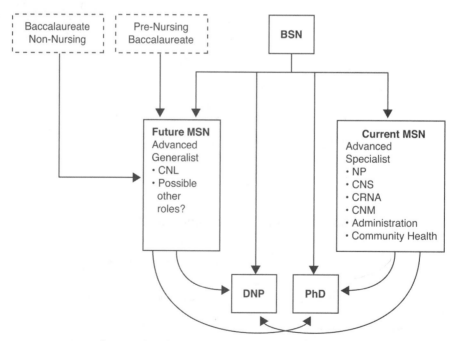

FIGURE 16-2 Educational pathways.

In this educational model, as envisioned, master's education programs would prepare advanced generalists in nursing. This may include education tracks preparing Clinical Nurse Leaders. Other possible tracks may include preparation for middle management roles.

Research-focused education programs that award a PhD, DNS, or DNSc degree, prepare graduates for research careers. Graduates of these programs may assume positions in academia, practice, policy, or administration. The primary focus of the PhD or other research-focused programs is to prepare individuals to advance the science of nursing through the generation of new nursing theory and knowledge.

Doctor of Nursing Practice programs prepare graduates for a variety of roles with an emphasis on nursing practice. DNP is the degree title awarded and does not indicate the graduate's specialty area of practice, which includes any of the APRN roles, or may include health policy, informatics, organizational leadership, or community health nursing. Entry into a DNP program may be post-BSN or post-MSN. During the transition to this new model of nursing education, many DNP students who choose to advance their education will have already completed an MSN program in one of the APRN roles. Curricula will need to be individualized to the student's previous educational background and clinical experience.

Nursing Curricula Interfaces

End-of-program competencies for the BSN, MSN, DNP, and PhD nursing programs are not discrete but overlap and build on each other. How each degree program curriculum, or end-of-program competencies, interlocks is depicted in Figure 16–3. The specific areas of overlap in competencies and content are dependent upon the individual's previous educational background and clinical experience. For example, an individual who holds an MSN degree with preparation as a CNL or an APRN will already have attained many of the end-of-program competencies expected of the DNP graduate. On the other hand, an individual who enters the DNP program immediately after obtaining a BSN will need extensive graduate-level preparation in an advanced area of nursing practice. Likewise, areas of overlap between the DNP and PhD curricula may exist, depending upon the area of study, research, and practice.

Preparation for Faculty Roles in Academia

Consistent with expectations in other disciplines, the appropriate preparation for nursing faculty is at the doctoral level. Expectations for nursing faculty should not differ from those of other disciplines within the academic community. Graduates of both research-focused and practice doctorate programs are eligible for full participation in a faculty role consistent with the institution's criteria. Education is a discipline itself. Additional coursework or opportunities for obtaining pedagogical expertise may be provided as part of the doctoral program or through a mentoring program for new faculty. Nursing education is not an appropriate area of focus for either the PhD or DNP degree. Rather, the primary area of preparation in a doctoral nursing program should be in an advanced area of nursing practice or nursing research.

Summary

Nurses, more than any other health professionals, have constant contact with patients and opportunities to influence outcomes of care. Nurses provide services across the continuum of settings from critical care, senior day care to school health facilities. The IOM and other well-respected

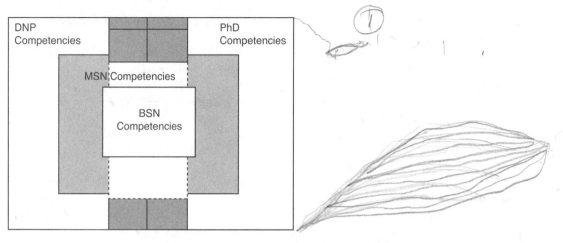

Indicates areas of overlap between the PhD and DNP curriculum

Indicates area of overlap between the MSN and DNP/PhD

FIGURE 16–3 Designing nursing curricula and interfaces of nursing competencies.

interdisciplinary groups have urged all health professions to redesign the way future practitioners are prepared. Current and projected changes in an increasingly complex health-care system, and the nursing profession's potential to influence health-care outcomes have created a powerful mandate to prepare a highly and differently educated future nursing workforce. Nursing also must participate in and lead the redesign of care delivery models. New practice and education models are needed to attract highly qualified and professionally motivated individuals to the profession.

This vision presented is just one possible model for future nursing education. This model includes a minimum of a baccalaureate degree for entry into professional nursing practice, graduate level preparation in an advanced generalist role, doctoral preparation for practice in all nursing specialties, and research-focused doctoral preparation to expand nursing knowledge and scientific base. What may occur in the future cannot be predicted and will be dependent upon the nursing community as a whole.

A future nursing education model requires an evolution and expansion of nursing education at all levels of practice. The nursing profession cannot afford to be the least educated profession at the health professions' table. Nursing cannot rely on past experiences and current practices. An open, thoughtful, and creative dialogue is needed to achieve this new model of nursing education, for which the ultimate goals are an expanded highly educated nursing workforce, increased access to high-quality care, and improved health-care outcomes.

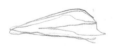

Aiken, L. H., et al. (2001). Nurses' reports on hospital care in five countries. *Health Affairs, May/June, 20* (3), 43–53.

Aiken, L. H., Clarke, S. P., Cheung, R. B., Sloane, D. M., & Silber, J. H. (2003, September 24). Educational levels of hospital nurses and surgical patient mortality. *Journal of the American Medical Association, 290,* 1617–1623.

American Association of Colleges and Universities. (2004). *Taking responsibility for the quality of the baccalaureate degree, report from the greater expectations project on accreditation and assessment.* Washington, DC: Author.

American Association of Colleges of Nursing. (1996). *The essentials of master's education for advanced practice nursing.* Washington, DC: Author.

American Association of Colleges of Nursing. (1998). *The Essentials of baccalaureate nursing education for professional nursing practice.* Washington, DC: Author.

American Association of Colleges of Nursing. (2003). Working paper on the clinical nurse leader role. Accessed at **http::/www.aacn.nche.edu/CNL/.**

American Association of Colleges of Nursing. (2004a). Series of motions taken by the AACN board of directors. Accessed at **8MembersOnly/pdf/Spring04Dialogue.pdf.**

American Association of Colleges of Nursing. (2004b). *The position statement on the practice doctorate in nursing.* Accessed at **http//www.aacn.nche.edu/DNP/DNPPositionStatement.htm**

American Association of Colleges of Nursing. (2006). *The essentials of doctoral education for advanced nursing practice,* DRAFT February 2006. Accessed at **http://www.aacn.nche.edu/DNP/pdf/ Essentials2–06.pdf.**

Batalden, P. B., Nelson, E. C., Edwards, W.H., Godfrey, & M.M., Mohr, J. J. (2003). Microsystems in health care. Part 9. Developing small clinical units to attain peak performance. *Joint Commission Journal on Quality and Safety, 29*(11), 575–585.

Berlin, L. E., Wilsey, S., & Bednash, G. D. (2005). *2004–2005 Enrollment and graduations in baccalaureate and graduate programs in nursing.* Washington, DC: American Association of Colleges of Nursing.

Buerhaus, P., et al. (2003). Is the current shortage of hospital nurses ending? *Health Affairs, 22*(6), 191–198.

Buerhaus, P., Staiger, D. O., & Auerbach, D. I. (2000). Implications of an aging registered nurse workforce. *Journal of the American Medical Association, 283*(22), 2948–2954.

Department of Veterans Affairs. (1998). News Release: VA commits $50 million to new national nursing initiative. Washington, DC: Office of Public Affairs News Service.

Institute of Medicine. (1999). *To err is human: Building a safer health system.* Washington, DC: National Academy Press, p. 1.

Institute of Medicine. (2001). *Crossing the quality chasm.* Washington, DC: The National Academies Press.

Institute of Medicine. (2003). *Health professions education: A bridge to quality.* Washington, DC: The National Academies Press.

Johnson, W. G., Brennan, T. A., Newhouse, J. P., Leape, L. L., Lawthers, A. G., Hiatt, H. H., & Weiler, P. C. (1992). The economic consequences of medical injuries. *Journal of the American Medical Association, 267,* 2487–2492.

Joint Commission on Accreditation of Healthcare Organizations. (2002). *Health care at the crossroads, Strategies for addressing the evolving nursing crisis.* Chicago: Author.

Kimball, B., & O'Neill, E. (2002). Health care's human crisis: The American nursing shortage. Princeton, NJ: The Robert Wood Johnson Foundation.

Leape, L. L., & Berwick, D. M. (2005). Five years after to err is human. *Journal of the American Medical Association, 293*(19), 2384–2390.

Mohr, J. J., Barach, P., Cravero, J. P., Blike, G. T., Godfrey, M. M., Bataldrecen, P. B., & Nelson, E. C. (2003). Microsystems in health care: Part 6. Designing patient safety into the microsystem. *Joint Commission Journal on Quality and Safety, 29*(8), 401–408.

Spratley, E., Johnson, A., Sochalski, J., Fritz, M., & Spencer, W. (2001). The registered nurse population, March 2000. Findings from the national sample survey of registered nurses. U.S. Department of Health and Human Services, Health Resources and Service Administration, Bureau of Health Professions, Division of Nursing.

Stewart, I. M. (1953). *The education of nurses.* New York: The Macmillan Company.

REVIEW QUESTIONS

- What implications do you envision for the nursing profession? For health-care outcomes? For the health-care systems?
- Identify how changes in nursing education relate to changes in other health professions' education.
- Discuss what the impact would be on nursing practice and the profession if no changes are made to the current nursing education model.

CRITICAL THINKING EXERCISES

Dialogue with a variety of stakeholders in nursing education and identify critical curriculum revisions that need to occur to address the concerns raised in the IOM reports.

Review materials on the AACN Web site (http:www.aacn.nche.edu) on the CNL or the DNP; describe the impact these initiatives may have on nursing education and practice.

Interview several stakeholders, such as employers of nurses and health-care consumers, to identify professional nursing role competencies they see as critical for the future health-care delivery system. How do these compare to those proposed by AACN in the *Working Paper on the Clinical Nurse Leader Role* and the *Essentials for the Doctor of Nursing Practice?*

INDEX

Page numbers followed by a "t", "f", or "b" indicate tables, figures, or boxes, respectively.